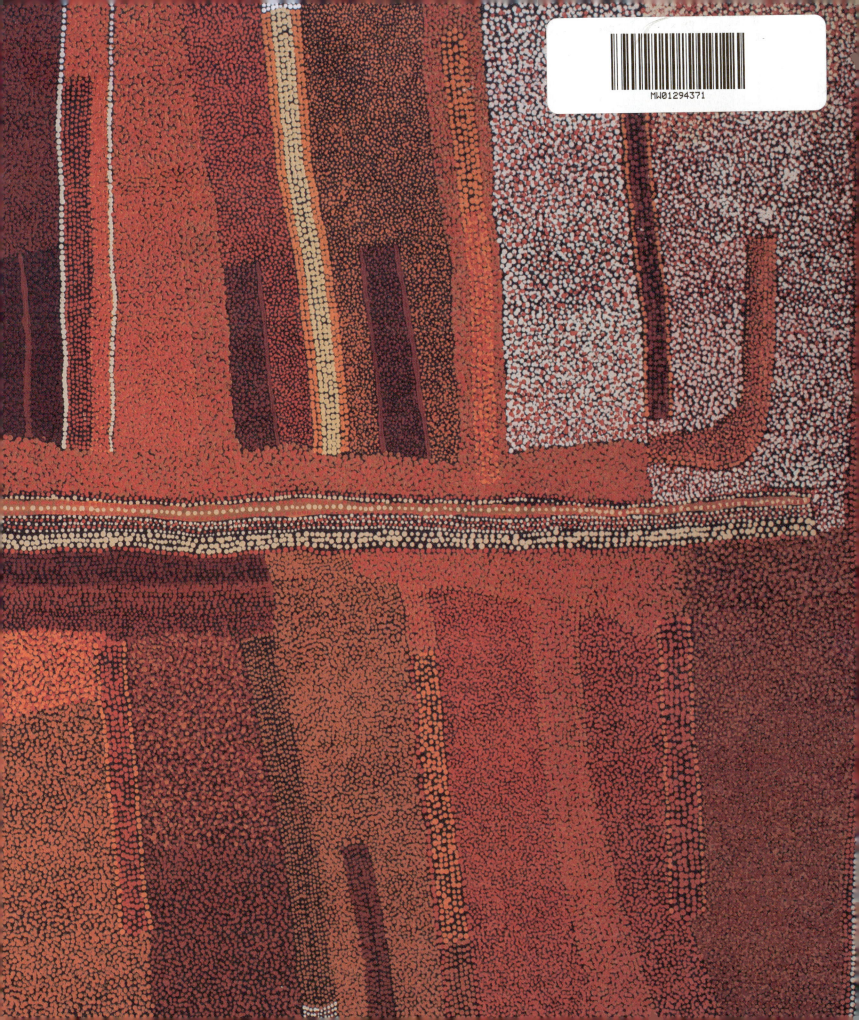

# TRADITIONAL HEALERS
*of Central Australia:* Ngangkari

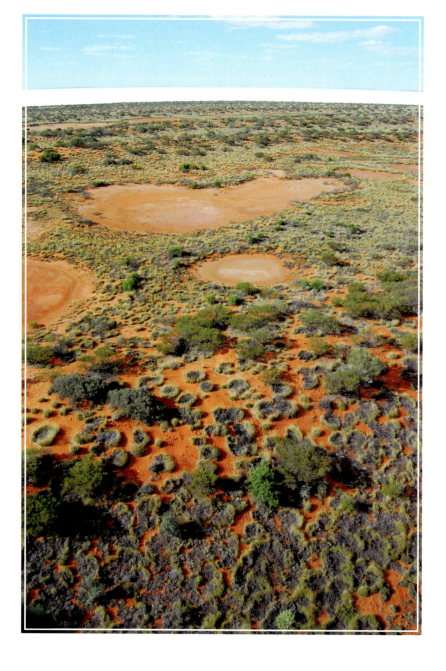

# TRADITIONAL HEALERS
*of Central Australia:* Ngangkari

 Ngaanyatjarra Pitjantjatjara Yankunytjatjara Women's Council Aboriginal Corporation

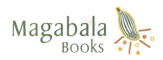

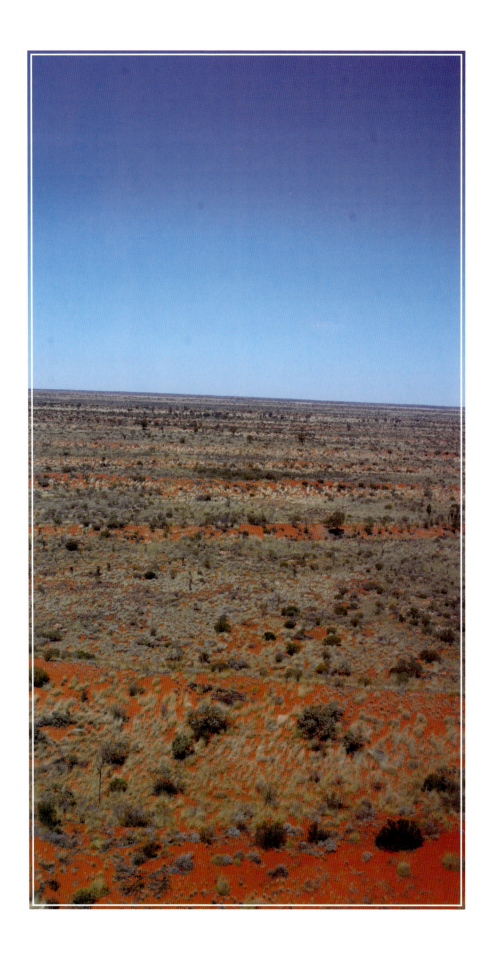

In memory of Rupert Langkatjukur Peter

1941–2012

Number One Ngangka<u>r</u>i

*You've got to remember that this is the tradition, this is the knowledge and Law.*
*It's something that has been held onto which came from the days before there were hospitals and other*
*forms of doctors. We were responsible for looking after all the people. We have held onto that knowledge ...*

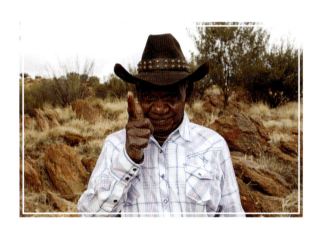

First published 2013 by Magabala Books Aboriginal Corporation, Broome, Western Australia

Website: www.magabala.com   Email: sales@magabala.com

Magabala Books receives financial assistance from the Commonwealth Government through the Australia Council, its arts advisory body. The State of Western Australia has made an investment in this project through the Department of Culture and the Arts in association with Lotterywest.

Copyright © Ngaanyatjarra Pitjantjatjara Yankunytjatjara Women's Council Aboriginal Corporation, 2013

All rights reserved. Apart from any fair dealing for the purposes of private study, research, criticism or review, as permitted under the Copyright Act, no part of this publication may be reproduced by any process whatsoever without the written permission of the publisher.

Design concept Tracey Gibbs, designer Margaret Whiskin

Cover concept by Rhett Hammerton

Printed in China at Everbest Printing Company

Compiled by Penny Watson with Rupert Langkatjukur Peter, Toby Minyintiri Baker, Andy Tjilari and Angela Lynch

Translations (from Pitjantjatjara, Yankunytjatjara and Ngaanyatjarra to English): Linda Rive, Patrick Hookey, Elizabeth Marrkilyi Ellis, Suzanne Bryce

Glossary: Linda Rive

Ngangkari interviews and recordings by Angela Lynch, Patrick Hookey, Linda Rive, Suzanne Bryce and Penny Watson

Photography: Rhett Hammerton and others as credited in captions

All historical image research conducted via Ara Irititja Archives. Ara Irititja is an Anangu-owned community-based knowledge management system. The Ara Irititja project team identifies records and electronically copies material and information about Pitjantjatjara Yankunytjatjara people (Anangu) and is committed to repatriating historical material to Anangu via the interactive multi-media archive database. For further information or to make a donation please contact:

John Dallwitz, Coordinator, Ara Irititja, Pitjantjatjara Council Social History Unit, PO Box 1234, Marleston SA 5033

National Library of Australia Cataloguing-in-Publication entry

Traditional healers of the central desert: Ngangkari/Ngaanyatjarra Pitjantjatjara Yankunytjatjara Women's Council Aboriginal Corporation (NPY)

9781921248825 (pbk)

Healers–Western Australia

Aboriginal Australians–Health and hygiene

Ngaanyatjarra (Australian people–Medicine

Traditional medicine–Western Australia

362.849915

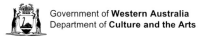

NOTES TO THE READER

The profiles of the following people have appeared previously in *Ngangkari Work – Anangu Way,* Ngaanyatjarra Pitjantjatjara Yankunytjatjara Women's Council Aboriginal Corporation, 2003: Andy Tjilari, Rupert Langkatjukur Peter, Jimmy Baker, Dickie Minyintiri, Harry Tjutjuna, Whiskey Tjukanku, Nakul Dawson, Arnie Frank and Jacky Giles, as has material from Josephine Mick's and Arnie Frank's in the Wangkanyi section.

Some material by Andy Tjilari and Rupert Langkatjukur Peter in the Wangkanyi section has been drawn from audio recordings published as: *Speaking up about Mental Health* – (Audio CD) Rupert Peter and Andy Tjilari, NPY Women's Council, 2009. Translated by Patrick Hookey.

*Names of people and places*: The names of people in this book are spelled correctly using Pitjantjatjara orthography and as specified by each individual for this book. However, some people's names have been and are spelt differently elsewhere.

CAPTIONS

Front cover, photographs and composite image Rhett Hammerton; endpapers, Bernard Tjalkuriny, *Kaliwani*, 2011. Acrylic on linen, 200 x 120 cm: photograph Amanda Dent, © the Artist, courtesy Tjungu Palya; back cover, Sally Hodson; p. 2 (opposite title page), Sally Hodson; p. 3 (title page), composite image by Jo Boniface, backgound photograph by Steve Strike and hands photograph by Angela Lynch; p. 4, Sally Hodson; p. 5, Rupert Langkatjukur Peter, photograph Rhett Hammerton; and p. 7, Rupert Langkatjukur Peter giving a healing treatment to Timothy Young, 2011, photograph Rhett Hammerton.

> HOW DO YOU PRONOUNCE NGANGKARI?
>
> **NUN-ka-ree**
>
> For more information see 'Spelling and Pronunciation' p. 266

> ACRONYMS AND ORGANISATIONS
>
> **APY Lands** Anangu Pitjantjatjara Yankunytjatjara Lands
>
> **NPYWC, NPY Women's Council** Ngaanyatjarra Pitjantjatjara Yankunytjatjara Women's Council
>
> Nganampa Health Council
>
> **RFDS** Royal Flying Doctor Service

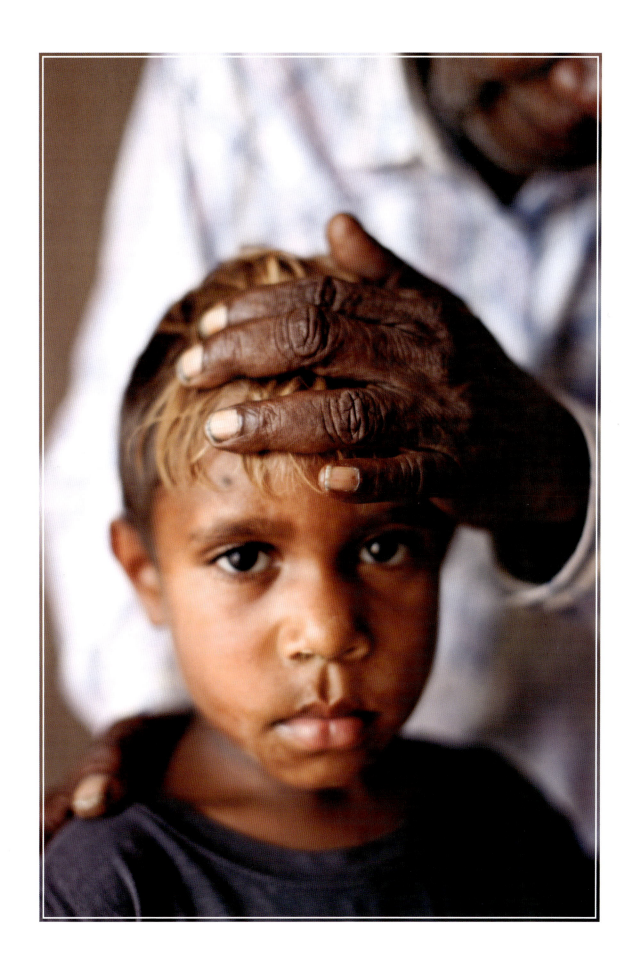

# Contents

Foreword — 11

Alani – Introduction — 15

Ngangkari

   Andy Tjilari — 23

   Toby Minyintiri Baker — 29

   Rupert Langkatjukur Peter — 41

   Naomi Kantjuriny — 47

   Ilawanti Ungkutjuru Ken — 55

   Maringka Burton — 67

   Pantjiti Unkari McKenzie — 77

   Sam Wimitja Watson — 85

   Josephine Watjari Mick — 99

   Jimmy Baker — 107

   Dickie Minyintiri — 113

   Tinpulya Kangitja Mervyn — 119

   Bernard Tjalkuriny — 127

   Whiskey Tjukanku — 137

   Harry Tjutjuna — 141

   Nakul Dawson — 145

   Arnie Frank — 147

   Wakupi Clem Toby (Dalby) — 151

   Martin Wintjin Thompson — 159

   Jacky Tjapaltjarri Giles — 163

   Ngulitjara — 165

Wangkanyi

    Changing World      173

    Ngangka<u>r</u>i Work      181

    Kurunpa – Spirits      191

    Grief, Death, Dying      205

    Substance Abuse      213

    Mental Health      227

    Working Together      239

    Recognition and Equality      247

    Children and Youth      251

    Future Ngangka<u>r</u>i      259

About Ngaanyatjarra Pitjantjatjara Yankunytjatjara

      Women's Council Aboriginal Corporation      263

Spelling and Pronunciation      266

Glossary      267

Acknowledgements      271

NPY Women's Council Region Map      272

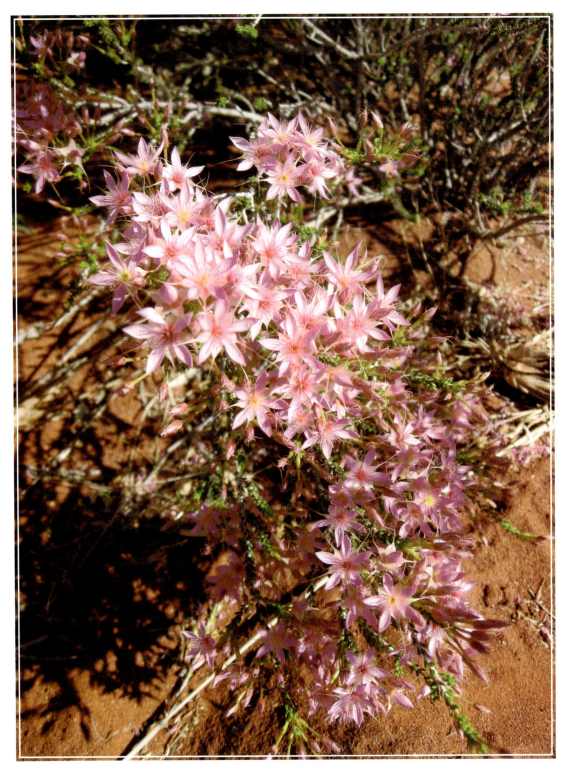

PHOTOGRAPH SALLY HODSON

# Foreword

It is both a privilege and honour to write the foreword to this most extraordinary book. The knowledge, wisdom and skill of our traditional healers is becoming increasingly recognised within Australia as well as internationally and it is with great thanks to the hard work of the Ngaanyatjarra Pitjantjatjara Yankunytjatjara (NPY) Women's Council for bringing into focus the work of our healers – not only for the direct benefit to the health and well-being of the community but to ensure that health practitioners are being educated in understanding and working with traditional healers to improve health and mental health outcomes. The work of the ngangkari throughout the Lands has been remarkable and this book goes some way towards furthering their work as well as providing an invaluable resource for the rest of the nation.

Aboriginal people within Australia are the oldest continuous living cultural group in the world. There is good reason why this is so. It has often been noted that at the time of colonisation, Aboriginal people were thought to be healthier than most Europeans. It was not by luck that this finding was possible. Aboriginal communities throughout Australia have had their own systems of health care and of healing methods for many thousands of years. Traditional healers are an essential part of life, family, community and culture, and have ensured the healthy development and well-being, as well as the recovery and healing, of our peoples since the beginning of time. In addition, traditional systems of governance and Law, kinship and skin groups, belief systems and custom provided for a life based on respect for relationships with all things in the universe. The connection to country as a source of health and renewal provided balance and sustainability. Being part of the landscape allowed for a continuity of existence across time. This strength of culture has been evidenced through the resilience and survival of Aboriginal peoples despite many generations of profound adversity and will continue to provide avenues for healing, recovery and well-being into the future. Some of the most innovative and effective health care systems are increasingly recognising the value of Aboriginal ways of understanding life and healing.

As a young Aboriginal girl growing up in Perth many years ago, both my grandmother's and mother's healing ways had always fascinated me. They were so knowledgeable about so many things and yet there was no recognition of this most important and valuable knowledge system within western education or health systems.

After completing my training as a doctor and psychiatrist, I was keen to incorporate Aboriginal ways of knowing and being into my work, recognising the limitations of western methods in healing and recovery. This was especially true in regard to mental health problems and social and emotional well-being issues I had encountered working with our countrymen. This journey subsequently led me to meet and work with the traditional healers employed through the NPY Women's Council.

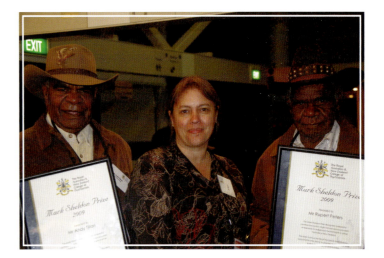

Ngangka<u>r</u>i Andy Tjilari (left) and Ngangka<u>r</u>i Rupert Langkatjukur Peter holding their awards and Dr Helen Milroy (centre), who nominated them for the Royal Australian and New Zealand College of Psychiatrists (RANZCP) 2009 Mark Sheldon Prize in recognition of their 'noteworthy contribution to Indigenous mental health.' The ceremony was held in Adelaide, South Australia, 2009.
PHOTOGRAPH ANGELA LYNCH

Our very first encounter occurred at a national psychiatric conference in 2000 where Mr Tjilari and Mr Peter were presenting their work in regard to Aboriginal mental health. I had never felt so proud – seeing our countrymen speaking out about healing – and I knew in my heart, my grandmother was also there watching in spirit.

Over the past twelve plus years it has been a wonderful journey of discovery and partnership, showcasing Aboriginal healing and knowledge to the health and mental health community both in Australia and around the world. The importance of their work has finally been recognised in our healers receiving both national and international awards for their significant leadership and contribution to mental health.

As our understanding of traditional methods increases, it is easy to see some of the overlaps with more recent developments in mental health care. Family-centred care – recognising the vital importance of attachment systems, holistic approaches and long-term support – are well recognised in Aboriginal systems.

There are also many parallels with methods often employed in psychotherapy such as developing trust, being held in mind (or spirit), developing shared understanding, meaning and use of metaphor. Traditional healers often have extensive knowledge of family and belief systems, can give culturally appropriate interpretations to symptoms and provide healing treatments. They also support each other in their practice, commit to lifelong learning and pass on their knowledge for the next generation of healers. The true potential of our Healers is yet to be fully realised.

This book is a collection of stories and profiles of many of our traditional healers throughout the Ngaanyatjarra Pitjantjatjara Yankunytjatjara Lands. It is a wealth of information about traditional healers and their methods that will be a vital resource for health practitioners around Australia as well as internationally. It is also important to recognise the privilege readers have in being able to learn and understand the many teachings in this book. The knowledge contained within should be treated with due respect. I would also like to express my gratitude for the generosity shown by the many contributors and their willingness in showcasing how healing our way continues on as it has done since the beginning of time.

As I was quoted by Mackean in the *Medical Journal of Australia* some years ago:

> *Healing is part of life and continues through death and into life again. It occurs throughout a person's life journey as well as across generations. It can be experienced in many forms such as mending a wound or recovery from illness. Mostly however, it is about renewal. Leaving behind those things that have wounded us and caused us pain. Moving forward in our journey with hope for the future with renewed energy, strength and enthusiasm for life. Healing gives us back to ourselves. Not to hide or fight anymore. But to sit still, calm our minds, listen to the universe and allow our spirits to dance on the wind. It lets us enjoy the sunshine and be bathed by the golden glow of the moon as we drift into our dreamtime. Healing ultimately gives us back to our country. To stand once again in our rightful place, eternal and generational.*

Healing is not just about recovering what has been lost or repairing what has been broken. It is about embracing our life force to create a new and vibrant fabric that keeps us grounded and connected, wraps us in warmth and love and gives us the joy of seeing what we have created. Healing keeps us strong and gentle at the same time. It gives us balance and harmony, a place of triumph and sanctuary forevermore.

Dr Helen Milroy
MB BS CertChildPsych *W. Aust.*, FRANZCP

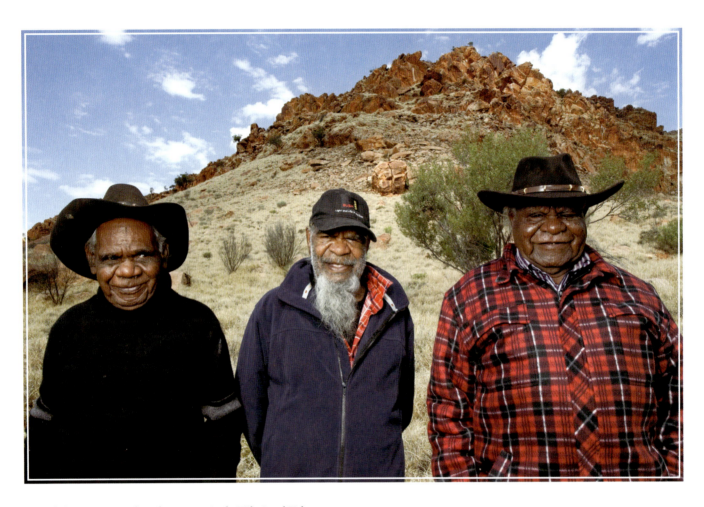

From left: Rupert Langkatjukur Peter, Andy Tjilari and Toby Minyintiri Baker, 2011. PHOTOGRAPH RHETT HAMMERTON

*We hope that our people in the future will realise, 'Hey! These named ngangka̱ri have done a marvellous job of recording our traditional culture!' It makes us proud and happy to think about these ngangka̱ri tjukurpa, belonging to all ngangkari.*

# A_la_ni – Introduction

Welcome to our new book. Given that we were once, only recently, naked spear-carrying people, and now that we have exchanged our spears for a new way of life and have almost forgotten how to pick up our spears and go hunting for meat, we are still very new to books. All we knew once was our spears and spear throwers.

Our people everywhere have always followed the instructions given out during our public speeches, early in the mornings. We used to listen to alpiri speeches every morning, just before dawn, in the early dawn light. Alpiri is the time when people talk, just before the sun comes up, early, as soon as the dawn's breaking, when you can see the ground in the early morning. People used to talk about where we would be going hunting, and they would name the places we'd be going to, and which kind of meat we'd be going for, and so we'd be able to prepare our minds for the day. All children would hear the speeches. As soon as dawn was breaking, people would start talking. We'd wake up to the sound of people giving speeches during the alpiri time. During alpiri speeches everybody would be advised as to which way they would be going, and of the hunting strategy for the day, and who would be going on the advance party to assess the hunting, and if they were going to go for one day or for a few nights and maybe keep going and then come back a few days later, or a month later. Some speeches were made during the night when people were lying down semi-asleep and so, of course, they'd hear all the speeches, and so in the morning, what was said would be discussed further.

Now we have this book, which is something that resembles our own alpiri speeches. We have opened up our lives to you, spoken our own alpiri speeches and put them into this book, for white people, and for you, to read. We never knew about books or paper before, never! All we have ever had are paperbark trees. We called the papery bark from the paperbark trees nyiri, which is the same word for paper and book. Paper and books come from white people, not us. We never wrote our Tjukurpa – our story, history, Aboriginal Law, 'Dreaming' – down before. Paper is now part of our lives, and so now we have written our own nyiri – our own book.

This is our own version of alpiri that we have spoken about, written into this book, and you may now read our stories about ourselves. This is the first time people like us have collected our stories together and written them down on paper. They are all in one place on this paper, and you can read our Tjukurpa that appear like written alpiri. We do have our Pitjantjatjara Bible, of course.

We did know how to communicate by making marks, of course, which we called walkatjunanyi. When travelling, we would make marks on the ground to say, 'We are heading off over in that direction!' and we'd scrape marks on the ground to tell them to join us later at a certain point. We would make a number of similar marks reminding them not to delay in joining us. We'd use our feet to make the marks on the ground. Tjinangku – we'd write with the feet.

We'd communicate these sorts of things: 'Go around that way and camp overnight. The following day keep going to that important big place, because that is where we want to meet up with you next!' or 'Women and children come along now!' or 'We have already gone on ahead!' 'We've gone in that direction!' We'd mark the ground in a straight line with the foot. We would mark the ground with our hands too, to leave a message for our families, instructing them about where we were heading. We still do this. Our families still do this. So we were almost writing, poor us! We were writing, but not on paper! Today we go by the whitefella Tjukurpa. Telephone. We use whitefella telephones to say, 'We are going in that direction!' Or we write it down on the paper.

So the notion of writing on paper is a very new one, but here we are with our own book. People can choose which part they wish to read. All the people who look at this book will be able to understand us more, and we are happy about that. We are really happy to offer a number of ngangkari people's stories.

The stories are about how we all walked the land, how we all lived, how we took our spears and hunted our meat, and how we cooked it, and how everyone sang inma, ceremonial song, all the time to the children, and how we lived our lives like that. Stories of our way of life are all here in this book. We naked children were always dancing! We adored dancing! We were naked, but who minded? We sang all the time. We'd be playing and we'd hear the melodies rising up and we'd know there would be inma in preparation. In the early evening the inma would begin and everyone would gather around for the dancing and singing and we would watch it. We have so many stories about our traditional life because our lives are so rich.

We have carried on with most of our traditions as well, and so we are able to talk about them with clarity and familiarity. We've told you a lot about our lives in our new book, so when you open it and read our first words in this opening section, you will read these words that we are speaking now. We are writing down new stories this time, new stories, different from the ones in our previous book *Ngangkari Work — Anangu Way*, now out of print.

Spoken Tjukurpa from we ngangkari are inside this book. It contains Tjukurpa about the healing touch of the ngangkari and stories about how ngangkari came to be – as well as many other stories, stories about the campfire, living beside the fire, in shelters made of branches and beside windbreaks, living inside beautiful warm and comfortable wiltja – shelter, or cool and shady wiltja. Our shelters protect us from the elements and keep us dry from the rain. Our grandmothers would ensure they were well maintained. We would sleep warm and cosily inside, next to the warm embers of the fire. We were well looked after children. We were healthy – ipilypa.

Everyone was healthy because of ngangkari. Ngangkari would arrive quickly when summoned to a sick child. If the child had, say, sore ears, the ngangkari would work quickly around the ear area of the sick child, in the comfort of their own wiltja. The ngangkari would remove the badness and banish it from the home wiltja. Ngangkari are skilled at recognising and banishing mamu, away from the home wiltja. Mamu are harmful spirit beings – a dangerous spirit force or energy

Children would respond well and bounce back to health quickly. The ngangkari would regularly follow up with the healing breath – the blowing treatment – afterwards. The blowing-breath treatment is the finishing touch to any treatment. The parents would be relieved and happy about the treatment and ngangkari would always be praised and thanked, sincerely. This is how we lived, how our grandfathers lived.

In our first book we spoke a lot about achieving acceptance and recognition in the western medical world. Many ngangkari have already given a number of their stories in that first book. That was a great book, with great stories. We knew that it would bring us out into the open, and it did. People understood us a lot more after that first book came out. That's why we told the stories, for people to read. We put a pair of hands on the front cover to show that ngangkari work primarily with the hands. Ngangkari are gifted with healing hands. Mara ala – healing hands. Mara nyangatja mapan tjara – these hands hold mapanpa.

These hands work with the spirit. Inside these hands are mapanpa. The hands touch the sick person. The person being touched is always happy to be given the healing touch. The family members are happy too. Ngangkari make people happy. People freely watch a ngangkari treatment and they are always thrilled to see ngangkari at work. They place their absolute trust in ngangkari and ngangkari deliver results.

We used to carry mingkulpa – wild tobacco – around in the old days, but how did we do it without pockets? Well, we bundled our mingkulpa up inside emu feathers. We would rub the mingkulpa on rocks and make it just right to take in the mouth. This is something we all enjoy. A ngangkari will also carry mapanpa around in that same emu-feather bundle. The ngangkari would always have his bundles with him. Of course all men had their bundles of mingkulpa! You don't need to be a ngangkari to have an emu-feather bundle. Women and men all had to carry their mingkulpa somehow. Women were very good at bundle – making. After all, they'd be making manguri – headrings – all the time. They'd make beautiful manguri in order to carry their water bowls safely back home, balanced on their heads. We Anangu have got many different tools. Ngangkari have many tools of their own, and most of the time these tools are quite public and can be seen by others.

In this new edition, we are making public some more stories, newer stories and newer information about ourselves, in the same way that a ngangkari will open his feather bundle and reveal his mapanpa.

People can read about us, and our communities, and hopefully understand that there are ngangkari in many communities – that we are many rather than few. We hope they will be happy about these stories. We want people to enjoy our stories. We ngangkari have not spoken like this before, this is the first time in history that we ngangkari have revealed so much about ourselves. Our forebears never spoke publicly like this before and in this book Toby speaks for the first time ever about his own life.

Ngangkari have had varied lives, and this book is full of ngangkari lives and stories. Our own people can read these stories and we hope they will derive a lot of joy and pride from knowing what strong Law we have and what strong culture has come down to us from our forebears. We hope they will be happy and proud to read about their own people – their own ngangkari.

These stories are all ngangkari stories. All ngangkari follow ngangkari rules. We are strict about following our Law. We work according to the ancient Laws and rules of our ancestors. We work with our special perceptions, our eyes and our hands. We see everything and we are always ready to help. We see mamu. Ngangkari know everything, proper ngangkari.

We can help depressed people by talking to them and speaking to them straight, to help them move forward from their poor mental state, and we continue talking and talking to them to help them regain their equilibrium. It is like this: 'You might be depressed from something that has made your life go wrong, why have you allowed it to mess up your life?' and they'll say, 'No, it is because my wife has been swearing at me and I have been angry and because of that I have been depressed and sad'. And so we'd say, 'But you have no reason to be so sad, you should be happy, don't be sad, be happy and think about your family. Be happy within your family. Perhaps you have to leave your wife, if she is ruining your life, you need to get happy and find happiness. Choose your heart! How can you live with a sad kurunpa? With a healthy kurunpa you will live a happy life.' Like that. We counsel people, yes we do.

We work our way through to the start of the problem. 'Are you sad because of the arguments?' They'll say, 'Yes, there have been arguments directed towards me and because of that I have been depressed.' So we advise them, 'You must continue to talk to ngangkari about this and we will treat you for your inner depression'. So they continue to see a ngangkari and the ngangkari has a look and gives them a healing treatment and brings about inner harmony. 'Your argumentative inner-self is not good for you but now you are less angry, you will be happy and live a happier life'. We work often like this, on happiness.

Helping people with mental health problems is the same as that, we are very effective. We also work on the circulation flow, which is one thing ngangkari highly value as a treatment. Ngangkari open the flow again, and people quickly improve, and everything is soon better.

When someone is right at the end of their life and in palliative care, then it is too late. It is too late for the dying person, and they know that. So all we can do is wait, but that is good too. Perhaps the dying person is an old man, and if so, the relatives accept that. We are all happy that they have lived a good life, and there is no argument and everyone's satisfied that everything that could be done was done. The person passes away with dignity and everyone is OK about it. Ngangkari have a job to do then, but it is too late for the dying person. Nobody is worried that he is departing because we know he has had a good life and has been a successful hunter and has lived a long and healthy life and now it is his time to depart. The whole family is happy and proud of him and some of the younger people are hoping to receive the bequest of his kurunpa.

This is how all our grandfathers died. They died in good circumstances, and died of old age. Of course everyone is very sad that they are losing him but they accept that death is a fact of life. What is the point of worrying too much? Listen, you are not to worry too much. Move forward. The surviving widow is still broken-hearted when her man dies and she cries aloud and her kurunpa inside is crying too. They think about him all night. People can't forget him. They will cry and be sad. They will wait for a couple of weeks for the kurunpa to be gathered and placed inside the surviving widow.

It makes us proud and happy to think about these ngangkari Tjukurpa, belonging to all ngangkari. All the ngangkari know the rules. Ngangkari are very intelligent people. Ngangkari have a lot to consider. They use their foresight, their eyesight and the touch of their hands. That is how they work. We hope people will enjoy reading the new stories in this book because they are good stories and tell the clear story. Most of them are new stories, which are placed next to some of the earlier ones. We also have paintings of Tjukurpa, culture, country, travel and mamu. All the paintings have Tjukurpa in them.

We are really happy with our new series of stories. They are only open ngangkari stories. These stories are only the ones allowed to be open and public. Our sacred Law is for Anangu only. We do not speak about our sacred stories. People can read this without fear, even children can read this book without fear. This book is for Anangu to read about ngangkari and for them to be proud they have their own healers. They can read in this book about our own inma. They can read the stories about how children became ngangkari and perhaps they may wish to become ngangkari themselves. We are proud of all the people we have healed.

We tell how we live and work because it is only ngangkari telling their stories in this big new book, bringing their important stories out into the open. It is them to whom we give credit. They'll have the pleasure, seeing people read it and see the realisation dawning – 'Oh! So that's it! These stories are all by ngangkari! This is marvellous, these stories are marvellous!' The stories are all by ngangkari and they are all good. They are all important ngangkari thoughts. We hope that our people in the future will realise, 'Hey! These named ngangkari have done a marvellous job of recording our traditional culture!'

Andy Tjilari, Rupert Langkatjukur Peter and Toby Minyintiri Baker

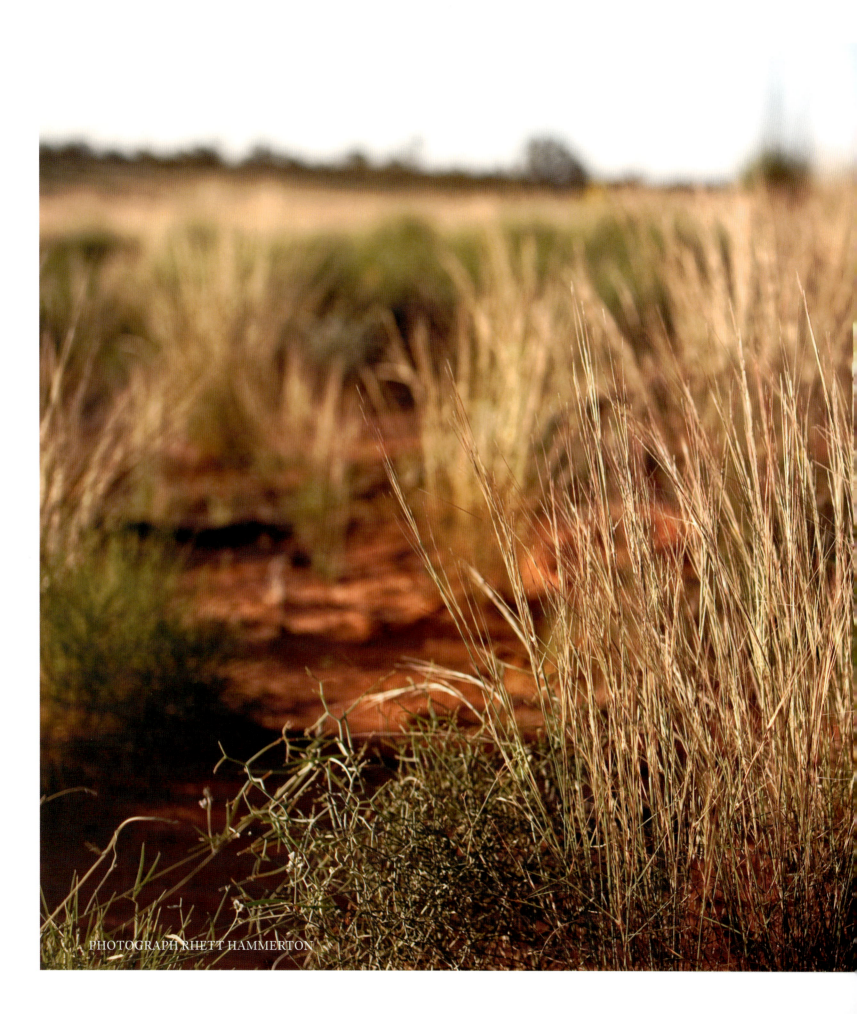
PHOTOGRAPH RHETT HAMMERTON

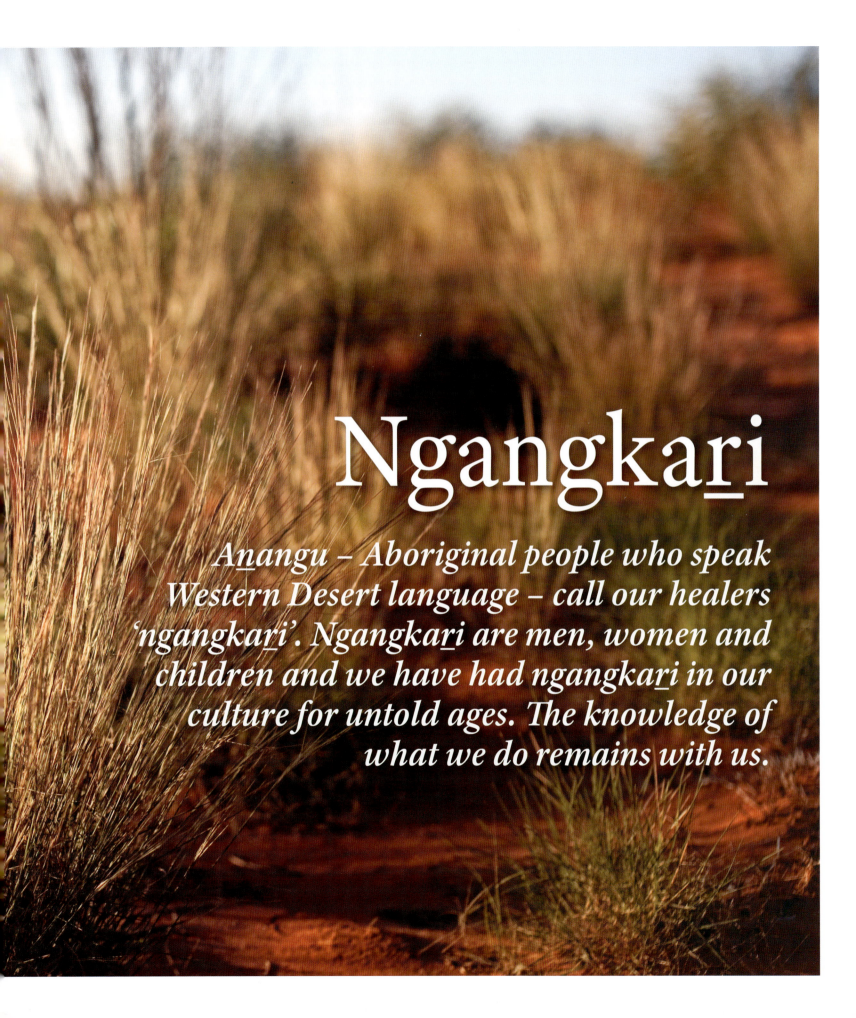

# Ngangka_ri_

*A_n_angu – Aboriginal people who speak Western Desert language – call our healers 'ngangka_ri_'. Ngangka_ri_ are men, women and children and we have had ngangka_ri_ in our culture for untold ages. The knowledge of what we do remains with us.*

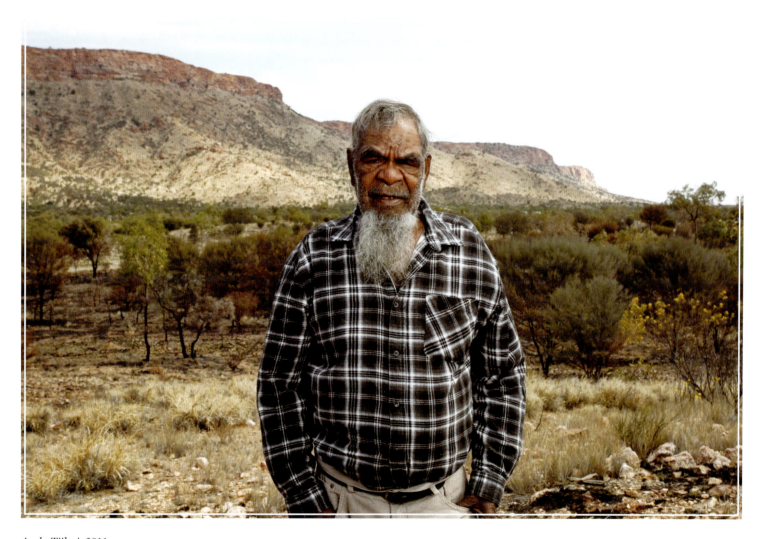

Andy Tjilari, 2011. PHOTOGRAPH RHETT HAMMERTON

# Andy Tjilari

When I was growing up I used to have three grandfathers, who were all ngangka<u>r</u>i. The first one was my mother's father. The second was my father's father and there was a third, who was another one of my father's fathers (my grandfather's brother). So I lived with these three ngangka<u>r</u>i. Well, actually there were four, because my father was a ngangka<u>r</u>i as well.

Grandfather used to say, 'Oh, don't you think that we ought to give our grandson here some of our mapa<u>n</u>pa, ngangka<u>r</u>i sacred tools? Shouldn't we give him some of our sacred tools so that he can become a ngangka<u>r</u>i himself?' After he had spoken like this, they thought about it and talked about it among themselves. They decided, 'Yes, alright. We will.' So my grandfather said to me, 'Grandson. Come over here. Come and sit down next to me and listen carefully.' So I came and sat down next to my grandfather. My grandfather asked me, 'Do you want us to give you ngangka<u>r</u>i power, so that you can live your life as a ngangka<u>r</u>i? You'll have to help sick people, and heal them, whether they are men, women or children.' I replied, 'But grandfather. I am not a ngangka<u>r</u>i. I don't know how to.'

He replied, 'Well, if you want to, I can give you some power right away, and you can make a start on your life as a new ngangka<u>r</u>i. What do you think? You tell me. Don't forget, if you do become a ngangka<u>r</u>i, the power will stay with you all your life and you'll never lose it, or be able to throw it away. So if I make you a ngangka<u>r</u>i now, you will always be a ngangka<u>r</u>i.'

My father was observing all of this. He told me that the way I would have to heal people would be to pull the sickness out of their bodies in the form of pieces of wood, or sticks, or stones, things like that. This is so that people can actually see with their own eyes the sickness that is removed from their bodies. This is the commonly accepted way we ngangka<u>r</u>i do our work. It is so that people can see us taking their sickness away from their bodies, which gives them a sense of removal. My father told me I'd have to make sure I showed them what I took out, so they could see it, before I disposed of it.

I said to my father, 'But how? How am I supposed to do that? I don't understand how ngangka<u>r</u>i work. How could I ever be able to do that?' He replied, 'Don't worry, we'll show you. It won't be hard once you know how.' So I was shown. I was given the power of a ngangka<u>r</u>i by all my grandfathers, and I still have that power today. They taught me everything I know. They didn't tell me how to do it. They showed me. They also placed inside me the sacred objects I would need to be my tools for working as a ngangka<u>r</u>i. These are called mapa<u>n</u>pa. Nobody else showed me or taught me but my grandfathers and father. I didn't learn from any books or papers.

In the past, many children became ngangka<u>r</u>i at a very early age. Children who took an interest in the healing arts often asked to be given power and to receive training. Often this training took place, as it did for me with the other ngangka<u>r</u>i, at a distance from camp. The ngangka<u>r</u>i would light fires at a separate camp and they would wait for the spirits to bring them special powerful tools. The ngangka<u>r</u>i would stay in that camp and would sleep there too. During the night, when they were all asleep, all the ngangkari people's spirit bodies would start to rise up from their sleeping bodies and soar upwards. Now you know how people fly around in aeroplanes and drive around in cars? Well, for Anangu, and for ngangkari, when they are asleep at night, their spirits move around in a similar kind of way. The ngangkari could be men, women or children. Their spirit bodies begin to fly around and to visit the sleeping spirits of other people to make sure all was well. They would say, 'All is well among our people tonight.' They would place mallee eucalypt leaves around the camp.

The spirit of a sick person is usually too sick to fly properly, and often crashes into trees. This is when the ngangkari's night time work is very useful, because they will see the injured spirit holding onto the trunk of the tree, or rather, not on the trunk of the tree, but fallen on the ground at its base. The ngangkari will come up and rescue the spirit. In doing so, he is able to recognise who it is and will say, 'Oh, this is such-and-such. He is not well. Poor thing, he needs help here.' So he'll pick up the spirit and take him to the body and ask the sleeping person to wake up. 'Wake up. Your spirit is not well. Sit up and I'll put you to rights.' The person will sit up, the ngangkari will replace the stricken spirit, and all will be well again very soon. By the next day, he will be quite better. This is a very special skill which we ngangkari alone have. This can be referred to as 'Ngangkari tjutaku Tjukurpa' – Ngangkari Law.

While all the ngangkari are gathered in the special camps, hundreds of mapanpa will come flying in. Mapanpa are special powerful tools. Hundreds and hundreds will come in and the ngangkari discuss them as they arrive. They have a lot to talk about, as you can imagine. Meanwhile the mapanpa are hitting the ground with small explosions, 'boom, boom, boom!' The ngangkari dash around collecting up the objects; kanti that look like sharp stone blades, kuuti that resemble black shiny round tektites, and tarka – slivers of bone. Each ngangkari gathers up the pieces he wants. These pieces become his own private property. This, too, is Ngangkari tjutaku Tjukurpa.

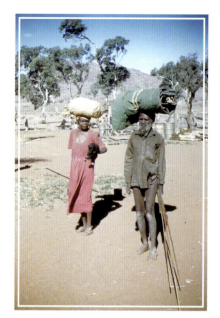

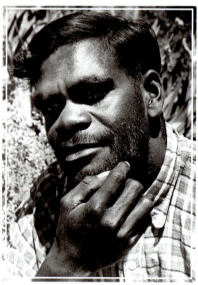

Top: Tommy Urutjakunu and Anawari Ingkatji (Andy Tjilari's parents) setting out on a journey from Pukatja, 1960.
PHOTOGRAPH BILL EDWARDS, ARA IRITITJA AI-0013203

Bottom: Andy Tjilari, an elected church leader, in Pukatja (Ernabella), South Australia, 1952.
PHOTOGRAPH HAMILTON AITKIN, BILL AND ALLISON ELLIOTT COLLECTION, ARA IRITITJA AI-0019251

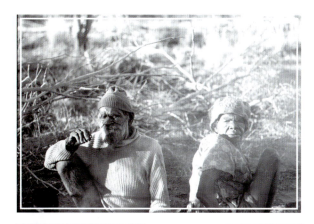

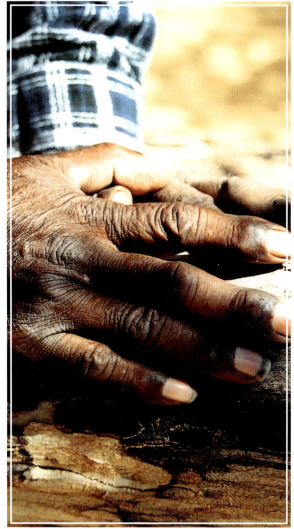

Top: Tommy Urutjakunu and Anawari Ingkatji (Andy Tjilari's parents) beside a smoky fire, 1975.
PHOTOGRAPH PETER BROKENSHA, ARA IRITITJA AI-0027778

Bottom: Andy Tjilari's hands. PHOTOGRAPH ANGELA LYNCH

I was taught this as a child, and one day my turn came, when I was told, 'Child, come with me.' I went with father. He said, 'Push your hands into the ground.' I was frightened! I thought there must be a mamu – negative spirit force – in there or something! But I did as I was told and I pushed my hand into the ground. I didn't know it at the time, but there were mapanpa buried in there. It was a mapanpa hole. I felt something in there. 'What's this?' I pulled out the mapanpa. It was a mapanpa in the form of a sliver of bone, quite big. Father looked at it and then gave it to me, saying, 'This is your own mapanpa now. You keep it now.'

Ngangkari use their own mapanpa to do their healing treatments. It could be a tarka, kuuti or kanti. The mapanpa live inside parts of ngangkari's bodies, such as the palm of the hand. Sometimes the hands feel as if they have been speared by the power of the mapanpa.

I realise all this sounds very different to all you doctors and nurses who have studied so hard at university to get where you are today. You have studied so many books. But consider that we are nevertheless working towards the same goal of healing sick people and making them feel better in themselves, as you are. In that way we are equal. We are the same.

When Anangu are terribly ill with a life-threatening illness, we understand that sometimes it takes a doctor to do a full operation to save their life. Yet that sick person's spirit may still harbour something that will continue to affect their recovery. So ngangkari can help on another level that you modern doctors cannot.

There are some very powerful spirit figures in our culture called Karpirinypa. Karpirinypa give ngangkari gifts of mapanpa which help in the healing process. Powerful healing forces from our mapanpa can bathe a sick person in a healing energy. The forces seek out mamu, or the malignant forces that cause the sickness in the first place, and destroy them. You'll see nothing from the outside, but the healing is taking place on the inside. This is our usual healing method.

A normal kind of ngangkari treatment comes from the hands, where the main power is. Power! Power! Ngangkari power enters the sick person, and the sickness is extracted in a physical form, so that the sufferer can see with his own eyes what it was causing his pain. The healer can either throw the object away, or bury it somewhere. Again, this is Ngangkariku Tjukalpa, or ladder to the stars.

I am not saying only I do this. No. All ngangkari in the east, west, north and south have these powers. We are everywhere. Ngangkari are everywhere, and we are men, we are women and we are children.

We did not invent any of this yesterday, either. All this Tjukurpa – story, history, Aboriginal Law, 'Dreaming' – comes from ancient days. Because it is so old, it will never die. Ngangkari power will be around forever.

I am now going to talk about mamu. There are many mamu, some who crawl about the trunks of trees and others who walk along the ground. Some mamu look like dogs. Other mamu look like emu – Karpirinypa is one of those. Karpirinypa walks around, closely resembling an emu, and
he is the owner of a great number of mapanpa, kuuti, kanti and other types of stones and blades. He carries them around with him, and when I was a child, he gave some to me.

While he would probably never hurt a child, he was perfectly capable of causing injury to a man. Despite that, he gave both my grandfather and I many mapanpa. I have held on to mine all my life. This occurred on our country out west. In order to prevent me from losing my mapanpa, back in the days before pockets, my grandfather made me special emu-feather bundles to carry them around in. From that time forwards I became a holder of mapanpa, a Mapantjara, walking naked on the land. Grandfather gave me the bundles and I took great care of them.

The mapanpa were so closely associated with the emu that he would come around at night and make noises exactly like an emu does. Ngangkari men would travel west and, while sleeping and resting on those journeys, would hear him coming along, making noises like an emu call. He was named Karpirinypa; indeed, they were all called Karpirinypa.

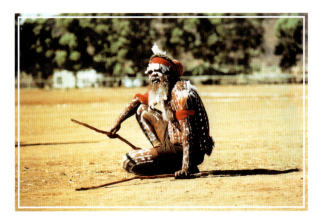

Above: Andy Tjilari performing the Wati Kirkinpa Inma at the opening of the new Pukatja football oval, South Australia, 1992. PHOTOGRAPH MAGGIE KAVANAGH, NPY WOMEN'S COUNCIL COLLECTION, ARA IRITITJA, AI-0035327

Opposite page: Andy Tjilari, *Ngangkariku Tjukalpa*, 2011. Acrylic on canvas, 25 x 30 cm. PHOTOGRAPH RHETT HAMMERTON.

*Ngangkariku Tjukalpa (Ngangkari's ladder to the stars): All the ngangkari sleep in their wiltjas, shade shelters, at night. They seem to be asleep, but really, they are listening. At once, they all rise up together and glide into the night sky, like eagles soaring. They are on a marali journey – spirit journey undertaken by Ngangkari. They soar higher and higher, journeying along a ngangkariku ladder. Ngangkari call this ladder a tjukalpa. Tjukalpa is the same word for ladder, and the Milky Way, and this is where they are heading, to the stars. Their journey takes them from their camps and waterholes to the stars, where special ngangkari healing work begins.*

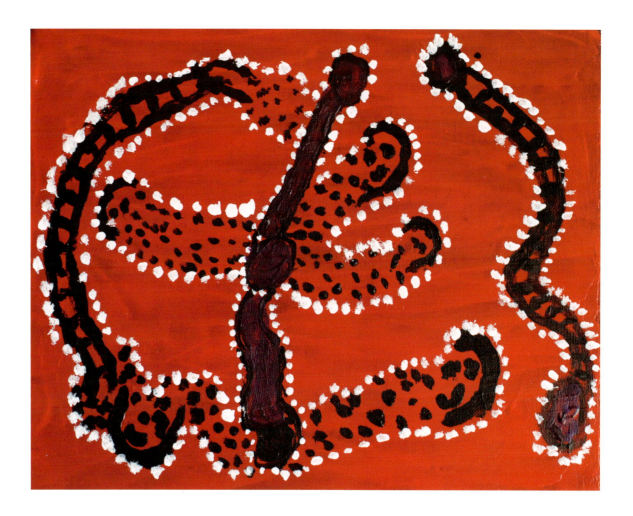

Karpirinypa they were called, and when they came close to the men they would angrily hurl objects at them and knock them down. Those Karpirinypa Mamu Men were really dangerous and fierce. They'd hurl things at men, or try and chop them, or thump them.

But the ngangkari men would hear them coming. They'd hear them talking as they came closer, and would easily recognise them from their emu-sounding voices. The men would go out to them, and they'd take the boy ngangkari with them, and circle around and call, 'They are here! They are getting too close to the people!' They'd be all around, making those noises, but when spotted, we'd all be given mapanpa.

Yet I, a mere child, did not fear them, because they would always give me more mapanpa of all types – kanti, kuuti, tarka – all kinds – and I'd then give them to my grandfather. 'Grandfather, put these inside emu-feather bundles!' In this manner, I received my gifts from the emu. I always gifted some to my grandfather because I loved him so much.

We were still naked people then, with no other way to carry things like that but in emu-feather bundles. This story I am telling comes from the early days, when ngangkari were made in this way and many mamu walked the earth, not just one, but many. Mamu in the shape of dogs, mamu in the shape of emus, such as Karpirinypa.

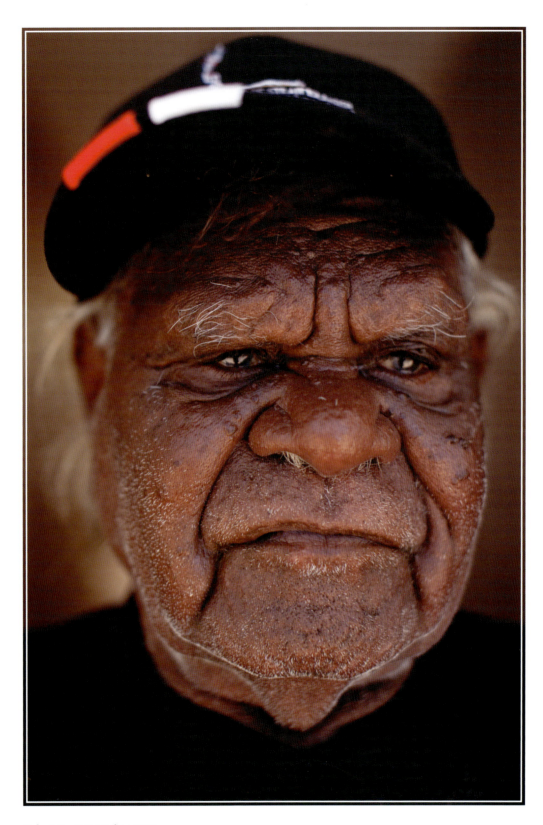

Toby Minyintiri Baker, 2011. PHOTOGRAPH RHETT HAMMERTON

# Toby Minyintiri Baker

The name that I was born with was Minyintiri. My grandfather gave me that name, Minyintiri. When white people came into our Lands, I was given the name 'Ginger' and later on 'Toby'. They are both new names that I was given.

I was born at Irurpa down from Kanpi in the hills. Irurpa and Kanpi are on the ridge there. Irurpa is my grandfather's home and my father's home. Tommy Tjuwintjara was my father. My mother's country is quite close but my father's country and his father's country is Irurpa. We lived on the ridge country around Irurpa and Kanpi. Irurpa is up on a hill not far from Kanpi. It's a spring in the river that's in the hills. It's a creek that comes down from the ranges there.

I was born at Irurpa but my pulyi, fell off at Kanpi. Pulyi is the umbilical cord that falls off by itself, or is cut off by the women if it is too long and gets in the way. Where your umbilical cord comes off is called your home. Everybody has an umbilical cord.

My grandfathers were all healers. They were all ngangkari. They knew all the Tjukurpa. I learnt from the ngangkari Tjukurpa when I was growing up, when I was a child. Traditionally our grandfathers got their Tjukurpa from the spirit and their daily plans from those important stories that were handed on during a time similar to the alpiri public speech time.

We know the Tjukurpa, and the stories, and we know we can get mapanpa from the Tjukurpa and through the stories. You're born with the power or you can get the mapanpa through somebody giving it to you, somebody can put it in your hand and then you get it. Others get the power through words, when somebody says something and you can get power from something, from words. There are different ways to become a mapanpa person – from your Tjukurpa, through the spirit when somebody gives it to you, and through language. There are lots of stories that ngangkari keep secret, which we are handing down to the next generation.

If somebody is sick they will search for a ngangkari and that ngangkari will heal the sick person. The men used to tell the mothers, 'If your child is sick, take it to a healer and they'll heal and fix the child'.

Our fathers and the other men before them were very powerful ngangkari healers. My father's brother, Nuyumpakunu, was a truly powerful ngangkari and he used to give treatments at Kanpi and at a place called Ularipa. I was given powers by the men and I had healing powers given to me by my father's brother. Nuyumpakunu gave me powers and taught me the rules. He gave me the gift of healing powers. I had the gift and the powers then.

When I was a child and holding Dad's brother's mapanpa I used to heal people because I had the ngangkari power. I can lay hands on people, wirulymananyi, and sometimes my mapanpa can send illness out from a person's body – it can do it separately from me. I haven't got total control over it – it can do some things on its own, if I can't actually get it with my own hands.

Our tjamu – grandfathers – give us lots of stories. They gave me stories and told me everything about our land and our people. My own father didn't have mapanpa, but my other father, Nuyumpakunu, my father's brother, he was a mapanpa man and he's the one who gave me my mapanpa. I still have my mapanpa within me. I followed my grandfather's ara, tradition, his Tjukurpa, his kuka – meat –and everything, but it was my father's brother – Nuyumpakunu – who gave me the mapanpa. He gave mapanpa to a number of children.

Before, when we used spears, some ngangkari used to catch a lost spirit with their miru, their spear thrower. If the spirit landed on the spear thrower then they would bring the spear thrower towards the person's body and place it against the person's body, which would allow the spirit to go into the body. These are advanced techniques. The healer didn't place his hand on the spirit after it landed on the spear thrower. There was once a really powerful healer that lived to the east of us. There was a man who died, and this healer from the east brought him back to life. He used his spear thrower to bring that man back. He was a really powerful healer.

When someone has died, the spirit has already left the body and there is no breath left in the body, but the spirit is still there close by. So we bury the body, during the first funeral service, and we stand a digging stick or a spear above the burial site. For a woman, we put a digging stick, a wana, above the body; for a man, his kulata. They used to leave the spear or the woman's digging stick above the burial site, the kurulpa. The kurulpa is a grave. A kurulpa is a mound on top of the body, which is in a hole. You dig a hole and you lay the body in, and then on top of the body you put lots of sticks. You put sticks on top of the body, sticks and leaves, and maybe sometimes rocks, and then you cover it with dirt – that wood and grass mound is the kurulpa.

The spirit of the deceased person stays around with the body and people could hear it. The spirit can travel around. The spirit goes off and eats foods like caterpillars and insects, and maybe other things. It can hear the noise of people calling out. When Anangu are shouting out to each other in the bush, calling out 'Paa! Paa!', the spirit will hear them and it will answer them. The spirit will go down the spear or down the digging stick, it will travel down the spear and into the body, and it will go 'Brrrrrrrrr,' and then the people know that the spirit has come to rest. So the spirit travels down the spear or the wana, down to the kurulpa, which is the logs and sticks, then down to the person that's underneath it, to the body of the deceased.

During the second funeral ceremony the spirit from the deceased spouse is collected and given to the bereaved wife or husband. They used to do lot of ceremony when the wife came. There would be a group of healers who would surround the kurulpa to assist in getting the spirit, the kurunpa from the kurulpa into the widow, the living widow who was left behind by the deceased. I'm a widower and I've got my wife's spirit here inside of me. She is gone but I have her spirit with me still.

A long time ago people used to gather pii. Pii is the 'skin' of a caterpillar nest. Pii is the actual outside of a nest which the caterpillar makes to live in – the yuunpa. That's what you collect and you remove all the kuna, or droppings, of the caterpillar out of the bag and you clean it and you put it on burns. Once that

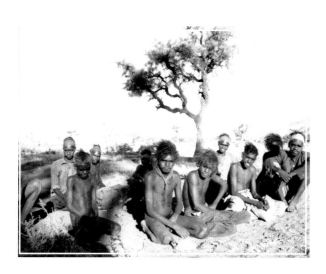

Toby Minyintiri Baker (centre, left) sitting with other nyiinka (segregated young men) at Pukatja (Ernabella), South Australia, 1944–48. PHOTOGRAPH RICHARD BROCK, ARA IRITITJA AI-0027577

happened to me, near Kanpi. I was playing and I burnt my arm. My mother and father put a pii on my skin when I got burnt and it was like a bandage. And later on I started scratching so they said, 'Take it off now, take the pii off.' And so they took it off and my skin was fine underneath. It had all healed! There's a lot of pii. The wanka itchy grub's nest that they make, that's the pii. And all the kuna, the caterpillar's kuna, you remove that and what you have left is just the nest and that's the pii.

One morning I was playing, and I fell into the fire on a spinifex clump. We were playing and lighting fires, the way that kids do, and jumping up and down from trees. I fell out of the tree into one of the spinifex clumps that was burning. Mum and Dad put the pii on me like a bandage and four days later when the bandage fell off I was better. Something in the pii reacts with the burn and causes it to heal itself. That's our own medicine, and it is a very effective medicine. The caterpillar's nest works by melting into the skin and healing it. In that pii, the caterpillar's bag, the nest, there are medicinal properties that heal a burn.

For the skin or ears there's another medicine we use. This is the milk that is found in the stomach of a baby rabbit. It is squeezed out and put on the head. If a child has sore ears and the mother is lactating, she can also squirt breast milk into the ear. The mother's breast milk has medicine in it.

A powerful medicinal plant that's used all the time is irmangka-irmangka, *Eremophila alternifolia*. You collect the leaves and pound the leaves up and make it into oil, which is very fragrant and beautiful. Eucalyptus trees have a nice oil too. A lot of the trees make nice oils for making medicines, whilst others are poisonous, such as walkalpa – the highly poisonous emu poison bush. You mash the walkalpa leaves and put it in the waterhole – an emu drinks it and dies. The emu drinks the water that is left out for it in a rockhole. If a person drinks it they'll die too, like the emu.

When my aunty Anilyuru was still alive, she took us to Ernabella Mission. She was my father's sister-in-law. That's my aunty, she's passed away now. She's got a lot of grandchildren living today at Watinuma. A lot of her grandchildren live there. I don't know what year that was. I was a small child, and there were no houses anywhere – except Ernabella probably had one or two very small houses. There were a lot of camels around, but not many houses. There was a sheep station near Indulkana called Muruly, and there was Ernabella Mission, and those two places had the only buildings that existed in our world at that time. People used to get dingo scalps in exchange for food. They sold the scalps to white people. Our fathers used to work on the sheep station but my mother had died long before, when there were no houses at all, long, long before, when we were still living in the bush with no clothes.

When I was a big boy I started work. One day I was fixing a tyre. I was working and then a whitefella stole me, he hid me away and made me work for him. When we were fixing the car he sent my brothers off, and then he took me away. He took me in his car. I was a really lively child and I could work hard, and that's why he stole me to work with him. That man got me, and then he said, 'Oh, he's my son', and looked after me and grew me up and made me work on the station. And that woman who was his wife was like a mother to me. She was like a mother to me. My own real mother had died a long time ago.

I lived there for a long time at that station, living in a tent. I was working on that old station, Wanukula – Mulga Park Station. There was a big waterhole there named Wanukula. Wanukula was the first place, south of the current Mulga Park homestead. I worked with the white people on their station, and with a fella called Ted Pukuti from Mulga Park. We worked together on a sheep station. Then we moved to the new station at Mulga Park with that man who stole me, and we lived there with Ted Pukuti. We moved from that old place Wanukula, to the new place, because there was more water there. There are a lot of rockholes around there, Wanukula and many others.

A white person named me Toby. Lots of men like me were given the name of 'Toby' or 'Ginger' for some reason. I worked everywhere as a station hand, helping out where I could. I worked as a stockman with the white people. We travelled around and I gave healing treatments as well.

I was a very young man when I saw the Maralinga bomb smoke. It came up as far as Ernabella. There was dust everywhere. It was everywhere – on the leaves, on the grass, on the trees, on the bark. That was the mamu, we call it mamu, and the irati, the poison, and from that time everybody was falling down and dying. Only old Trudinger, who was the superintendent at Ernabella mission during the time, and the few who were helping him were digging pits and laying all the dead people in lines and burying them. They didn't have one cemetery – they just had one long line where they buried everybody.

Many people died. My aunty died, Pikulpa's mother, at Wamikata. My uncle died. We buried him. And then my Aunty Anilyuru, my father's sister, the one who took us to Pukatja, she died. I became really sick too and I was just about to die. I screamed, 'That big hole there's been dug for me, for them to bury me!' There was a grave already prepared for me. Somebody made a big fire and my father's younger brother went and got all the intestines out of a fox, the muturka. He minced the fox's intestines, minced it with the liver, and he covered me all over with the paste, and then I was laid on hot fire ash. I was screaming, 'Oh!' I nearly died, but God kept me alive and saved me.

My family took me back to Ernabella to try and get me some medicine. We got to Itjinpiri, near Ernabella, and I was walking in the front, staggering along. I was just walking like a dead man.

Opposite page: Toby Minyintiri Baker, *Puyu Pakala*, 2006. Acrylic on canvas, 131 x 96 cm.
PHOTOGRAPH COURTESY MARSHALL ARTS, © THE ARTIST AND TJUNGU PALYA

*Piti tjuta (all the rockholes). Each rockhole has a wanampi (rainbow serpent) living in it. This country stretches from Uluru to the Western Australian border and down to Watarru. Wanampi tjuta (many rainbow serpents here). One lives at Malara, two at Piltati, and others at Kunytjanu, Mutitjulu and Watarru. The two women at Piltati are sitting by the fire performing a sacred ceremony. They are calling the smoke up. Puyu pakala (the smoke is rising) from each of the waterholes. Smoke coming out everywhere.*

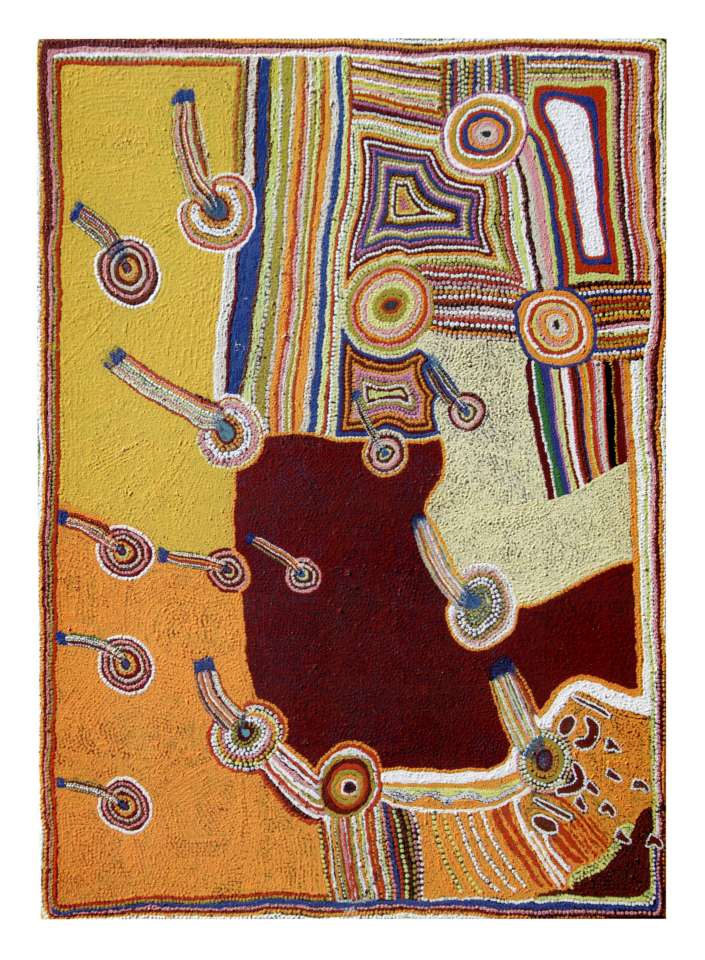

I was very sick from the Maralinga ira_ti_ and a lot of other people were dying around me. Then I looked down. 'Eh? Something fell!' And I looked – there was a lovely bottle that looked like gold, shiny. A voice said to me, 'Drink it! Drink from that bottle which looks like gold!' My father said, 'No! Don't drink what's in the bottle! Don't drink that! It's rotten! It's an old something inside that bottle!' Yet I drank it! It was sweet. I threw the bottle away. I lay down, and my father was crying. I was really on death's door, lying there. Then I woke up and I said, 'Hey, where's that bottle?' I was looking for that bottle that had something gold in it. 'I threw that bottle here; where is it?' It had disappeared! Nothing! There were no marks on the ground, nothing!

I got back up and we went on to Ernabella and arrived there in Ernabella Mission. I saw a lot more people who were sick, sitting, lying down, sick and really weak and frail. Then I saw my Dad's uncle was lying there, and an uncle and a grandfather and an older brother. I sat next to the fire and my father's brother, Nuyumpaku_nu_, was marching around talking really angrily, in a rage for somebody to help me. And I was saying, 'Why's he doing that?' But he was telling another ngangka_ri_ to strengthen me. The ngangka_ri_ strengthened me and he said, 'Oh this one's alright, he has mapa_n_pa inside him that's been protecting him!'

There were lots of people talking about their family members who had died and they were weeping. People were dying right there while we were sitting there. It was really bad, that Maralinga bombing, you know. We were just sitting there and people were dying around us. People were telling us about who had died – it was a great tragedy.

The Maralinga bombings that came brought a mamu, a totally different kind of mamu that killed everybody. This was a mamu that came raining down from the sky like a rainstorm. We used to see it every night. We used to look at the sky, which looked terrible. The sky never looked how it would normally look before. It looked red. It was hideous, ugly, proper red. The sky used to be red every night – it was absolutely awful. A lot of people don't know about Maralinga. It was a nasty thing that killed a lot of people, really nasty. Anybody who wasn't there will never know just how frightening it was. The Maralinga ira_ti_ – the nuclear fall-out from Maralinga – that was a big ira_ti_ – a dangerous invisible poison, which killed everybody's spirit. I nearly died but I was lucky. I survived.

The ira_ti_ from Maralinga went into people's breath inside their bodies and stopped their breathing, and they died. I know, because I nearly died. I was there, ready to die. I was ready to die and I came back to life because I drank that gold liquid in that bottle. The ngangka_ri_ couldn't heal anybody. None of our techniques worked. It wasn't anything we were used to. It was outside our experience. There was nothing anybody could do. The ngangka_ri_ couldn't heal anybody. They couldn't see anything or touch anything in anybody. It was like water, like saliva that came into a person's body. It was like a strange water or saliva that killed people. Everybody was u_l_iringanyi, pakuringanyi. This means being too weary and close to death with an illness that affects everything.

I drank from that bottle, which had something gold inside it. God made me drink it. He gave that to me and kept me alive. I never knew what the story was behind that bottle, and I can only assume it was God.

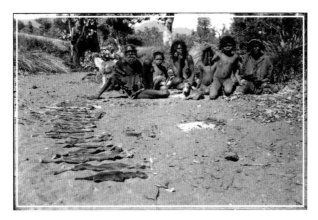

Left: Toby Minyintiri Baker has identified Tommy Tjuwintjara Baker (his father, far left) and Kunytjiriya (his mother, far right) with himself the smallest child (next to his father) and other members of his family (including siblings Jimmy Baker and Tjuwilya Baker) beside dingo scalps, Pukatja (Ernabella), South Australia, 1942.

PHOTOGRAPH HARRY BADENOCH, LEN YOUNG FAMILY COLLECTION, ARA IRITITJA AI-0030739

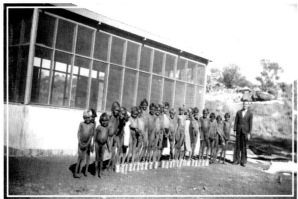

Left centre: Teacher Ron Trudinger and students stand beside the first school building at Pukutja (Ernabella), South Australia, 1940.

PHOTOGRAPH STEPHEN WARD, BLUE FOLDER 032, WARD COLLECTION, COURTESY STREHLOW RESEARCH CENTRE

Left below: Toby Minyintiri Baker identified this image as a copy of a photo given to him by Dr Duguid years ago. 'Native guide and son', South Australia, 1939.

PHOTOGRAPH DR CHARLES DUGUID, COURTESY SOUTH AUSTRALIAN MUSEUM AA 79/1/381

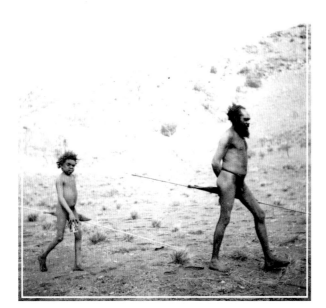

Later, when white doctors like Dr Duguid arrived on our Lands, they brought their medicines and treatments, which were different to the ngangkari medicine. People still got sick and still needed to see ngangkari though. Doctors can work with open sores and put medicine in and heal them, whereas ngangkari work with the invisible, and with the spirit. We used to say, 'Yes, they're giving them medicine for the sicknesses that they see, but ngangkari are working differently. We're working with the invisible, with what we can see with our ngangkari eyes'. So we worked separately, in the clinic or in the camps, yet the two styles of healing were working together really well. There was a famous blind ngangkari living in Ernabella at that time, Ngulitjara, who was my uncle.

There was a photograph of my father and I, taken at Kanpi. Dr Duguid gave that photograph to me, but I lost it a long time ago. Dr Duguid gave me a lolly, which I didn't like because I didn't know what it was! I was walking along with my father carrying our bundles of spears. They took a photo of my father and I with our bundles of four or five spears and spear throwers – we call that bundle a tjilira. We were both carrying the same set of tools.

Dr Duguid was riding a camel and we took him along with us for a while and then we left him. There are a lot of photographs taken by Dr Duguid. Dr Duguid was a good man.

There was a long period of time in my middle years where I'd lost my powers. I lost my power because I ate some emu fat. One day, when I was an adult man and a father to my children, living in Finke, I ate some emu meat and emu fat. Ngangkari mapanpa don't like emu fat; they get annoyed by it. When the mapanpa smells it, they flee and never come back. They go away. My mapanpa fled back to where they came from. That's when I lost my powers. I ate the emu fat at Finke, and that's why I lost my powers. Later I lived at Pukatja for a while, but I didn't do any healing there because I didn't have the powers any more. I knew a lot about ngangkari work, but I didn't do any healing when I was living at Pukatja.

My father's brother, Nuyumpakunu, was the one who originally gave me the mapanpa, and he would have had the power to get my mapanpa back and replace it inside me, but sadly he had died a long time earlier in Pukatja, and so he wasn't around when I lost my powers. He was a big, important, extremely powerful ngangkari. So my powers were lost because I ate the kalaya kanpi, the fat of emu. But I still had some powers left. This can happen to any ngangkari who might eat emu fat or echidna fat. Not just me.

One night, Rupert took me down to the ngangkariku iwara, to a sacred place, where only men can go. Women can't go there, only men. I went on a marali, on a spiritual trip, a sacred miilmiilpa ngangkari trip, on the one that's only for men. This is a really sacred journey. And that's how I got some more of my powers back. I hadn't lost all of them – there were some left, because I got mine from that Tjukurpa that was in my body. It was always there but I had lost parts of it.

I didn't have the power for a long time, but I learnt again from Langkatjukur Rupert Peter. Langkatjukur taught me, and so did Andy Tjilari. They used to take me on the ngangkari iwara, down the ngangkari road to where ngangkari travel. I got my powers back again when still living in Finke, but a lot of what happened to me is secret and sacred ngangkari business and I cannot talk about it.

Rupert and Andy took me on the marali and allowed me to get more of my powers back, and my powers have increased. I can do more and I help out more. I can help them do healings, whereas before I didn't. They retrained me after I got my powers back.

Langkatjukur Rupert Peter borrows my mapanpa sometimes. I've got two mapanpa within me. Sometimes when Rupert's working I work with him. I can close the healing with my mouth, because I've got the closing power in my mouth. It goes from my mouth, and I put it out and blow on my hand, on my thumb, and then I place it on the body and that's how I close it – that's the closing. That's one of the closing healing techniques that you can have mapanpa for – the power from the mouth, the breath. When we say puuni, we are saying the word for 'blowing', that's the word we use – puuni. This is really miilmiilpa – it's really, really sacred. It was never spoken about before because it has songs relating to it; it was never told in the past to outsiders. Before, when I didn't work with Andy and Rupert, when they didn't take me on the marali, I couldn't have assisted in doing the closing-up technique. Rupert does his work and I do the closing up.

Toby Minyintiri Baker, *Wati Kalaya*, 2011. Acrylic on linen, 116.5 x 90.5 cm.
PHOTOGRAPH AMANDA DENT, © THE ARTIST AND TJUNGU PALYA

*This is Wati Kalaya (Emu Man) and Wati Kipara (Bush Turkey Man). They are making kali (boomerangs) and that kipara hit that kalaya right there in the chest. That's him lying down there, that's my brother. After that the kipara went around behind all the kalaya tjuta and started to whistle and all the kalaya children got scared. 'What's that, who's whistling? Must be mamu (evil spirit)' and they got really scared and ran off, all the way to Watarru.*

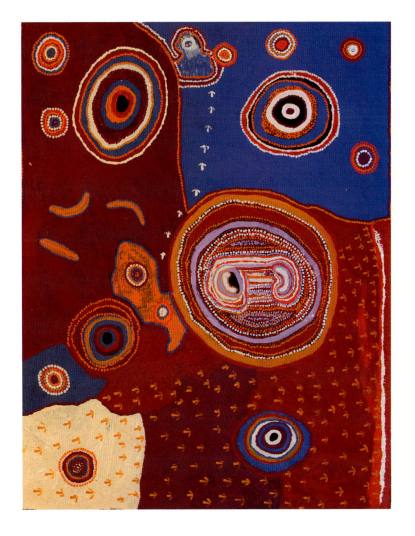

I've got my mapanpa back now, of course, and I'm well. I have my Tjukurpa, my mapanpa and my kurunpa (spirit, will, self) which I got from the Tjukurpa. It's still here today, I've still got it. I've got my mapanpa, it's inside my abdomen. I was very sad for a long time about the loss of my first mapanpa.

Once Rupert Peter lost his key and he couldn't find it. So what Rupert did was he got my mapanpa from my abdomen and he sent it out to look for the key. It found the key and brought the key back to him! My mapanpa went to where his key was and it got the key and brought it back! My mapanpa is still here in my abdomen and Rupert can come and get it. If you send my mapanpa off, it can do like find lost keys!

I only got to work with Rupert Peter just recently, and I have worked as a ngangkari for the NPY Women's Council in the last few years, after Andy Tjilari left. Rupert Peter said to me, 'You have healing powers, you have mapanpa and I can see you have the closing mapanpa skill,' and he said, 'Come with me'. Rupert's got the extraction technique for getting the sickness out and I have the technique for closing it up so the sickness doesn't return. He tells me where I am going when we're working together. I can work with the tendons, pulyku. I can see inside and I can lipulankupai (make things level', harmonise, equalise, balance) – it is similar to wirulymankupai, a healing treatment.

I can work with the tendons, moving the tendons. By moving my hand along it I am ensuring that the tendon starts working properly. From the point of the ear along the neck down, from the bottom of the ear that goes along the neck that goes down to the body, that's the tendon that we work with to make sure that all's well. We work with the tendons by putting our hands on one and running our hands along it. We're treating it to bring it back to its optimum working level after something may have been blocking the flow of blood. Any blockage will stop the flow and cause dysfunction and sickness.

Ngaalypa is the breath of life. Without the breath, without breathing, and without the spirit, you cease to be, you're dead. No spirit, no breath – no breath, no spirit. If a spirit is away from the body for too long, it turns and it starts growing hairs on it and that person turns into a mamu. That's why you have to retrieve it quickly and put it back into the body where it belongs, back in the person that it belongs to.

With the spirit you breathe, you're alive, but without the spirit, you die. Only with the spirit can you breathe. Everybody is the same. Without the spirit you're dead, just to be buried. Breath is a sign of life and keeps the spirit there.

Everybody is born with a spirit, and breath. The breath comes in at birth. A child is a living child when it has a spirit and movement. A child is born with a spirit and with breath, and it needs the mother, the mother with the breast milk. Some people think a child has no spirit, or maybe that the spirit comes in later, but every baby is born with a spirit. Without breath, spirit and life, a child doesn't live. God gives everybody a spirit, and gives the child spirit. We have all got a spirit.

You know a car, we put a battery in and it comes to life? It's like that! We all have a spirit. Everybody has it. Even snakes! All lizards, rabbit-eared bandicoots, kangaroos, all animals have it. A dog has a spirit and breath. All animals have spirits. When you spear something for meat, it dies because it hasn't got the spirit any more. Without it there is death. We're alive because we have that spirit. But if we didn't have a spirit we'd all be dead, long ago. That's why ngangkari always think about the spirit. We always recognise the spirit first. We always search for the spirit and place the spirit in its correct place if it is misplaced. Were you born without a spirit? No, you weren't!

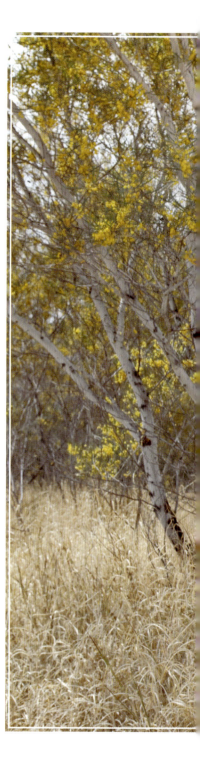

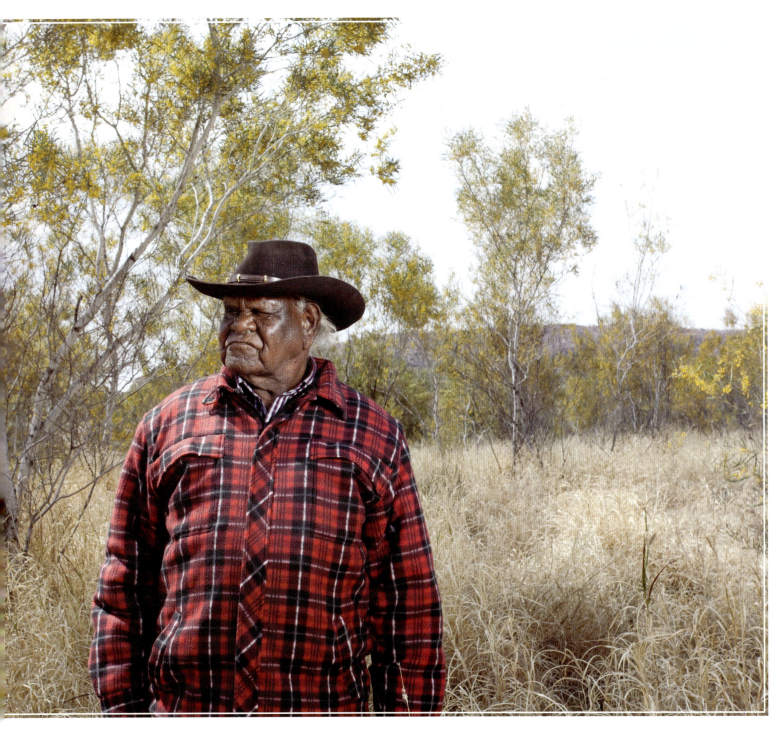

Toby Minyintiri Baker, 2011.
PHOTOGRAPH RHETT HAMMERTON

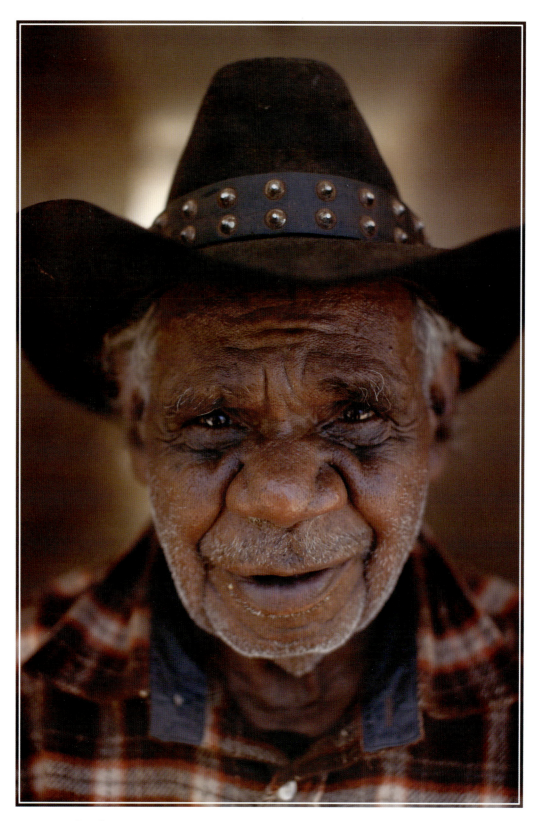

Rupert Langkatjukur Peter, 2011. PHOTOGRAPH RHETT HAMMERTON

# Rupert Langkatjukur Peter

When I started out as a ngangkari I was only a small child. I used to live with all my extended family. My grandfather was a ngangkari. He was my mother's father. I was always watching him work on sick people. I used to run and fetch things for him, and do things for him. I was always nearby. One day, as he was about to do some powerful work on a person, he told me to go away and not to look. He said, 'Child, go away. I don't want you to see what I am doing here.' But I told him that I wanted to watch him and help him with his work. I told him that if he wanted I could fetch things for him. I stayed and watched him closely.

As he was working I looked carefully at his hands. At one point I saw something come into his hands. I wondered, 'What is that he has there?' I was intrigued. I hung around really close, pestering him to show me what he had. But he told me again, 'Child, go to your father. Quickly. Don't hang around here.' So I went to my father, but I kept peeking over to see if I could watch my grandfather working. I couldn't see what was going on. Later on, I asked him, 'Grandfather, what was inside that person's muscles? What was that dark thing, that blackish thing?'

My grandfather told me – and he was the number one, too – that something had been lodged inside that knot of muscle. He'd looked and searched and he'd found what he was after. Then he took it out and cleared out all the space, widened the space, and then threw away the black object. He cleared out all of the things that were inside. He also went up and down the spine carefully looking for foreign objects that may have been lodged in there too. He took whatever it was from the sick person's body. He took it outside. He carried it away, all the time thinking about the state of the person's spiritual well-being and their spirit.

When Anangu go up to a ngangkari and ask, 'Please give me a healing treatment. I've got a raging headache', the ngangkari usually replies, 'Alright, but you'll need to wait for a short while and then I'll see you.' This is because a ngangkari can get a better diagnosis and a more effective healing treatment if he is able to see them and treat them at night first from his marali – his spirit body. If he just rushes in too quickly, he runs the risk of making mistakes. Ngangkari don't work too quickly for this reason.

Just say a sick person approaches a ngangkari around a certain time of day. The ngangkari won't know the exact time but he'll look at the sun and he'll say, 'Come and see me tomorrow when the sun is in the same position again.' The sick person will reply, 'OK, no problem', and he'll go and sit in the shade for the rest of the day. That night, the ngangkari will go out in his marali spirit body and heal the sick person through his spirit body. Meanwhile the sick person will be sleeping in his wiltja – his shade shelter. By the next morning, he'll be well again. But he'll still go and see the ngangkari. He'll watch out for the time, but he won't be looking at his wrist. He'll be watching it in the way all our predecessors have been watching the time for generations. He'll be watching the progression of the sun across the sky. When the sun reaches the appointed time, he'll go to see the ngangkari again.

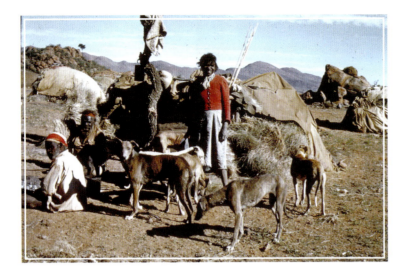

Left: Rupert Langkatjukur Peter's family (from left): his father, Rupert Peter Senior, his uncle Charlie Aluritja and his aunt Murika Aluritja, Pukatja (Ernabella), South Australia, 1950–59.
PHOTOGRAPH SHIRLEY GUDGEON, ARA IRITITJA AI-0005931

Opposite page: Rupert Langkatjukur Peter at Pukatja (Ernabella), South Australia, 1950.
PHOTOGRAPH RICHARD SEEGER, COURTESY MUSEUM VICTORIA (XP944)

When he arrives, he'll sit down next to the ngangkari. The ngangkari will ask the person if he is better. He'll suddenly realise that he is better and say, 'Hey! How did that happen? I was feeling really sick, but now I am not! I got better just by being here!' All the ngangkari has to do then is to balance up the sick person to make him totally better. He'll touch the area that was causing the pain and the sufferer will be sick no more. If the ngangkari doesn't get the chance to give a complete and thorough treatment, he won't be quite as successful in healing the sufferer. What works best for him is to look over the person both outside the body and inside, where the spirit dwells. Ngangkari are particularly effective when working with children this way.

Ngangkari clean blood effectively using the old methods. We take out the dirty blood by the mouth and spit it away, without damaging the body internally or externally. However, a blood transfusion sends old dead blood around the veins of a living person, and we are not happy about that. It is dangerous. When a ngangkari uses the suction method to clean out blood, he would never swallow it. He would always spit it out. Unclean blood is dangerous. We all know that. Where there are no ngangkari treatments available, I suppose a blood transfusion is the last resort and if it will save a life it must be alright.

Health clinics started up in this area because of sick people. They started up because of a need. But the old treatments have found it difficult to keep their proper place in the clinic environment. We have been working for many years as ngangkari. We started working as ngangkari when we were children, after we were given the powers from our grandfathers. As you know we specialise in treating people with mental health problems. We go around and see people after they contact us. When we see them we write the consultation down on paper forms that we send to Women's Council. This way of working works well.

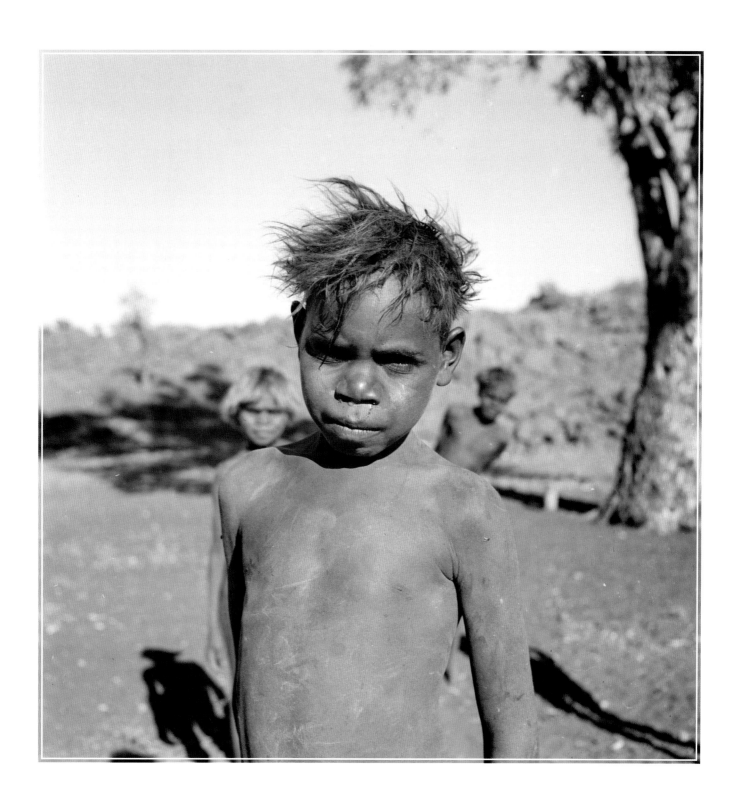

*Rupert Langkatjukur Peter*

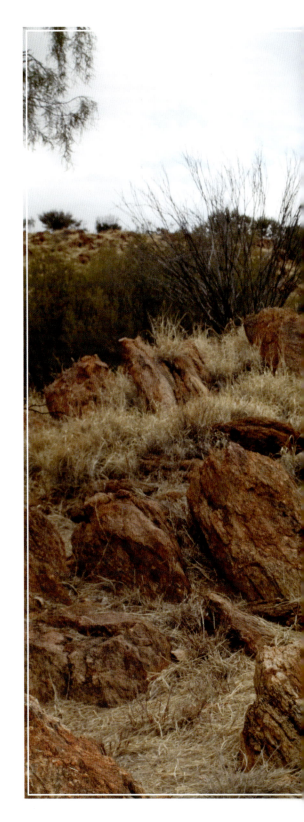

Rupert Langkatjukur Peter, 2011.
PHOTOGRAPH RHETT HAMMERTON

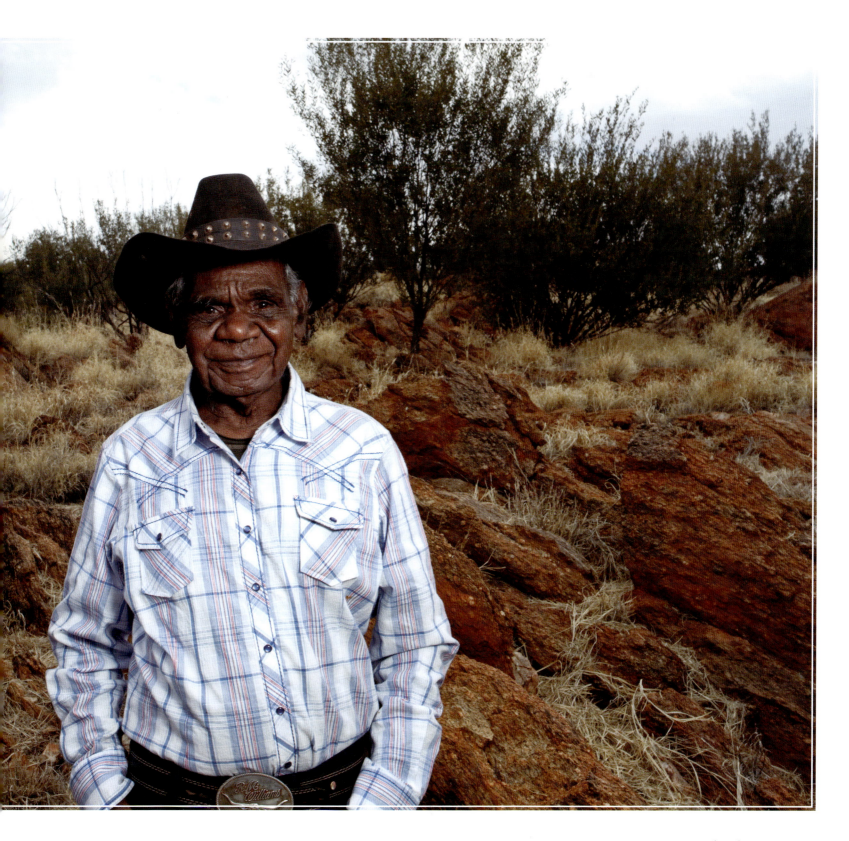

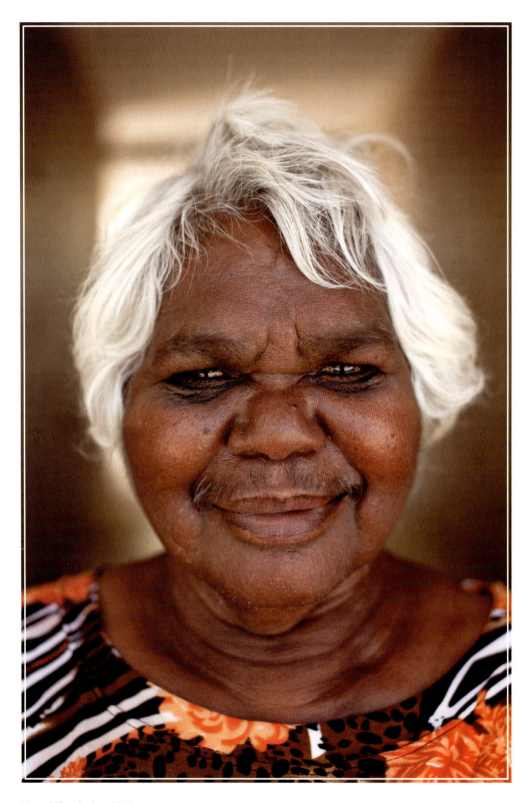

Naomi Kantjuriny, 2011. PHOTOGRAPH RHETT HAMMERTON

# Naomi Kantjuriny

My mother and father died a long time ago. My older sister was only young. My father's country is Kunamata. My father travelled across the country to marry my mother, and after they were married, they moved to Ernabella, where they lived for many years. But my father's real country is Kunamata, which is Ili Tjukurpa, which I, in turn, now carry, like a dream. Kunamata is a Fig Dream place, we call that Ili Tjukurpa.

Although I speak Pitjantjatjara, I was born on Yankunytjatjara country, at Victory Downs, and I lived in Yankunytjatjara places, such as Kulgera. My mother is Pitjantjatjara also and my father is from Kunamata.

When my father and mother were travelling east to move to Ernabella Mission, they carried my older sister with them. My mother carried my older sister down to Wapirka, where Victory Downs Station is now. She stayed there while my father went over to Ernabella. Mother stayed there because she was expecting a child – me. My mother is called Tinpulya. My older sister was the only child at the time, but then I was born at that same place, Victory Downs. I was a little girl at Victory Downs.

While we were there, so I've been told, my father died in Ernabella. My father went back to Ernabella alone because my mother couldn't travel due to expecting a baby, and that's when he was murdered. It is said that a kutatji executioner murdered him. So my mother was there living at Wapirka, with her two little daughters, me and my older sister, Tinkiri Goodwin. Tinkiri Goodwin Wangka is my older sister. My mother lived at Victory Downs with us two, when I was just a tiny baby. A white man came to see us, he was a policeman, and he told my mother, 'Your husband has died'. My mother was terribly worried and distressed. She had lost her husband just after she'd given birth to me.

My father had gone along that olden-time road towards Ernabella, and had died there, leaving us two daughters without a father. The policeman came and told my mother that her husband had died. So we stayed there for quite a while, because my mother was suffering from grief so badly.

After a while we returned to Yunyarinyi – Kenmore Park Station – and lived there for a while. Mother carried me, and my older sister walked. We had no donkeys to carry us, or any motorcar back then. So we lived at Kenmore then, until my mother Tinpulya returned to Victory Downs, while my sister and I stayed at Kenmore, where we began to grow up a bit. I was still only a very little girl then. There were a lot of Anangu living on Kenmore, though I've no idea about any whitefellas. I was too little, you see.

When we were a bit bigger, my sister and I went with our mother back to Victory Downs. My big sister was now old enough to start work on the station, and I was a big girl. We lived at Watju for a while and then we moved to Kulgera, where we stayed for a longer time, right on the highway.

Anyway, one day, a different man came into our lives, and he married our mother. He became our mama nyuyurpa, our stepfather, and he grew us up. He hunted for us and he hunted kangaroo meat for us. So we had a new father after our father died.

When I got a bit bigger, I was in the habit of travelling around by myself, while my mother and sister stayed home. I would travel around by myself, and then I'd go back to my mother and sister. I could never bear to stay too long in Ernabella, because I thought it was a horrible place then. I would go to Kulgera as well, and I remember seeing tourists travelling up and down that highway, but I was always scared of them, and I'd hide from them. It wasn't a real road, it wasn't a highway at all, but people did travel up and down that road. White people moved around the country with mobs of cattle and people were always on the move. Young men went off with the herds of cattle, working. I myself went off by myself again to Kenmore, and then I went back to Ernabella.

When in Ernabella, I went to school, where my teacher was Nganyinytja. There was a white woman too, called Miss Nicholson. But my teacher was Nganyinytja, an Anangu woman, who was quite strict with us! She'd smack us if we were naughty!

When I was living in Ernabella, my ngangkari powers were awakened within me. Nobody gave me them, they just came to me alone. I'd give treatments and healings and make people well. I would give ngangkari healing treatments and make people well, which is what the work of a ngangkari is all about.

In later years I based myself in Kaltjiti, where I gave many healing treatments over the years. We call a healing treatment wirunymankupai and I use what is called mara ala, which means open hands.

It was in Ernabella where I received the gift, which initially scared me! I'd walk around at night, and I'd be frightened of the power I had. This power just came to me alone. It was a gift for me alone. I'd wander around at night with my powers, and return to my camp early in the morning. All I could think was that I must have become a ngangkari for some reason. I was only a teenager at the time. I asked my mother, 'Mother, why do I drift around at night so much?' and she replied, 'You must be a ngangkari then.' My mother, Tinpulya, told me this. My reaction was, 'What?!' and she said, 'Yes, it seems that you have become a ngangkari all by yourself!'

I told my mama nyuyurpa about my open hands, and he was surprised because of my young age, but he said, 'When you are older, you'll be able to perform fully fledged healings', which made me proud. So I'd try out the healings, and train my hands to be open. I was still wandering around at night, and I think I'd do healings during those times. My mama nyuyurpa was a ngangkari himself and he could recognise what a ngangkari was; in fact I now know that he did give some of his powers to both me and my sister when we were younger. My mama nyuyurpa would give excellent treatments also, and he taught me a lot about the work of a ngangkari.

Interestingly, my older sister and I have exactly the same looks! We look the same! She is living on the machine now. She's on renal dialysis in Alice Springs.

I began healing people at a very young age indeed. Remember, this is what we call wirunymananyi, and I have been doing so ever since. We say wirunymankula waninyi – which means, to declare someone well and to banish the illness. The illness, or pain, can take the form of phlegm, or back pain, and this is what I specialise in. I used to ask my mama nyuyurpa, 'I can't understand why I am on the move all night!' and he told me, 'You are mara ala, and you are a ngangkari, and that is ngangkari practice.' 'Truly?' 'Yes,

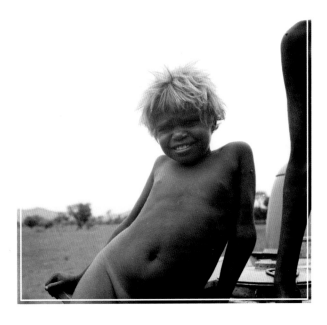

Naomi Kantjuriny, Pukatja (Ernabella), South Australia, 1951.
PHOTOGRAPH RICHARD SEEGER, COURTESY MUSEUM VICTORIA (XP 1071)

that is true.' So my mama nyuyurpa explained what was happening, and he guided me in my practice. He would talk to me about treatments and how to do them and he encouraged me to get better at it.

I was still nervous when I first started out though, but my relatives encouraged me also and helped me. This was many, many years ago. In the intervening years, though, basing myself in Kaltjiti, I have become a fully fledged practising ngangkari, and have healed many people, particularly children. I lived in Kaltjiti for many years.

My work was as a healer, mostly helping women and children. Women would come to me and tell me about their health problems and I would give them healing treatments. Very often they didn't need to tell me what was going on, because I'd know already. I could tell if it was a back pain problem or whatever. So I'd give the appropriate treatment and I know they were good. Women and children were healed by me countless times, especially children. Sick children would be brought to me and not long after their treatment they'd be saying, 'Right, I'm off to play!' and off they'd go!

In Ernabella, people would go and see the white doctors after they'd seen a ngangkari. They'd tell the doctor they'd seen a ngangkari already and the doctors encouraged this, because it made people stronger. The white nurses would be happy as well. The only difference was, they were on a salary and I was not. I would tell them that I didn't get paid for my work. Ngangkari have always worked for free.

People would become sick or ill or feel uneasy, and so they'd come to see a ngangkari. What we do, what I do, is to sit them down and to work on their bodies, wirunymankupai – and give them a healing treatment.

Soon they'll be telling me, 'Thank you, my abdominal pain has subsided, I feel better now'. So I will have given them a treatment on the stomach area, which soon makes them well. The touch of my hands has a healing effect. I give a firm, strong touch, and remove the pain and sickness, and throw it away, away from the sufferer. People will come to me and say, 'I am not well. I am suffering. I'm miserable and unwell', and so I say, 'OK, let's have a look at you,' and I touch them in particular areas and massage their pain, make their body feel centred and grounded. After their treatment they will stand up and tell me how they feel and, of course, there is always an improvement.

At night I see spirits. Kurunpa. The kurunpa spirits talk to me. Spirits separate from the body when someone is unwell or suffering and I see them. This is how I find out they are not well. I have dog friends that help me, as well. These dogs are my friends. At night I travel around by myself to make sure the women are alright. I see everyone at night, how they are, if they are alright. Sometimes it scares me but it is my work, I have to do it. I travel alone and that is what I do.

I specialise in children's health. Women will come to me and tell me that their child is unwell. I tell them to sit down with their baby. Their baby or child will often be crying, but I'll settle them down. They cry if they are in pain and they are frightened. I ask them, 'Where is the pain?' and they might say, 'I can't eat. I just don't feel like it.' I feel around the stomach area, around the abdomen, and I detect the exact location of the pain, and I draw it out, and whilst doing so I'll ask them, 'Can you feel this? What are you feeling?' and they'll tell me what's happening for them. I know they'll get their appetite back later. After their treatment, they'll be coming back to me and telling me what they ate! I tell them, 'Right, that's it. Feel better?' and they tell me, 'Yes, I feel better here in my stomach and I also feel better within myself', and I know they are cured.

Another example might be a woman might come to me and tell me she's had a headache for two days. I'll work on her and give her a treatment – wirunymankupai – and, you know, straight away she'll tell me that she is feeling better and her headache pain has disappeared. Some people enhance my treatment with pain tablets, taken afterwards, and when I later ask them how they are going, they always say they are much better and their headaches are gone.

I am an expert when it comes to healing headaches. My auntie Kunytjitja Brown came to ask me for a treatment for her severe

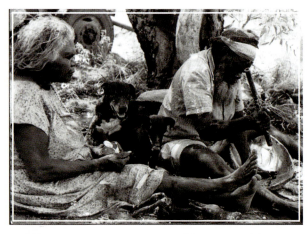

Top: Naomi's mother, Tinpulya Maniya, and her mama nyuyurpa (step-father), Jimmy Tjutjupai, making piti (wooden bowls) near Walytjitjata where the itara, or bloodwood trees, grow, in 1982. Suzanne Bryce recalls, 'They lived at Putaputa and had a garden. Jimmy Muntjantji and his family lived there too. The community was small and they lived there to look after really important Law country.'
PHOTOGRAPH SUZANNE BRYCE, ARA IRITITJA AI-0025913

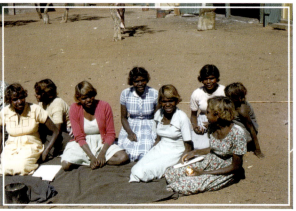

Bottom: Women sitting in compound, dressed for church, left to right: Lizzie Kayukayu, Tinkiri Goodwin Wangka (Naomi's sister), Dulcie Mintji Peter (deceased wife of Rupert Peter), Angkuna Tjitayi, Naomi Kantjuriny, Angkaliya Tulapa Brumby, [child obscured] and young Yukari Goodwin, in Pukatja (Ernabella), 1957.
PHOTOGRAPH BRUCE EDENBOROUGH, ARA IRITITJA AI-0004429

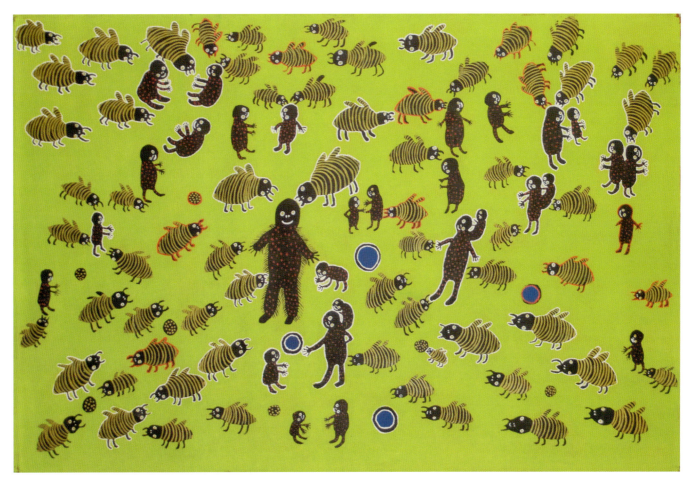

Above: Naomi Kantjuriny, 'Mamu', 2007. Acrylic on linen, 152.5x101.5 cm.
PHOTOGRAPH COURTESY THE ARTIST AND GALLERY GABRIELLE PIZZI

Right: Naomi Kantjuriny, Feather Basket, 2010.
PHOTOGRAPH BELINDA COOK, COURTESY TJANPI DESERT WEAVERS

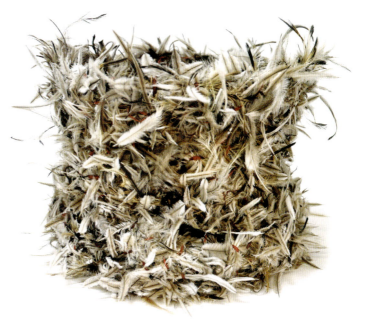

headaches, which I gave her, with total success. She and I had a drink of tea together afterwards because she felt so much better!

I work on bad backs. People who have a bad back come and see me and tell me how miserable they are. I feel really sorry for people when they have back problems, because it is a miserable and painful situation. I work on them hard, and make their backs better. I tell them to see a male ngangkari for those problems which require a man's special touch.

If drunken people want to see me I tell them to drink water and to go to the clinic.

Depressed people can feel a lot better within themselves after a ngangkari treatment. That's one of our specialities. Their spirits are out-of-sorts, and not positioned correctly within their bodies. The ngangkari's job is to reposition their spirits and to reinstate it to where it is happiest.

Some people ask me how I do the treatments that I do. I tell them that I have unique skills that are not easily explained, which I developed by myself. I travel at night and check on the health of people, and make sure everyone's alright.

After a treatment, it is our task to ensure the sickness doesn't return and pain doesn't return. So we have to dispose of the pain in our special way. Ngangkari know how to do this. We have special powers in our hands. I have very special powers in my hands, and I use those powers to heal people.

Our work is to mould the shape of the body so that it can accommodate the spirit properly. In that way, people are well. I ask people afterwards, 'Are you feeling better now?' and they tell me, 'Yes, I am feeling great!'

Ngangkari touch people. We touch, and that is our special art and our skill.

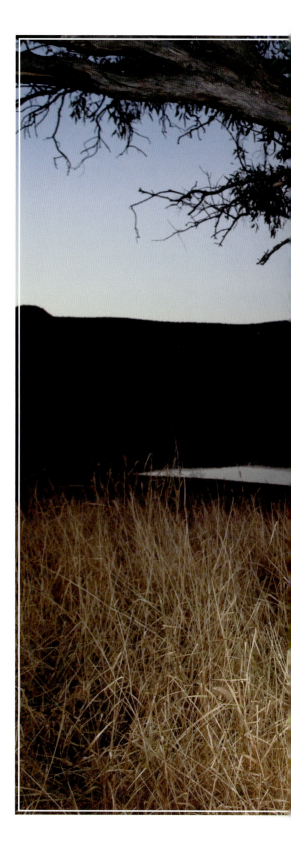

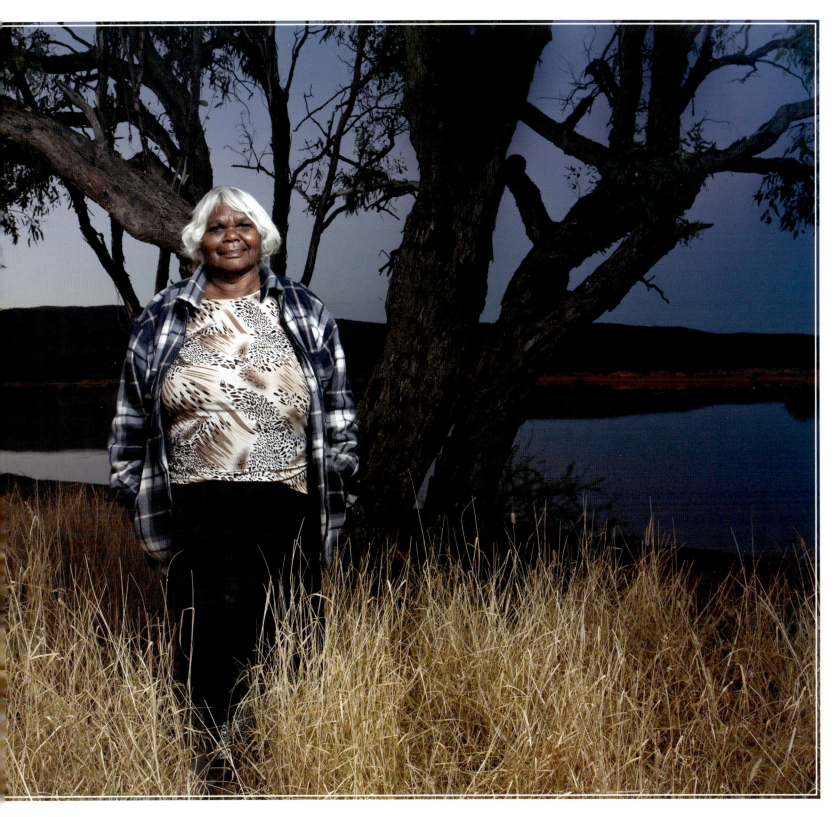

Naomi Kantjuriny, 2011.
PHOTOGRAPH RHETT HAMMERTON

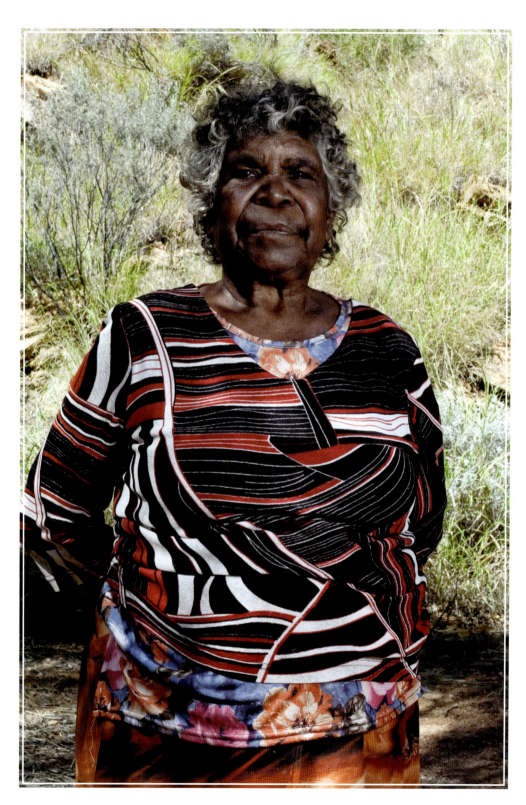

Ilawanti Ungkutjuru Ken, 2011. PHOTOGRAPH RHETT HAMMERTON

# Ilawanti Ungkutjuru Ken

I am very sympathetic – ngayulu ngalturingkupai – towards children who are very sick when they are sent away for medical care, when they are really sick. We help them out with our ngangkari skills. They really need our help.

I started working as a ngangkari publicly in about 1999, but before then I kept my ngangkari skills hidden. I didn't heal people in the open, I kept my treatments hidden for a long time. I've done a lot of healing work in my life, I've done a lot of ngangkari work, I've healed men, women and children. The children get well immediately after I've healed them.

I became a healer because my two brothers are healers, and I used to travel with them in what we call marali. My brothers used to take me travelling on their spiritual journeys. Tiger is one of my brothers, and he used to take me and others along with him. We used to join together and travel. After travelling with my brothers in the spirit realm, I learnt a great deal from that, about the spirit plane. I had the gift of healing within me but I didn't use it, because I didn't know how to initially. But I learned to use it after going on the trips with my brothers, even though I'd hide it. I'd heal people but I'd always say, 'No, I'm not a healer'.

I heal women and also men. In the beginning I used to say I didn't have any healing skills but my brother used to tell them that I was a healer because he knew that I had it within me and so I tried, I tried tentatively to heal people. In the beginning I was doing it quite shyly and I didn't boast about it, I just kept it to myself quietly.

One of the treatments that we perform is to heal the spirit, that's the main work we do. We ensure that the spirit is in the right place and is correctly situated in the body. I learnt that from healing my own children. That's how I learnt, from first healing my own children.

People used to tell me I was a healer and I was always quite modest and said, 'No I'm not!' But they said, 'But we know you heal people!' It is mainly the women who ask me to heal them. When I used to say, 'No, I'm not a healer', they always said, 'No, we've heard you're a healer!' and sure enough I'd heal them. This was at the NPY Women's Council meetings of women from the Western Australia, the Northern Territory and the Anangu Pitjantjatjara Yankunytjatjara Lands. I used to heal them at the NPY Women's Council meetings. I was quite bashful about my skills. But people used to say, 'You have the gift!' I do work well on women. I have been encouraged. I often doubted my ability, but I have been getting good feedback.

All my family used to say, 'We have seen you heal people and then they recover.' Other ngangkari get paid money for their work. They heal and they get paid for healing people, but I wasn't getting paid to do it. But people used to say, 'It's not a matter of payment that makes you a healer, you have the gift.'

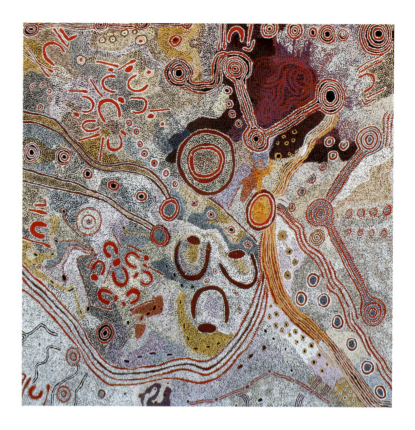

Ilawanti Ungkutjuru Ken and Mary Katatjuku Pan, 'Seven Sisters', 2011. Acrylic on linen, 2 x 2 m.
PHOTOGRAPH SKYE O'MEARA, © THE ARTISTS, COURTESY TJALA ARTS

I used to travel in the spirit with my kuta – my older brother – many times. Travelling in what we call marali. We used to take our children on these spiritual trips as well. I've got eight children including grandchildren and grandsons. They come with us too on marali. My eyesight is not as good any more so I probably won't be going on marali too often any more. It will have to be up to my grandchildren to carry on the ngangkari tradition in our family. They know everything about it, and they know the stories. One of my granddaughters has the gift, the ngangkari skill, and she does healing too. She heals people. Lisa Ken is her name and she heals children too. She used to keep her gift hidden – following in my footsteps obviously! She kept it hidden before, but now she heals openly as well.

I was born in Watarru. Tiger's mother is my father's older sister. So Tiger is my cousin, but I call him 'brother' in the Aboriginal way. Another of my brothers has passed away. Another of our family members passed away during that bombing, the nuclear bomb testing at Maralinga, after the puyu, smoke, came through Ernabella. My mother passed away near Fregon. My father passed away in Ernabella. My father's name was Matantji and my mother's name was Mauta.

My mother came to Ernabella Mission and she died from a disease, long before all the houses were built there. My mother was born in Watarru, and she brought me to Ernabella and to places near where Kaltjiti is today, when I was a child. We lived in Ernabella, and my sister Mary Katatjuku and I went to school in Ernabella along with our other sister, Kanakiya Tjanyari. My father married two women. First my father had one wife, and there was just my sister and I, and then he married another wife after that and had Kanakiya.

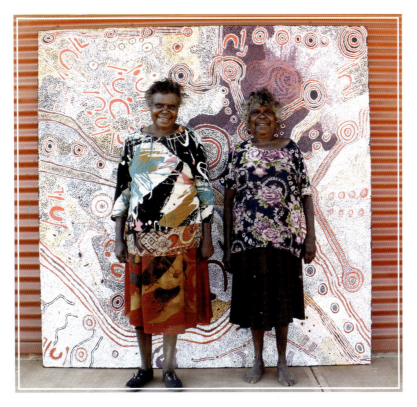

Ilawanti Ungkutjuru Ken (right) with her sister Mary Katatjuku Pan and their collaborative work 'Seven Sisters', at Tjala Arts, Amata, South Australia, 2011.
PHOTOGRAPH JOANNA BYRNE, COURTESY TJALA ARTS

My mapanpa lives inside my body and it has the power to take the badness away from someone else's body and destroy it. We say in our language that it 'eats it'. I don't really eat it exactly but I destroy the sickness and make it vanish. So when we heal with our hands we get the badness out. It's the mapanpa that helps us to grab what's invisible, that sickness in the body that we cannot see with our eyes, and take it into and through me, to where my ngangkari magic is within my body, and it devours it and turns it into nothing.

Another way I work is to get something out from a person who has had harm done to them. I do the healing, I take it out of that person, but I don't keep it inside me. It's not kept in me. I keep it in my mapanpa, and hold that in my hand while I am asleep. It might look like an evil bit of stick. Later on I will put it back in my hand and it becomes visible and then I can see it. But it's a force within me that's working, it's my spirit and the power. We are working as a team and that's how it works. So when I do the healing, when I get something from a person it's not visible straight away because my mapanpa, the magic healing power, works that way.

If somebody observes me with evil intent, my body becomes hot, as though I have got a real temperature. That is my body telling me to beware – our powerful selves and the mapanpa that belong in our body, the magical power, is telling us that it's a sign. My skin and face gets very hot when I detect it, and I don't feel well. It's a familiar feeling that I know, when I feel I may have a temperature, it is a warning that tells me something's looking at me or talking about me. My powerful inner self becomes fierce and dangerous and my mapanpa will show me if someone's talking about me or looking at me and it'll show me – 'See that person over there!' When I feel my body is on fire, and I have burning hot skin, when it feels like I am burning up, I see it, 'Oh it's that person there talking about me or looking at me the wrong way.'

Yesterday I did a big healing job, working really hard. I must have healed about seven women at the NPY Women's Council executive meeting! So I worked really hard, Naomi and I, working together. The women were all complaining of aches and pains. We were very busy on the Thursday afternoon and evening, and then again early in the morning on Friday.

One of the reasons that people come to us is when they are finding it hard to walk, or if they have lower back pain, aches and pains, knees, hips and pelvis, so we work with their energy. We are very much like physiotherapists in that respect. We refer to that style of treatment as wirulymananyi, which means 'making it smooth'. So with our hands we massage and stroke the painful area and allow movement to become fluid again, and the legs and joints to work better. Sometimes we feel something there. My mapanpa will seek whatever it is that's been blocking the movement of the person's legs. It'll get it and remove it, because it causes them to be tired and stiff, and we massage their legs and their joints. It's kind of like physio – we touch and work with the muscles. Sometimes I take something out from the body but my mapanpa destroys it. My mapanpa will destroy it, but if it's something really, really big that has to be seen with the eyes, that really needs to be dealt with, then it will show it to me by putting it into my hand. But when we work with people with their muscles and their legs, it helps that person, and heals that person. My mapanpa destroys it.

The other thing that we do when we work with the head is to blow onto the person's head. We call that puuni, which means blowing. We put butter onto their head and we blow on it and blow into their head and the person is healed instantly. I do that to my husband and he gets better, so it's good.

I don't search for kurunpa. I don't search and find kurunpa. Others do that, but I can just ensure that their kurunpa is in their body in the right place. I can work with the kurunpa if it is in a different position. It might not be in its normal place so I get it and put it back in its normal place and touch it in a way that brings it back to its strong power. You can feel around, you might feel it at the back and then you bring it round to the front because that's where the kurunpa sits, just in the front here just at the top of the abdomen near the breast bone there – in the stomach area near the breasts, that's its home there. There's a nest that the kurunpa has! That's the home, that area.

Your kurunpa helps your tendons and muscles work properly, and it helps you to show the way. If you haven't got your kurunpa in your body, your body and your legs freeze. You can't walk and you can't see. You start vomiting. Those are the symptoms of a person whose spirit isn't working at its optimum. Some ngangkari can see clearly if a person's kurunpa is not in that person's body, they can search and find a person's kurunpa – they will look for it, find it, bring it back and put it back into that person, back into the correct location.

Wherever a person is, the spirit will follow. If a sick person is taken somewhere the spirit will follow but it doesn't really connect with the body, it's just hovering in the distance there, not strong enough to make that final distance to the body. So we ngangkari find the spirit and put it back in the body, we do that. I've seen that being done often, I've seen other ngangkari getting the spirit and putting it in the person's body and that person instantly being revived. I can see people whose spirit isn't within their body or in the right place and if their spirit is not healthy I sometimes try to get their kurunpa – but my mapanpa it's not so skilled in that particular area. I've tried to find a lost kurunpa and grab onto it but my mapanpa lets me down! There's probably a reason for that.

My father's name is Matantji. He was a ngangkari and he used to use his miru, his spear thrower, to capture lost kurunpa. His powers were so strong that he would capture the lost kurunpa and return it to the sick person. His mapanpa would bring the kurunpa and place it on his spear thrower and then he would pick up the kurunpa and then place it back into the person's body. That person would get well immediately. He could also get his mapanpa and send it off to work on its own. He would hold out his miru and his mapanpa would come back and land on his spear thrower. So when he searched for a person's spirit he would get his mapanpa from his body and send it off and he'd hold his spear thrower out and the mapanpa would travel around looking for the sick person's lost kurunpa and when it was found, the mapanpa would bring it and put it on the spear thrower and he would catch it. Sometimes if his mapanpa wouldn't come back onto the spear thrower he'd know that it was close by so he'd walk around in that area and he'd feel for his mapanpa. It's the body that tells you. It's like taking your own temperature – the ngangkari knows where his mapanpa is just from feeling his or her own body. The ngangkari's body tells him or her by becoming warm or hot when walking around. If they walk in a certain direction and begin to feel warm then he or she knows they're on the right track to finding his or her mapanpa and the sick person's kurunpa.

I used to watch my father doing this healing process many times. But my own healing technique is different to his. My healing techniques are with the hands and the blowing on the head, and placing hands and blowing into the heads of people. My power goes in through the air that goes in through the head, and it heals people.

There were a couple of times when I went and did some work for a doctor, who told me, 'This patient is not alert, their eyes are closed and they are not moving.' The patient was a child. I placed my hands and worked with them, played with my hands and instantly the patient became alert, and started moving around and looking about.

Many of my family members possess mapanpa and are shy about using their healing powers publicly – including me – and we have kept it hidden for a long time. I've got two mapanpa. One is the fire and the other is the eagle – they are my two mapanpa. The waru is from my home Watarru. Watarru is fire dreaming, Tjukurpa, dreaming. Waru is fire. Walawuru is eagle.

Some of my technique is kumpilpa – this means it is hidden. My mapanpa will get a kurunpa on its own, but it is invisible. It goes through my body, and through my hand, and when I put my hand onto a person, it might get something, but it's invisible. It's invisible and it goes into my hand and into my body. My mapanpa devours it and sometimes it places it into my hand. After I've gone to sleep I might wake up and see something that is in my hand. If that happens, I know how it got there and I know I have healed

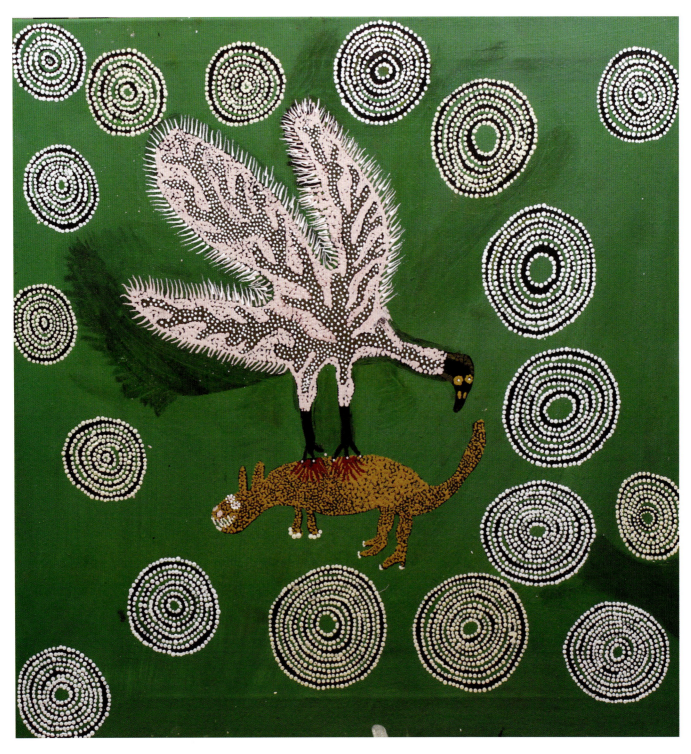

Ilawanti Ungkutjuru Ken, *Tjulpu (Eagle)*, 2011. Acrylic on linen, 101.5 x 101.5 cm.

PHOTOGRAPH SKYE O'MEARA, © THE ARTIST, COURTESY TJALA ARTS

somebody with the help of my mapanpa. After that happens, there's a period of time where I spend some time sitting quietly, so as to allow that process to occur.

Sometimes my brothers and other family members travel on marali together. Sometimes certain groups will only travel together because they all have the same type of mapanpa. My brother gave me his mapanpa to use, when I was a child, but I told my brother, 'Please take your mapanpa back!' I said, 'I don't want your mapanpa!' So he took his back and then he gave me a separate one because my mapanpa is only for me. He was going to give me his own one, but I said, 'No, I don't want yours, I want my own to keep!' Poor thing – my older brother is sick now. He's not one hundred per cent in the brain any more, poor thing.

I was asleep and dreaming when my brother gave me the mapanpa. You know when you are getting an injection and something is coming into your body? Well, it was like that! I screamed out with fright in my dream because something was being put into my body – it was the mapanpa! I screamed out loud! I was a big teenage girl when this happened. When I was a teenager, I rarely tried to heal people, but sometimes I would just feel for illness by placing my hand on their body. Just by putting my hand on their neck, shoulder or head for a few seconds, I could give them pain relief. So that's what I used to do before, when I was younger.

Sometimes, if ngangkari are not very strong, strong power can hurt or destroy them and can give the ngangkari a heart attack, or something akin to an electric shock. This is if the power has come from negative forces. Some objects can be powerful, depending on the power behind it. There are different levels to the power. The most powerful is the one that gives the ngangkari a real kick, which can hurt that ngangkari and hurt the mapanpa inside.

Sometimes we ngangkari can put our mapanpa inside a person, and the mapanpa stays in that person's body and destroys everything bad within that body. Afterwards, when its work is done, it comes back to the owner. This happened to me once. There was this man who placed his mapanpa in my body and I felt so wonderful! When his mapanpa was inside me, and working, I felt really, really good! After it left I still felt really good! I felt so healthy!

A long time ago I worked as a health worker in Amata. I used to go for courses to Adelaide training to be a health worker. I used to learn about lots of things to do my work as a health worker, watching doctors work. We used to work together. I learnt these skills at the hospital. We learnt there in Adelaide at the hospital during the course, gaining skills. We did a lot of observations of how doctors and nurses did their work and we learnt about how we would work back in our communities. We learnt things like, if there's an accident, what we were to do, how to assist people who have had a car accident, or if a child breaks their arm, how to fix that. We learnt how to speak with patients, after car accidents, to make sure we don't move them, about moving them safely and giving them water – or not giving them water – and making sure that the nurse passes on that information to the next nurse for their next stage of the treatment.

My work as a health worker was a lot about looking after sores: cleaning sores, putting ointment, bandages or bandaids on them. And we learnt what to do when people suffered a head wound: how to clean the wound and how to put stitches in, if stitches are required. The nurses used to teach us that before you do anything you've got to wash your hands and put your gloves on; for example, before cleaning a wound. They taught us about getting the needles and giving injections: how you give the injection really carefully, not too fast, and make sure there's no air inside the needle.

I was already married with children when I was doing this work. I was working as a health worker. We had a lot of people working with us – nurses who helped us with our work and our onsite training. When I worked as a health worker I wasn't working as a ngangkari, because, although I had the gift, I hadn't used it, so during that time I never did any ngangkari work, I was just learning the whitefella side of nursing. It was only many years later when I went back home to the bush that I started doing ngangkari work, working with my hands and doing the healing and massaging and that side of things.

There was a caravan that we had, and Sandra Ken, who was a nurse, ran it, and we were learning nursing, working from that caravan. During this time of my training I didn't tell anybody that I had ngangkari skills because I was still thinking, 'No, I'm probably not a healer,' but I still used to quietly heal, without telling anybody, I used to heal the children. I never told anybody but I used to see the kids were getting better and I just kept it quiet, just doing the whitefella nursing work.

There was an army medical team that came to Amata, once. They put a big tent up and we got other people from other communities to come there, and we worked together there, looking at people's eyes, checking people's eyes. And during that time I was helping assist the doctors by interpreting for the old people. I used to interpret for the whitefella doctors as well.

I was working at Pipalyatjara with Sandra Ken during the time when they had a small shop and clinic. I worked at Amata when all my children were small and I also worked at Pipalyatjara because some of my children lived there as well. When children are sick I go to them or the sick child is brought to me. People would be brought to the clinic and I'd do my healing on them.

We used to ring for the Royal Flying Doctor Service (RFDS) if a child was seriously sick or if we had a pregnant mother. I used to drive them to Irruntju, that's where we used to put our patients on a plane – in Irruntju – and they'd go off and be taken to see the doctors in a bigger town.

I don't remember other ngangkari working at Amata clinic when I was working as a health worker, there was nothing. There were ngangkari in Amata, but they weren't working with the whitefella medical staff. There were ngangkari doing work outside of the whitefella health system. They didn't work in the clinic – they were separate, they were doing their work just with their families outside of the clinic area.

The ngangkari used to get involved when patients were sick. They'd come in and heal, but this was a long time before it was well known that ngangkari worked together with the doctors. It's only in recent times that ngangkari have been working together with the health practitioners in this area. Some patients know when they are healed by a ngangkari and they tell the doctors they have been seen by an Anangu healer and this is what they got out of me. So they're giving that information to the doctors.

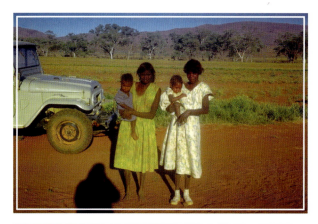

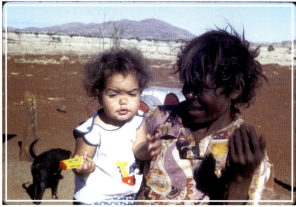

Top: Inpiti Winton holding her daughter Margaret Manantu (left) and Ilawanti Ungkutjuru Ken holding her daughter Sylvia Ken in Pukatja (Ernabella), South Australia, 1966.
PHOTOGRAPH DON BUSBRIDGE/BETTY CULHANE, ARA IRITITJA AI-0022715

Bottom: Ilawanti Ungkutjuru Ken holding her niece Rebekah Ken at Putaputa (near Pipalyatjara), South Australia, 1976.
PHOTOGRAPH NOEL WALLACE, NOEL AND PHYL WALLACE COLLECTION, ARA IRITITJA AI-0048171

There are some people who say they're ngangkari but they're not true ngangkari. You know, they'll go and do a healing, and they'll get a rock and show you, and say, 'Oh, look, this is what someone made you sick with'. That's been known to happen, and that's not right.

When a sick person comes close to me the hairs on my body will stand up on end and that's an indicator that the person next to me is sick. That's how I know, and sometimes I will heal them after that. My mapanpa will usually tell me what's going on, by the hairs on my arm rising – that tells me there's a sick person close by. Then I see that person. So the hairs rise up on our arms. Our mapanpa shows us or tells us somebody close by is sick, and we can see it too. This happens with Josephine too. My mapanpa will see it. It'll see somebody sick and then let me know by making the hairs on my arms rise and it'll tell me that that person has come to be healed.

My mapanpa can tell me if something's happening to my son. When anything to do with my son happens, my mapanpa will let me know. Certain parts of my body will pulse. We get a feeling in the arm or on the knee, or on the back and our body feels warm. This is referred to as nuunpunganyi.

A sick child will cry and resist and won't want ngangkari to help because they are in a lot of pain.

Sometimes we can heal people while we are sleeping. Our mapanpa does the work while we're sleeping and the sick people are asleep as well.

When people lose loved ones, the stress and the worry becomes so great that it fills up in their body. And sometimes a ngangkari can capture that deceased person's kurunpa and place it in a family member, and that helps the recovery process. That can help a person who has got a lot of worry from losing a loved one.

When a person is worrying greatly and is down, a ngangkari can get that kurunpa, that spirit, and lodge it inside another family member temporarily to build it up. The kurunpa is reinvigorated by being with another family member, and so when it is replaced in the owner's body, she is stronger and healthier immediately.

In the past ngangka*r*i did do that kind of healing often, getting the person's spirit and putting it in another person to strengthen, and then putting it back. There was a lot of healing happening when we were children, because our family was a family of healers, and so they gave many healing treatments. They used a lot of techniques that aren't practised any more. Sometimes in the old days they would take a person's kurunpa to a certain spot – for example, on a mound or somewhere like that – to become happy again, and then put it back in the person. Nowadays we also use the church for ensuring that the spirit remains happy.

For people who have lost a spouse, the bereaved person can inherit the kurunpa of the spouse who has passed away. Ngangka*r*i do a lot of work reuniting kurunpa, in order to help the person that's still alive, the one left behind, to be strong and happy again. Sometimes ngangka*r*i put the kurunpa into a surviving brother, a nephew or a niece.

Ngangka*r*i find the kurunpa and find the family member and put the kurunpa into them. I can see the spirit, I can see a kurunpa but I can't get it. I can't. If it is outside someone's body by itself, then I am unable to get it. But I can work with it when it's inside a person's body.

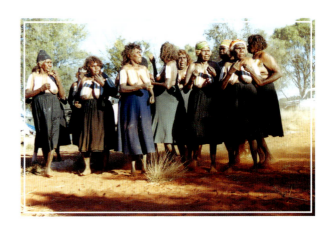

Above: NPY Women's Council members, from left (front row facing camera): Nura Rupert, Molly Miller, Ilawanti Ungkutjuru Ken, Nyinku Kulitja and Nancy Miller, performing the Seven Sisters Inma at the NPY Women's Council twenty year birthday celebrations, Ka*n*pi, South Australia, 2000. It was at this gathering that the women decided to perform this inma for the Sydney 2000 Olympic Games Opening Ceremony.
PHOTOGRAPH LIZA BALMER, NPY WOMEN'S COUNCIL COLLECTION

Opposite page: Ilawanti Ungkutjuru Ken, 2011.
PHOTOGRAPH RHETT HAMMERTON

A lot of people now have illnesses and medical problems, they've got diabetes and they've got asthma. They say, 'I'm sick. I can't walk!' So we do our special healing touching and laying of hands, and we tell them, 'You are not exercising! You've got to get exercise! Your muscles have become tired because you're not walking around! And your breathing, you need to breath better.' This is what I say to them, 'If you've been sitting around at home all day, and you can't walk, you must try! Don't just sit and work all day, you'll get stiff and tired!' I say, 'You should go for exercise for a little while! It will help! Go out digging for honey ants or witchetty grubs, or go hunting for goannas!' Yes, that keeps your body good and healthy and physically well, and that's why some people's muscles are loose. If you sit at home all day, or sit somewhere at work, without a lot of movement, say, if you are painting, if you are sitting still painting, that's no good for walking. It makes you stiff. It gives you problems. I find that that happens when I sit and paint all day, it happens to me too.

I teach my grandchildren to go out hunting and learn to hunt animals and learn to get honey ants and witchetty grubs. They can do the hunting! One of them got a perentie the other day. My granddaughter killed a perentie! I take all my grandchildren out with the teachers. I go with the teachers and do a lot of bush tucker teaching to the children, and I tell them about bush foods and our meats. And we tell them about whitefella foods and products that are no good for them. We want to make sure that they eat good

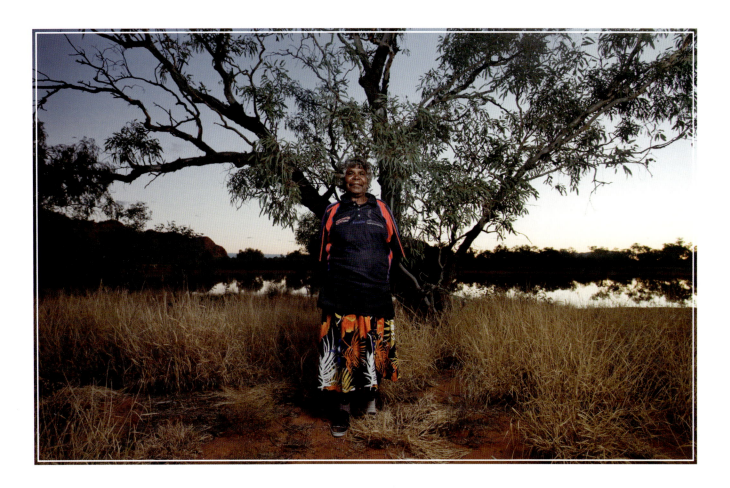

food, and not do bad things. We tell them about what is good and bad so that they can make good choices when they become older, when they become adults. And even for men to cook food, when they become a man they don't need to rely on their women folk to cook meals.

There are a lot of bad things that young people these days have to think about. Smoking and drinking, those are the really bad habits that affect people. But in the old days people used to walk for a long way and kill animals and do the hunting and they kept fit that way. They'd cook the animal, cut it up and share it with their family. But young people don't do that today. They don't do that. But you can learn how to kill the animal, make the fire for a kangaroo, dig a hole and fill it up with wood, burn it, cool it and then when the fire has died down then you cook it in the proper way.

This is the reason that I am contributing to this book; so that our knowledge can be shared. I can become well known in the ngangkari area and the healing world, and people who don't know about ngangkari can learn about us.

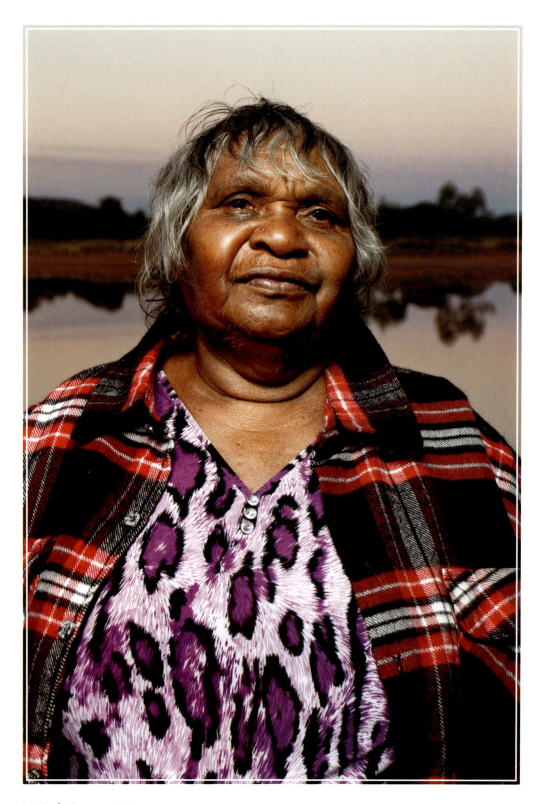

Maringka Burton, 2011. PHOTOGRAPH RHETT HAMMERTON

# Maringka Burton

The name Maringka was given to me by my big sister and the name Burton is our family name, which we have had for a long time. My father's name was Charlie Tjalkuriny. He was also known as Charlie Burton. The name Burton was given to our uncles. My mother, Naputja Yanyi, was also known as Yanyi Burton. They all got that name Burton. It is an English name. The Burtons are a big family now, and we are all a very happy family.

My father's traditional home is where a warmala traditional army came from. The warmala were waiting at Uluṟu to spear someone. They went to Muṯitjuḻu waterhole, and after they speared the person, they went back home to Malaṟa, and then after that they travelled down to Kunytjaṉu, where they waited some more. My father used to tell me these stories and I'd have to listen and learn. Now I am older I know the stories, and I paint the story elements in my paintings. I will never forget my father's stories. Rene Kulitja's old father used to dance all the dances for that inma (ceremonial singing and dancing), for that Warmaḻa Inma, which is a 'dodging spears' dance.

My father was Pitjantjatjara and my mother was Ngaatjatjarra, from the west. My father's traditional home is at Malaṟa, to the east of Pipalyatjara. A long time ago, my father journeyed to Papulangkutja and married my mother, who was from there. They spent their days walking and hunting around in the bush, as married couples do, and I was born in the bush near Anumara Piṯi, south of Irruntju. I don't know the exact date of my birth, but I think the clinic staff can estimate it.

We used to travel around a lot as a family group. We travelled around to many places because my mother's family wanted mother to see it, and so we travelled this way and that, and we also went to my father's country. We walked around a lot on foot. We went everywhere.

My mother and father lived at Angatja, Nyapaṟi and Malaṟa, with their three girls and three boys. That is where we used to live long time ago. Now there are only five of us still left alive. One has gone.

My mother used a mimpu to carry our water in. A mimpu is like a big deep bowl. They would make a mimpu using a sharp stone and a large piece of wood from a tree. We never got sick, except only once, Lynette got sick. When we were living at Nyapaṟi, Lynette got sick when she had been travelling on a marali journey, but when she came back down into her body, she didn't enter her body safely. She fell, not far from her body. That's when she got really sick. My father healed her. Her spirit fell next to her bed, next to father in his windbreak. Father healed her because he could see she was badly hurt. She was a really powerful ngangkari. You can ask her about it. She had fought with a big waṉampi rainbow serpent. Another time, when she was a child, she was walking along and she collapsed the tunnel of a big serpent with her foot, and that waṉampi died when Lynette stepped on its tunnel, and collapsed its burrow.

My mother died a long time ago and my father used to sleep next to us, and when sick people used to come looking for him I used to tell him, 'Father, here's someone looking for a healing treatment'. I would watch him work, see what he did, and watch him closely when he was extracting badness from the person's body, and throw it away. I loved it. I was fascinated, and I'd copy what he did, pretending to go and throw away the bad stuff, when he did! I observed my father's practise for years, and I became very knowledgeable. I was like his personal assistant! I was only little!

People used to praise him when he healed them. They'd say, 'Oh, thank you, Tjamu!' if it was a grandfather relationship, or whatever relationship he was to them, they'd say, 'Oh, thank you, Uncle!' or 'Thank you, Father!' or 'Thank you, Brother!'

I was very close to my father and we used to live together in a tight family unit at Amata and Ernabella. When I was a teenager, my father was becoming quite elderly, and one day, I asked him, 'Father, I want to inherit your mapanpa, because I want to follow in your footsteps and be a ngangkari like you.' He agreed, saying, 'Yes, it is true I am getting old now'. However, he didn't bestow his mapanpa on me at that point, but later on he did.

My father had been a ngangkari his whole life, and his mapanpa had been given to him by his father. When he finally did give me the mapanpa, I became mara ala – meaning, my hands became open, my forehead became open, and I could see everything differently. I was able to travel into the skies with other ngangkari, soaring around in the sky, travelling great distances, and coming back home in time for breakfast. Ngangkari travel around in the sky, just our spirits travelling, while our bodies remain sleeping on earth – our spirits join

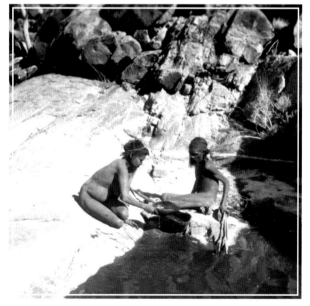

Top right: Charlie Tjalkuriny Burton (Maringka Burton's father) carrying his dog, Pukatja (Ernabella), 1933.
PHOTOGRAPH HERBERT HALE, HALE COLLECTION, COURTESY SOUTH AUSTRALIAN MUSEUM, AA124

*My father was a ngangkari who was ninti pulka and he gave me mapanpa tjuta*. Maringka Burton

Right: Yanyi Burton and Charlie Tjalkuriny Burton (Maringka Burton's parents) using a piti (wooden dish), to collect water at Aliwanyuwanyu, South Australia, 1940.
PHOTOGRAPH CHARLES MOUNTFORD (MOUNTFORD SHEARD COLLECTION), COURTESY OF THE STATE LIBRARY OF SOUTH AUSTRALIA, PRG 1218/34/1217B

*A long time ago, my father journeyed to Blackstone and married my mother, who was from there. They spent their days walking and hunting around in the bush, as married couples do.* Maringka Burton

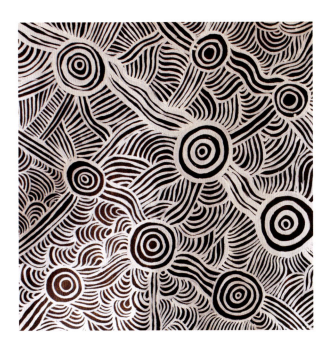

Maringka Burton, *Ngangkariku Road*, 2011. Acrylic on canvas, 67 x 55 cm.
PHOTOGRAPH RHETT HAMMERTON © THE ARTIST, COURTESY IWANTJA ARTS AND CRAFTS

*My father showed me this ngangkari road, it's about ngangkari, and he gave me all my mapanpa tjuta.*

together and travel. My father taught me that. He taught me everything, carefully and slowly.

Later, we moved to Amata. Amata is just a recently established community but in the old days there were no buildings. We did a lot of walking around, living in the bush. Amata, Pipalyatjara and Kalka were all established during similar times, but Amata came first.

We used to go for holidays with my family a long way from the communities, and the white people used to follow us with the ration truck, bringing rations to big camps like Yulpartji near Amata, or Angatja or Nyapari or Murputja. They'd bring food to us there and give us our food ration in exchange for dingo scalps. All that flour and food! We'd be out hunting, living in the bush, and we children would all be playing together, and my father would get dingo scalps and trade them for food. The Uniting Church people were there at Ernabella and they used to take the dingo scalps in exchange for flour, sugar, sweet tinned milk, golden syrup and tins of meat. There was no money around in those days.

I know that a lot of our people are on dialysis now. It is from that sugar we ate back then. We all know this now. We didn't know it before, though. It is the sugar that's creating havoc in our bodies because we have had too much sugar and that is what happens if you have too much sugar – it just wrecks your body. I am sad about it because I am at risk too.

It is a shame because we have always had wonderful traditional bush foods. We ate foods with minimal sugar – tjala, honey ant, and maku, witchetty grubs, and all the different berries – ili, wild bush figs, and wiriny-wirinypa, edible bush tomato. We had many fruits, and those fruits and nectars were really healthy, and didn't do our bodies any damage. There were only really strong healthy foods for us, with great nutrition. We had many different grains like wangunu, naked woollybutt grass, and we had other fruits. We had so much food!

We had all the bush medicines like irmangka-irmangka, which is made into a drink, and wakalpuka, dead finish bush. Bush medicines were used by everybody, it wasn't part of the ngangkari's specialised work – everyone used medicines from the bush regularly. We used the bark on the roots of the wakalpuka bush for a splint if a child broke their leg or arm. We would make a splint using the bark as a bandage. We put our medicines into a wira bowl. We'd put the skin of the nest of the itchy caterpillar onto burns and itchy sores. You take the nest and remove all of the droppings from the inside the nest and clean it and wash it and then you put it on the skin. It was a fantastically good treatment for burns, rather like doing a skin graft! If somebody scratched and itched, we'd put it on that as well. Everybody used these bush remedies

Right: Maringka Burton (left) and her best friend Niningka Lewis catching maku thrown from the tree by some boys (out of frame), Pukatja (Ernabella), 1959. PHOTOGRAPH IAN SPALDING, ARA IRITITJA AI-0023947

*We lived for a long time in Ernabella too, and I spent some of my childhood there, became a teenager there, and I went to school there.*

Below right: Maringka and 'ma*l*pa winki!' (a whole lot of friends). From left: Maringka Burton, with milpatjunanyi, storytelling wire, around her neck (storytelling wire is used as a rhythmic tapping and drawing device to tell stories in the sand), her ma*l*pa wi*r*u, best friend, Niningka Lewis, Mantatjara Wilson and Kunytjitja Armunta Yipati Brown, standing beside the manse at Pukatja (Ernabella), 1959.

PHOTOGRAPH ALLAN WILSON, ARA IRITITJA AI-0005976

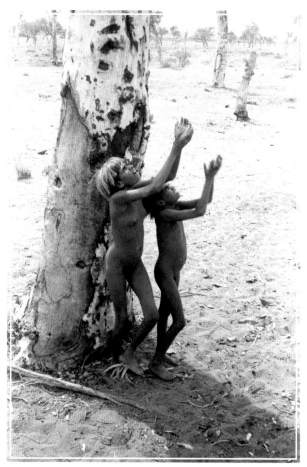

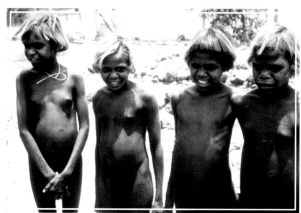

and everybody knew what to do for what ailment, and everybody knew how and where to get that medicine.

We lived for a long time in Ernabella too, and I spent some of my childhood there, became a teenager there, and I went to school there. My father used to heal many people when we were living in Ernabella. He was a beautiful man, was my father. When he became too old and was ready to leave this world, that is when I asked him to give me his mapa*n*pa before he departed this life. My sister Lynette was already a ngangka*r*i, she had become a ngangka*r*i as a child. She was already a very strong, powerful healer. Without doubt, her healing skills were equivalent to my father's skills. Little sister Lynette used to travel with our father on his spiritual travels.

My mapa*n*pa live in my body. I am a painter, and when I paint, my mapa*n*pa move right up into my shoulder and sit up there, out of the way. If somebody comes to me, needing help, I would have to ease my mapa*n*pa back into my hands again. Sometimes I would push them from one arm to the other. When I am giving a healing treatment, I push with my left hand and I extract with my right.

It was only when my father bestowed his mapa*n*pa upon me that I became a real healer, and open to that world. When something enters the body and hurts it, like pu*n*u, or splinters – you know bits of wood that go into the body – which we call pu*n*u, well, we get them out of the body because they are the

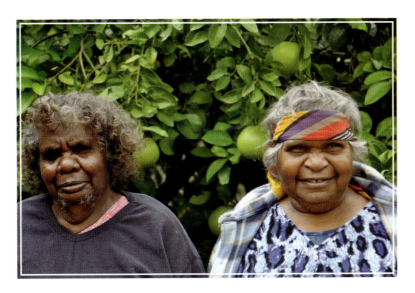

Malpa wiru, best friends, today! Niningka Lewis (left) with Maringka Burton, 2011. PHOTOGRAPH ANGELA LYNCH

ones that make a person sick in the body and in the mind. Punu causes sickness of all kinds, and it may only be a splinter or a fragment.

I work on the head a lot and I heal people if they've got a headache – when they say they've got a sore head, they cry if they are in a lot of pain or if they are having agonising thoughts and they are crying out for help. Sometimes people have bad thoughts that cause them a great deal of anxiety and pain. Sometimes that work is better done by the male ngangkari, for the men. Men help other men when they're sick. I only do their headwork if they ask, but I don't work with male bodies, you understand, not the rest of their bodies.

But a big part of my work is with the head. Sometimes other healers may send things into their heads and sometimes we have to get the thing that's been sent from another ngangkari into another person, such as a fine sliver of wood, a fragment of wood, like a splinter. We will get that thing and return it to its owner.

I get to go to various NPY Women's Council meetings: general meetings, Law and Culture meetings and executive meetings. Kanakiya, Pantjiti and I find we are very busy at those meetings, attending to women's business. We work together on women's issues and we specialise on women's bodies and problems. The work we do is the equivalent to the way the male healers specialise with the men. Sometimes when we do a healing treatment on a woman there can be a group of us healers working on the one woman. There can be two or three of us working on one woman at the same time.

If there is something serious like a car accident and we are called to attend, we go straight there without delay and we just go straight in to the scene of the accident. People have been hurt and the terrible shock of an accident shakes the kurunpa out of a person and so we go there to find the kurunpa and we bring it back and replace it. We do that as soon as we get there. We return it to the accident victim to help that person heal quickly, because without the spirit any bodily healing takes much longer. We are always there first because we live here, and ngangkari are always first on the scene, long before the Royal Flying Doctor gets there. When little children are involved, we are busy getting their kurunpa back immediately, because children who have been in car accidents are always damaged. Afterwards we attend the clinics, and when they call us, we do our work courageously without fear. We work in Mimili, Kaltjiti and Iwantja clinics, because we are asked so often to attend and be consulted.

I have also healed non-Aboriginal women. There was a woman once who had something happen to her leg. I worked on her leg, using the hands to massage the legs and muscles, and I healed her. We call that wirulymananyi.

In the past non-Aboriginal doctors would do their work, yet they didn't know about us traditional healers. They didn't know we existed. But our traditional healers were always busy healing people at home, looking after the entire community, while the doctors did their work in their clinic workplaces. But neither knew how the other one worked.

We are unable to do too much work with renal patients because their kidneys are no good and our treatments don't work on them, and, anyway, they are too delicate and are not allowed to be tampered with. So our healing techniques won't work too well on them, because their kidneys don't work. We never touch their kidneys. They are too vulnerable. But we do help with pain issues and discomfort, and we might do a little healing on their muscles and so on. We would love to have a renal machine in each of our communities, because we want our family members to be closer to their loved ones. We all want that.

I look after my sister. I'm her carer. I haven't put her away anywhere else, but I look after her myself. We take it in turns looking after her. I love my sister and I try to help her as best I can. She came in from Amata, and she has big worries in hospital right now. When I came to look after my sister she was so happy, you could see it in her body and her face, so I'm looking after her now. The spirit does get weak and sad when people worry for family and home – renal patients especially. And just by me being here with her, her spirit is happy just with the fact that I'm here with her. When I'm not here, she's not happy at all. You can see it in her face. I love my sister and I'd like to look after her for a long time. I like to look after my sister and care for her spirit. Many of the renal patients are doing really good things while they are here in town. Some do dot paintings and others make necklaces and this and that, keeping busy. But my sister here, she's not doing anything at the moment.

Dealing with the deceased, sometimes we can capture the spirit of the deceased and place it into the living spouse, which is a really caring and strengthening thing to do. You can really help a person by doing that. It is a really sad time

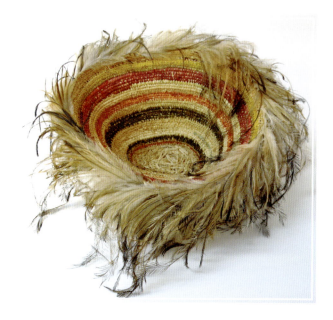

Above: Maringka Burton, *Basket*, 2010.
PHOTOGRAPH BELINDA COOK, COURTESY TJANPI DESERT WEAVERS

Opposite page: Maringka Burton, *Anumaraku Piti Tjuta (Edible Grub Burrow Holes)*, 2011. Acrylic on canvas, 101 x 101 cm.
PHOTOGRAPH RHETT HAMMERTON, © THE ARTIST, COURTESY IWANTJA ARTS AND CRAFTS

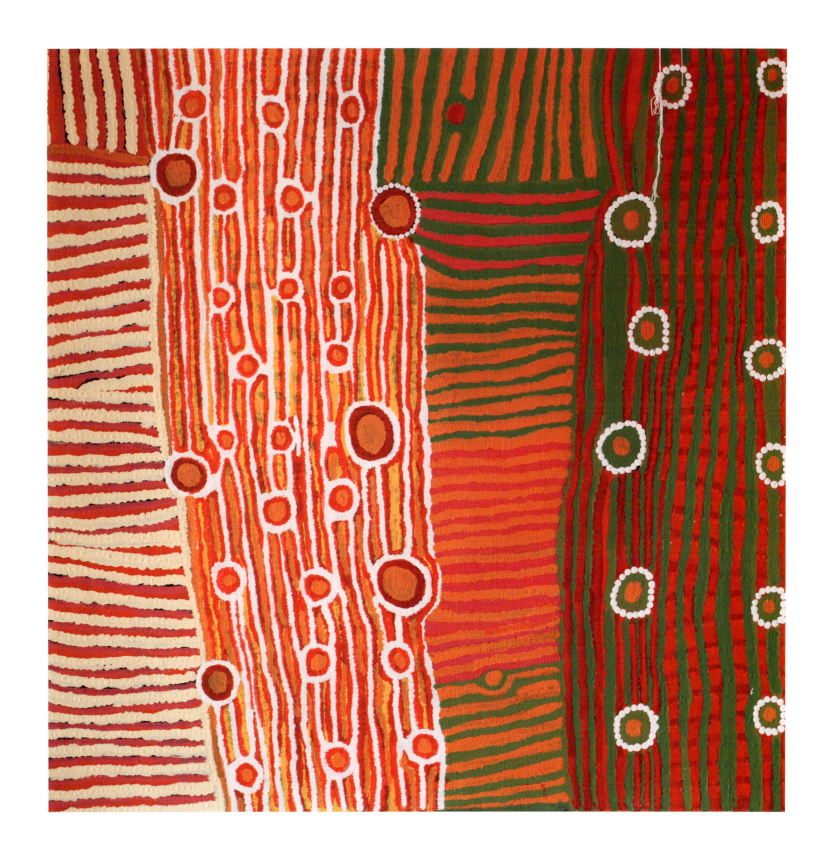

*Maringka Burton*

for the surviving spouse, so if you can join that deceased person's spirit into the one that's still alive it means they remain together until the other one dies away. If a woman dies away, the woman's spirit is put into the husband who's still alive. Sometimes if a son passes away, and the mother is really sick and bereaved, the dead son's spirit is placed inside the mother. In that way everybody is happier and it ensures that they get back to their normal health more quickly and are happier and healthier during their time of grief, because it is really terrible if somebody is too sad for too long.

My father used to use his spear thrower to call to the spirit of a deceased person to come. They do that with their mapanpa as well. They call to the spirit and it will come onto the spear thrower. Sometimes I can call a spirit with a branch. Using the branch I can usher it along, into the burial place, where the spirit should be. Sometimes the spirit will leave the body and leave the burial ceremony and travel around and make people sick. Sometimes, if I see that, I use a branch to brush it along, to brush it along so it goes back to the cemetery. But men, and only men, can call a spirit with their spear thrower, if a spirit from a dead person is drifting around where living people are, they can cause those people to become sick. That's why our work is to make sure that the spirit of the deceased stays with the body in its rightful place until it is dealt with.

We women ngangkari use the blowing technique on other women when they are having problems with their baby-producing organs. I shouldn't really talk any more about that, because it is women's only business, but it would be good to speak up about it, because it is our work, and others should hear about it. A lot of us women ngangkari do that kind of work on women. We want to ensure that our mothers-to-be are fit and healthy and so we do work on them to help them, to make sure everything is working perfectly. We want to make sure their baby-making parts are working, and the mothers' spirits are well, because we always work with the spirit. We always reposition their kurunpa in their bodies when they are sick.

I can't heal myself – ngangkari don't heal themselves. We can massage ourselves but can't heal ourselves. If we are unwell another woman can come and see to us. Most of the time when I am busy painting, that's the only time my mapanpa goes up from my arm to my shoulder and that's when I have got to push it back down to where the elbow is. See here on my elbow? That's where my mapanpa sits. I've got openings in my hand and an opening in the forehead. We say that ngangkari people are mara ala and ngalya ala, which means open hands and open mind. That's a term we use and when you hear someone say, 'Oh, he's mara ala,' that just tells you instantly that she's a healer, a traditional healer, a ngangkari.'

Opposite page: Maringka Burton, 2011.
PHOTOGRAPH RHETT HAMMERTON

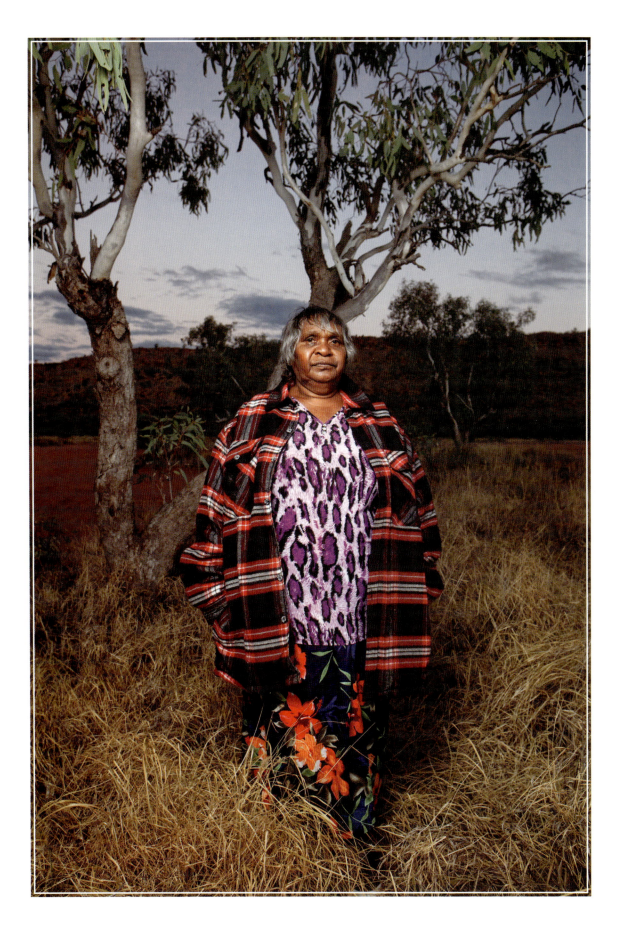

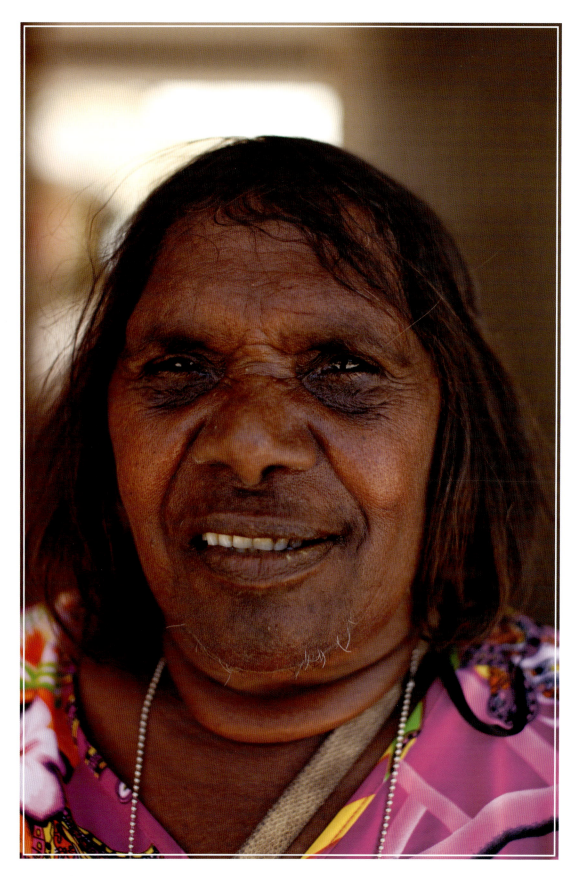

Pantjiti Unkari McKenzie, 2011. PHOTOGRAPH RHETT HAMMERTON

# Pantjiti Unkari McKenzie

I give healing treatments. I have always held onto my Tjukurpa – my story, history, Aboriginal Law, 'Dreaming' – and I've always seen things differently. I learnt a lot from observation, but my older brother was a ngangkari and he gave me some of his ngangkari powers. Two other ngangkari brothers donated some of their ngangkari powers to me that had come from Karylwarra.

My older brother, Sam Watson, gave me some mapanpa and so did a lady named Nyanyuma, many years ago, and these have been placed inside my body. In fact many years ago I healed myself with them, as I had a bad wound, and I caused my own mapanpa to enter the site with some force, very much like being speared with them, but there is not a single mark on my body to show any entry holes. I was quite ill with that injury but the mapanpa re-entered me and completely healed that major injury, and sealed up the entry points and I was whole again. Now I use my mapanpa to heal other people. I send the mapanpa outside my body through the same entry and exit points by opening up these points for the mapanpa to go out and do their work. Mapanpa all go out and come back in again, and so they are here in my hands. It opened by itself. Another elder ngangkari re-opened it for me. This happened after I had my children, but I have been a practising ngangkari since I was a big girl.

Nyanyuma gave me some of her ngangkari powers out of the kindness of her heart, intjanungku – so I could be a stronger practising ngangkari. Intjanuya ungkupai – things are given as a gift, without reciprocity. Intjanungku ungkupai. She gave them to me so I could be a better ngangkari. She knew I already had great promise. This woman wanted to help me be a better ngangkari, in case my children became ill or any of my relatives became seriously ill – I could help. This is what she told me. So she gave me a great number of powerful mapanpa and she placed them in my body. My older brother gave me the first lot. My older brother was the first and then the other brother was the second, and then Nyanyuma.

I work with women and children, and I also treat men if they are in need of a treatment and there are no male ngangkari available. If all the practising ngangkari are elsewhere then I am happy to give men healing treatments. This is an ancient practice and women have always helped the men, and the men have always helped the women. If all the male ngangkari are too far away to help, then the women will help, or if the men are nearby the men will help.

I was only a girl, a big girl, when I received my first mapanpa. This was a long time ago before any of us had ever been paid to give treatments. There were no other doctors around in those days. We were the only doctors then. We worked without any form of payment then and we worked out of the sight of white people. That was just what we did. It was normal back then. There was no such thing as money back then and so healing treatments were given freely.

My father was a ngangkari and my grandfather was a ngangkari. It is a tradition in our family that most of us would be practising ngangkari.

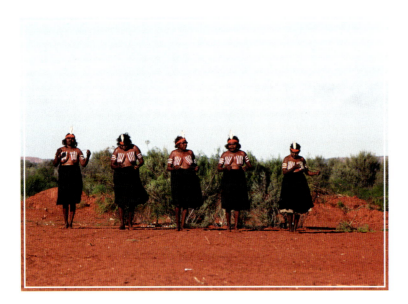

From left: Pantjiti Unkari McKenzie, Tjulkiwa Atira Atira, Nura Rupert, Tjuwilya Windlass and Nyinguta Edwards performing Inma Kungkarangkalpa (Seven Sisters Inma), Mimili, South Australia, 1989.

PHOTOGRAPH MARGARET DINHAM, ARA IRITITJA AI-0029081

We didn't see any conflict with our style of healing and the new whitefella doctors that came in because that kind of doctor does operations and so on. I give healing treatments to many children and adults. If anyone is sick and in need of help, I help them.

First I had training in how to open myself up to the power. My older brother helped me with that. Where the mapanpa are inserted is a sign of ngangkari powers. These flash and glitter. When I am asleep, they flash around, flickering light, glittering and flashing. They are ngangkari things, flicking and flashing. They flash in the same way that lightning flashes. Like lightning. Pinpantja, pinpapai, we call them. They are not eyes. I only see them when I am asleep, flashing and sparkling. Pinpantja. They flash just like diamonds. They are similar to diamonds. After I received those, I knew that I was a fully fledged ngangkari.

When I was just a young girl, I was already working as a ngangkari. I would give treatments to the other girls around me. We would go bush and I would give them treatments because I was too shy to do it in front of the other people. I couldn't bear for them to see me do it. So I hid with the girls, if one of them had, say, a headache, or something like that.

I do exactly the same as the men. I work on the spirit if it has been pushed to the side or if it is living in a tree. I get it back and give people back their equilibrium. A kurunpa will jump out of the body if someone is very ill or have had a shock. Everyone experiences this. We call this kurunpa wiyaringanyi. The kurunpa runs and hides in a tree. We recognise this condition and we feel the patient all over, and we realise they are empty of spirit. So we have to go and find the kurunpa, which usually isn't too far away. We look around, not far, and we might find it lurking inside a large clump of spinifex grasses, or perhaps it is hiding inside the leaves and branches of the person's shade shelter. We collect it and put it back.

In the days before white people, ngangkari looked after everyone. Whitefella doctors perform operations on people, and they give them needles, but Anangu ngangkari are quite different. We heal illnesses and upsets. All sorts of things can give someone an upset. Someone could have a fright from a dog,

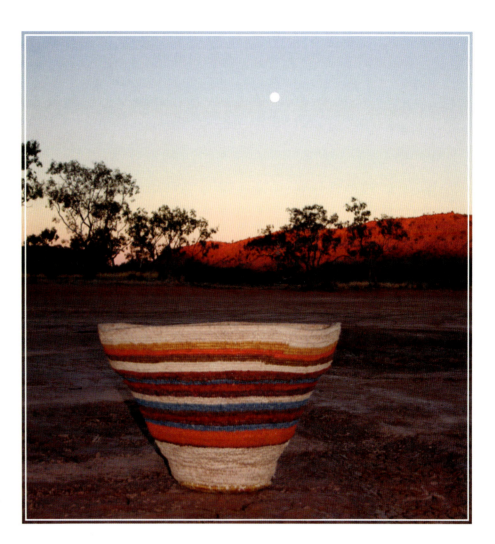

Pantjiti Unkari McKenzie, Basket, 2009. PHOTOGRAPH EMMA DIAMOND, COURTESY TJANPI DESERT WEAVERS

for instance. When children see something, something frightens them, like, they may see fighting, or something like that, they'll have a big fright and they'll be in shock. They'll be frightened and nervous. This will cause their spirits to leave their bodies, or become displaced, and illness presents itself in the form of diarrhoea. Their spirits will jump to the side and the child will be out of sorts.

Women ngangka*ri* and men ngangka*ri* are the same. They are exactly the same. Level. They work the same way. They are exactly the same, except of course, women ngangka*ri* usually specialise in women's health issues. This is because often sacred women's business is dangerous to men. Men wouldn't touch women if they thought they were going to impinge on women's business, so they just concentrate on the head, or the thighs or the feet. Women's bodies are really sacred to women. Women ngangka*ri* work on women's bodies. That is my work!

Say, for instance, if a woman is getting frail and thin and bony, we might lay her down on a bed and we'll get some fat, or butter-like ointment, and we'll massage her head and her abdomen, and we'll sing her a healing song, a sacred song especially for healing people. Women and men know this song. But it is a dangerous song nevertheless and it is closely guarded. There is always the danger that a dangerous, malicious man may try and steal this song, to do damage to a certain woman, and to make them sick. This is always the risk, so we only sing it in very safe and secure surroundings. If men are doing it, they will take the sick person a long way away and sing it there, just to be on the safe side. It is dangerous.

Women do the same. If the women are about to sing this song, the men say, 'You women, make sure you go a long way away before you start singing that song. Go a long way out bush, just to be on the safe side. Go to the other women! You are about to perform some business that should not happen near us men, so you'd better go and see the other women and go away together, safety in numbers.' So the women all go out together in order to sing the song safely. Men do the same, of course. When the song is being sung, we utilise the healing breath method. We breathe on the person, or blow on them, which we call puulpai. We have two essential ways of healing – ngangkari or puuni.

Men and women both use the healing breath. It is a ngangkari speciality and it works really well! It is a great way to heal and it works fast. The person gets well again and begins to put on weight again.

I never refuse anyone a treatment. If someone comes to me asking for help, I never refuse. I give them a treatment whatever the case. I always do what I can. Sometimes someone has been poisoned in a particular way, we call this poison irati, I feel sorry for them, because perhaps they have been bitten by a snake, or something like that. I have to kill that snake poison and kill that snake, because they are dangerous and because some poison lying around can enter the feet and go right up into the spine. The killing of the poison usually happens during marali. I use my own weapon. I have my own weapons that I use for these dangerous moments. I take them on my marali. My weapons are very old, and were given to me by my older brother, who got them from our father. I follow in my father's footsteps in that regard, as he was a very powerful ngangkari. My father's name was similar to Charlie Ilyatjari's and it came from Angatja area. My mother's name was Yangkuyi; she was not a ngangkari.

Women ngangkari always helped with birthing before. Women always helped each other. Listen, in the extreme case where a

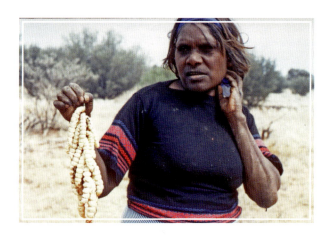

Pantjiti Unkari McKenzie with threaded maku, Pipalyatjara region, 1986.
PHOTOGRAPH SUZANNE BRYCE, ARA IRITITJA AI-0027374

*When no container is available women thread the maku together on a string made from a fine root of the ilykuwara. They pass the string through the tough part of the head, behind the chewing parts. The threaded maku are called maku wiliti.*
EXCERPT FROM 'WOMEN'S GATHERING AND HUNTING IN THE PITJANTJATJARA HOMELANDS' BY SUZANNE BRYCE, INSTITUTE FOR ABORIGINAL DEVELOPMENT, ALICE SPRINGS, NORTHERN TERRITORY

woman is having a very difficult birth and things are looking impossible, then a male ngangkari will come in and help the baby to be born. This is part of my work as well, birthing. Let's say a woman is in the bush having a baby and there is nobody to help, a ngangkari will help her in that case. He will help the baby get born. Ngangkari are highly skilled in everything they do! Men and women ngangkari are both the same, very skilled in anything medical. Women are ngangkari too, and very good ngangkari. Doctors may argue about treatments but ngangkari do not.

I have my own mapanpa. I keep them inside my arms. When I am giving treatments they move forward and assist me in the treatment.

Many problems we see today didn't affect Anangu before. Life was good then. We hunted our meat and speared it and the women dug holes to dig out grubs. We were all successful and excellent hunters and gatherers – kukaputju. Nobody had mental health problems then. There were no drugs, no marijuana and no alcohol. Anangu only had mingkulpa – wild tobacco.

When we used to go out riding donkeys when I was a girl, if another girl became sick and started vomiting, I would give a ngangkari treatment. We'd be going a very long way on our donkeys and we would camp out the night, foraging kampurarpa, bush tomato.

I was not scared the first time I went on marali, because other ngangkari took me and I was in safe hands. I still got a little bit confused though on one occasion, but my two uncles were there with me and they helped me through a tough patch. I was still learning. One time I crashed into the top of a tree and it made me really weak and I lost my appetite. I was given ngangkari treatments and I got better. It only happened the once.

Naomi, Ilawanti, Maringka, Kanakiya, Josephine and Janet Inyika are all women ngangkari. Wawiriya Burton, that old lady, she is a ngangkari. But there are many, many others. I don't know who they all are. I only know about the ones who work near me. We talk together, because we are a team. We also work as a healing team, healing as a group. We take it in turns to look at our people. Perhaps one of the others will see something I have missed, so it works well that way. Perhaps I will do the healing treatment and one of the others will help me. Janet Inyika helps me sometimes. We also have the chance to take a rest, when sick people are lined up to see us. One of us can have a rest while the other is working. We need to do that to recharge our batteries. We have power that needs to be recharged, just like you do with your batteries.

I have kuuti. Ngangkari use kuuti. Sometimes people complain that they have been struck by the force of someone's kuuti. A ngangkari will pull the kuuti out of their body and identify it, then someone will say, 'Oh look – it is my kuuti! It must have gone into you by mistake!' The person will not be feeling well so it is pulled out. Kuuti look like small black stones. They look like stones. Ngangkari keep them for themselves. They don't get sick when they get their kuuti and another ngangkari puts it into their body, where it then becomes a ngangkari tool. It lives there from then on.

We are ngangkari and we work together cooperatively. The role of the ngangkari is vital. We are putting our ngangkari Tjukurpa down on paper now. We are men and women. This is my Tjukurpa. What I am saying is open and public information.

I hope our young people will continue to want to be ngangkari in the future. I am holding onto my mapanpa for now, but my son is already working as a ngangkari and my daughter, Esther, is just starting out. She is really talented with young babies. But she's working in a private capacity only. I have given both of them tools.

I saw mamu all the time lurking in the trunks of trees when I was little. I was already working with kurunpa. If there were no senior men, I would work on people giving them healing treatments.

Without ngangkari, back in the past, Anangu would die without them, if they were too far away. Without ngangkari nearby, Anangu who were merely unwell would become critically ill, and die. If there were no ngangkari, then that is what would happen. But when there are ngangkari to help, then no problem at all! With ngangkari treatments a person is soon well again.

Ngangkari work with their hands. They work with the spirit in their hands. They take the pika, sickness, out with their hands. Others take the pika out with their mouths, sucking out the pika. They suck the pika out with their mouths. They suck out stones and the like with their mouths. Many healers give healing treatments with their mouths. I sometimes tell them – 'Don't suck too much out! Use your hands now!'

Ngangkari suck the stones out after touching the patient all over and feeling where the illness lies within, and then they suck the stones out of that spot. My older brother uses his mouth to remove stones and Andy Tjilari also does this treatment, but I do not, because I can't. I only know how to use my hands. The suction method is a men's treatment. Women, on the other hand, specialise in the blowing style of treatment, using the healing breath.

White people cannot give a ngangkari treatment with their hands like we do, and throw the sickness away.

I have spoken about ngangkari Tjukurpa – ngangkari Tjukurpa for you all to listen to. Ngangkari Tjukurpa for Anangu in the future to read and learn about.

And now we have got this new ngangkari book! And this is everywhere. Anangu will look at this book all the time. 'These are our ngangkari!' they will say.

This is for my granddaughter's granddaughter's little granddaughters of the future. For my granddaughter's granddaughter's granddaughter. For my granddaughter's granddaughter. This book is for my granddaughter.

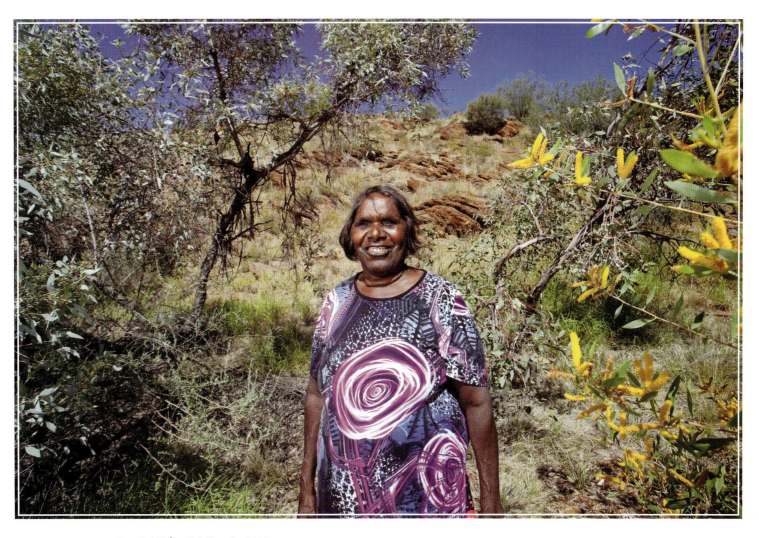

Pantjiti Unkari McKenzie, 2011.
PHOTOGRAPH RHETT HAMMERTON

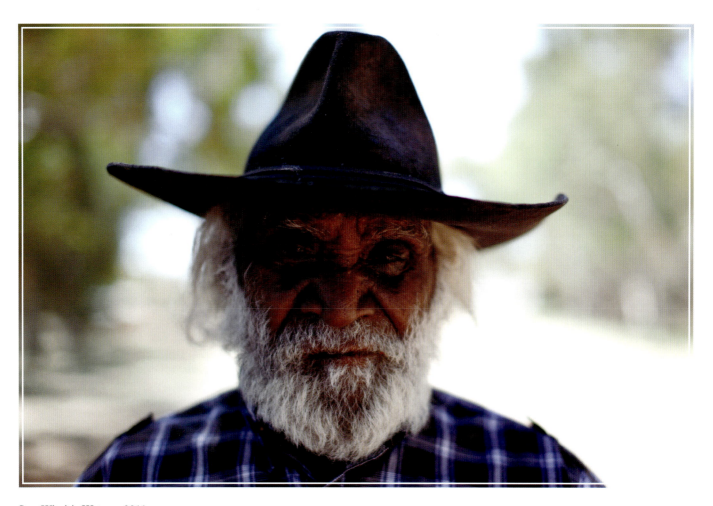
Sam Wimitja Watson, 2011. PHOTOGRAPH RHETT HAMMERTON

# Sam Wimitja Watson

I used to live out west at Warburton, and also in the Northern Territory, when I was a young man. In those days we didn't have any whitefella foods such as flour and tea, we only had bush foods, only kangaroo meat and water. I remember being photographed when I was a child, still completely naked. Nobody wore clothes back then. I was photographed by some tourists who were travelling through Warburton. After that time, my exposure to the modern world and white people was rapid, and it was around that time that I was introduced to clothes and put on trousers and shirts for the first time.

After that, I walked east to Ernabella as a young man, wearing trousers. Not long after I arrived there, a photograph was taken of me in Ernabella creek. I was already a man by then, but still single — no kungka, no woman! People were talking about me, saying, 'This is a man from Western Australia way. He's a western man.'

When I was a child my proper name was Wimitja. It wasn't until I arrived in Ernabella Mission that I was given the name 'Sam' after I became a wati, an initiated man, and then later I became 'Mr Watson'. I walked to Ernabella by foot. I decided to go to Ernabella Mission because I knew many members of my family were living there at Ernabella. When I got to Ernabella I was in shock to see all these naked people! People didn't have any clothes on, poor things! I'd been living in Warburton and everyone had been wearing clothes, and here I was in Ernabella and everyone was still naked! It embarrassed me so much to see them all naked. Children are OK, but the young women with their breasts all naked and the fully grown men embarrassed me, when I saw them naked! This was because at that mission it was believed that they should remain naked, and so they did. This happened in Ernabella.

Ilurpa is the name of the place where I was born. My parents were living in the bush and we lived entirely off the land: on the water, nectar, bush foods and bush meat. We lived by rockholes and water soakages. Ilurpa is a rockhole with a wanampi – rainbow serpent – in it. It used to have a wanampi in there but it is gone now. It left because the people left. Wanampi die when their owners leave. So it is dead now. It is not far from Blackstone. Whitefellas named Blackstone so that they would know which place they were talking about. But Ilurpa is my father's and grandfather's country, and that is where I was born. I've forgotten my grandfather's name, I can't remember. It was a different kind of name, but I've lost it now.

We still go to Ilurpa because there is good water there, and a tank and windmill. Of course back in the early days there was no windmill and we used to drink from the rockhole and the soak. My mother's country is Kirpiny, which white people refer to as Lake Wilson, which is near Pipalyatjara. My mother's name was Wipana. Her mother was named Kanmartjukunu and her mother's was named Kanmartju. They are Mai Ili Women, from Fig Country.

My father's name was Nyurpayakunu, and his language was Ngaatjatjarra, which is spoken around Ilurpa, near the Blackstone Ranges. My mother spoke a Pitjantjatjara dialect named Wiltjantjatjara, from east of Pipalyatjara.

I was born in the bush in the same way that my grandmother gave birth to my mother, in the bush. When my father became a man he went east and married a Pitjantjatjara woman – who was my mother. My father then had five children: first me, then Geoffrey, Pantjiti, Belle and Tjawina. My father had two wives actually, and we children came from the two mothers. I was the number one wife's son. She had three children and the number two wife had two children.

I grew up in the bush and I lived without any clothes, naked. All we had was kuka and kapi, meat and water, that's all. Ilytji is another word for puti or 'bush'. I was living in the bush and became a man there. After I became a free man I went to my father's country to the north and that's when the tourists took a photo of me.

I became a ngangkari because my father was a healer, a ngangkari pulka, as was my grandfather before him. My grandmother's name was Nyurpaya. I used to see mamu as a youngfella and I would take mamu out of children and other youngfellas. I'd kill the mamu or remove it from a person, release it and destroy it. It is common practice for fathers or grandfathers to give mapanpa and the power of healing to their children. You get the mapanpa through your family and through their Tjukurpa, and their home. That's where you get your mapanpa from, the home, and I got mine from Ilurpa. My father used to take me on the marali, and I learnt to be a good healer and I used to get all sorts of sticks and stones out of a person. When a sorcerer uses his magic in the wrong way to harm people, we ngangkari remove that harm. But I'm not as strong these days with my power, I'm getting a bit weak now.

I learnt with my father how to use the mapanpa. My father took me somewhere and I ate the mapanpa. In my case, I ate the mapanpa to become a big mapanpa person. My father took me to the mapanpa place where you eat it. The power comes into you when you eat the alu of the mapanpa. You don't chew it,

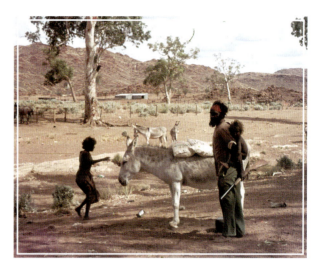

Sam Watson, carrying his son Peter Nyukuti Watson on his back, Pukutja (Ernabella), 1962–66.
PHOTOGRAPH MARGARET BAIN, ARA IRITITJA AI-0037140

Opposite page: Sam Wimitja Watson, Amata, South Australia, 1973–77.
PHOTOGRAPH BARBARA RIDLEY, BERT QUALMANN COLLECTION, ARA IRITITJA AI-0009633

*I walked east to Ernabella as a young man, wearing trousers. Not long after I arrived there, a photograph was taken of me in Ernabella creek.*

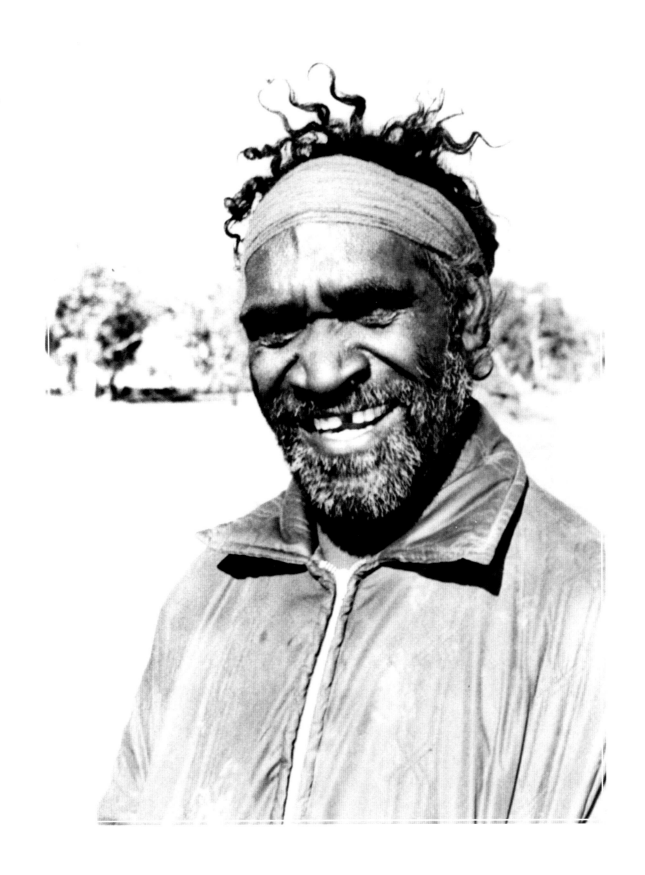

you swallow it whole. It is the liver of the mamu's food, the meat that they eat. We did this on that marali. Marali is a night journey, it's like foot walking but it's not, it's travelling through the sky. My kurunpa travels. You are travelling with your mapanpa. Some ngangkari can travel through the sky and sit up there. They travel at night and they stay there and then they come back before dawn to re-enter the body. I do that as well. My father took me on marali when I was a child so I didn't get scared. Marali is the travelling of the spirit. Sometimes another person can take you – it's like being on an aeroplane, flying around.

I still travel marali but I don't travel as much now. Sometimes I can, but not as much as I used to. We travel around and sometimes other ngangkari travel into a mamu's mouth, and the mamu gives them food and they eat it. The mamu are harmful spirit beings, invisible creatures of the night. When they do that, ngangkari increase their mapanpa's power. At dawn we arrive back into our bodies and go to sleep. We've got mapanpa in our bodies. In the old days nearly everybody had mapanpa.

I still travel on marali. I meet up with other ngangkari. I went north one time and met up with many other ngangkari. They were all naked, all these men and children ngangkari, all with different faces, and they were touching me and the next one would touch me and the next one would touch me, letting me pass.

I can get people's kurunpa and put them back into their bodies. If you haven't got a spirit, if your spirit's not in your body, you can die. We have power, like the power you have to drive that video camera with.

The mapanpa is mine, given to me by my father. My father gave me power with the mapanpa. It's like a light, it's like a power, and you get a kick, a bit like when people give you an electric shock to bring you back to life. That's what happens with ngangkari, they can give you a healing shock.

When you've become a fully fledged ngangkari, you can see lots of things. You see more mamu, creatures that appear at night. The senses in your body become stronger when you've got mapanpa – you have two hands with holes in the palms and you can see things and you can smell things, your sense of smell is stronger and you can feel things more strongly as well. We can smell sickness – we can detect sickness through our noses.

The mamu can see the ngangkari and it will leave in fright because they can see the mapanpa is more powerful than they are. They used to do that a lot in the old days. Ngangkari can see a mamu and frighten it and get rid of it. But now it's not common, you don't see a lot of mamu today. There used to be lots of mamu in the bush but since the church, bible and praying there are very few of them about. You don't see a lot of mamu about now, because they're gone. You know, in the old days when the people lived in the bush, the ones who didn't have clothes, my family, we used to see mamu all the time. We used to see mamu in the bush, everywhere, when I was a child and right through my life. You'd see them and most of the time the mamu wouldn't come close to me – they'd just keep on walking, walking past.

We have stories, Tjukurpa stories about dogs, Tjukurpa that are part of the land and the creation. But people also have dogs that are pets. My home's Tjukurpa is the rainbow serpent, the wanampi, similar in colour to the kuniya – a kind of python which doesn't bite – but it's the wanampi, the big rainbow serpent. There are other people who've probably got Tjukurpa – Dog Tjukurpa – but I don't, mine is the moving of the thumb, the wanampi. The wanampi, the hand sign for which is shaking the thumb, is different to the python. The hand gesture for the snake is moving the hand in a snake-like motion. I am wati wanampi, but I am friendly and kind. Where I come from there's a big waterhole where the wanampi lived and they used to touch it on the head in the old days. It didn't bite. The wanampi you can see.

At Ernabella Mission we men lived separately, on the west side. And I lived with all the ngangkari together. There were doctors living at Amata and they were like ngangkari too, they would heal the sick. The whitefella doctors came recently, they're new, but our ngangkari healers were around long before they came along. They saw white doctors at Ernabella Mission and Warburton Mission, but ngangkari doctors were around long before them.

I am a doctor, too, and I do healing. I heal people using all the different techniques. I use kuurtjankupai treatment method, which is the ngangkari suction technique, releasing the person's bad fluids for the patient to get better.

After I married my wife Monica, when she just finished school at Ernabella, we went to Amata. We had a child. My son was born in the bush. The clinic wasn't in Amata at that time. Amata was just a very small community with a few buildings when we had our first child. We lived at Docker River and we lived at Warakurna. I worked on some buildings there at Warakurna.

Healers can capture kurunpa and put it into a person. In the old day's mamu used to take the spirits of children. It happened to my brother. He went swimming and I said, 'Go home', but the next minute there he was, lying down, passed out, because his kurunpa had been taken. I told the mamu to leave and it went to the tree where other mamu were, and there were mamu dogs there. They were really, really evil and really hungry and used to eat constantly and they were the ones who used to grab the spirit first and eat that and then eat children. Mamu cats and dogs used to do that. Mamu cats and dogs used to eat children.

Now we're getting old, we're getting sicknesses like colds and diabetes and other diseases, we're getting old and slow. I haven't given my mapanpa to another member of my family yet because I'm still working using my mapanpa. I work as a ngangkari and have worked for a long time. Sometimes I heal. Even when I've got sore hands I still work healing, regardless of the pain.

A while ago in Kaltjiti we did a lot of big work because many of the people were really sick. Nearly everybody was sick and we went there and did a big healing. They're all really good now. A lot of people see me and they ask, 'Oh can you do a healing on me?' A lot of people ask me as soon as they see me, because they know I'm a healer, and they ask me, 'Oh can you heal me?' But I don't heal straight away on demand. But when it's quiet and one person asks me, I'll do it. There was also a woman who came to me who had bloating all over her body. I fixed her, got all that swelling down and she was good.

Somebody had a bad head from drinking too much. They had a headache, and you get that when you drink a lot. Your head gets sore and you also get sick, sickness that comes along after that, and we heal them for that. We push, we use our hands to push, push things out of the body, and it comes out. With your hand, this is how you do it, you push it, you pull it, push it down and then you grab it with your hand. That's with the mapanpa. You get it out with the mapanpa. The sickness is inside and you can get that sickness out, you can pull it out.

Sometimes if somebody's sick for a long, long time you can get really, really tired from being sick. And if you get too tired then you can die from that. But with whitefella medicine as well, a person can take it when the sister gives them a tablet or medicine and sick people can get well quickly.

Sometimes if you sleep in a place that was an old living place for others in the past, you can also get sickness that way. Spirits float about, resembling smoke, and the rocks nearby can all make you sick in the knee, in the hip, in the heart, or in the head, and a stick or a rock may become lodged in the body because of that place.

A kuuti is a stone, and a pika kuuti is a pika or a sore, it can get in the sore. And the spirit can become a rock and you can get that rock and you can put it in a container. My objects are all there in the clinic, you can see them! Those things in the bottle are neutralised. You won't get sick from looking at those objects and rocks if they are in a glass container. You won't get sick from looking at them because the sickness is all gone – it has been removed from those objects.

Kura kuurtjananyi is the sucking of bad blood. Kuurtjananyi was a common technique for healing, just to suck the blood out. You can also use the other techniques to get the rock or the stick out and after that you can apply suction to the area because the blood is still hot around that area where that object was. Kuurtjananyi. Kuurtjankupai is the suction method. Ask for all those bottles to be sent here and you can see all the rocks and sticks that I've got out of people!

Walatjunanyi is releasing or letting things go, similar to iyani, to send off or let go. You can get sickness out. Walatjunanyi is to send it off, release it and destroy it. I give the objects I have removed from the person to the clinic sister and they put it in a cold place, in the fridge, they are safe there, but sometimes that sickness can go back into a person, that stick or that rock. Sometimes if you give people you have treated their object, say, a rock or stick, and they take it home, they can easily get sick again. Sometimes people throw it in the toilet or they might put it in water or put it in dirt. I always tell them to put it where it's wet, in wet dirt. For example, if there's dirt where there's always water in a certain area, like from toilet or sewerage.

One time, years ago, somebody in Ernabella saw a whirlwind and mentioned that some people travel in whirlwinds and they said, 'Oh yes, that's Mr Watson travelling in that whirlwind!' Somebody said that in Ernabella. It's true, sometimes ngangkari can travel in a whirlwind. I'm still only a person, and I don't turn into a kupi-kupi! It is my kurunpa that can travel in a whirlwind. It's the spirit that can travel like that. The invisible spirit that can travel, the magic, mapanpa the spirit can travel.

Kuuti is a mapanpa. It's not a rock! Kuuti is like a bone, the white kurunpa. Kurunpa and kuuti is spirit. I got my mapanpa when I travelled with my father to a cave and we went in there and got my magic mapanpa, my magical powers, my magical healing powers. It was a long way west. I travelled there and got my mapanpa. My father gave me that mapanpa that time when we were travelling through that area. I was travelling above the ground and my father was travelling underground, below me. Some healers can travel under the ground as well as above.

Urkuni and ilani are two words that have the same meaning, which is to get out, pull out, to draw closer or to draw out. I used that healing technique when I was a child ngangkari, around the time my father went on the underground journey to get me the mapanpa.

My powers come from that place and I still have the powers I had when I was a child. When we see with our special sight, we can see things that normal people cannot see. We have an eye in the forehead. When our eye is closed we can't see anything. We can't see a person who is sick and we can't see any mamu. When we haven't got the opening holes in our hands we can't heal a person. But when our vision is open and the mouth is open for the kuurtjankupai treatment, that's when we can see mamu that are coming to bite and to kill and to eat women and children. Mamu can see our extra eye and they know that we are healers. How does our other eye and vision open and work? It's unexplainable. But our fathers and grandfathers can get you and press you in the forehead, and make your vision work. Our fathers and grandfathers do this just as it was done in the old days.

When I used to see mamu my body would show me. I used to destroy those mamu and make sure that they kept on going and did not come towards the people or towards me. Sometimes you can get things from your body and throw it out towards the mamu, and they can pick it up and eat it, and you can send them on along their way. I once ate the liver of the animal that a mamu was eating. That liver was burning and sizzling, because it was mamu food. I got it and I swallowed it and my ears popped open, the light came on and then the spirit came in. After that a ngangkari can see the mapanpa and the spirit world, that's what we do. We get our mapanpa placed in our hands and then we go home. That's how we get our mapanpa and that's why our ears can open too. When you're ngangkari you can hear. You can hear things that others can't hear. It is all because of the liver that was the mamu's meat, that they were cooking in the spiritual world on their spiritual fire, and that's what we eat, that liver. Our eyes and everything just burns, our ears pop open and our eyes pop open and our forehead opens up and we can see everything. Everything becomes close and clear. We think, 'Oh, my home's right here!' but really, it is not – it is really a long way away! Everything seems much closer because you can see everything so clearly and magnified when we get powers from the mamu's meat. We get the liver and swallow it whole. That is the mamu's meat, really, but the ngangkari who travel there to that spiritual land and the mamu's home swallow that liver before he can, and gain strong powers. After we swallow the liver we go back home and arrive there just before dawn. Mamu try to make me weak but they can't because my mapanpa always warns me of their presence, and keeps me safe.

Kuuti is similar to kurunpa. Fortunately kuuti and kurunpa can make you come alive, can make you into a person and it can make you well. We also call the mapanpa kuuti and it's the person's spirit. The ngangkari, the physical person, will go and get the spirit or kurunpa that's been devoured by a mamu and get it off the mamu and return it back to the person it was stolen from.

I work with the spirit or kurunpa. If the spirit goes to the back I can turn it around and make it go to the front. Why do they go to the back? Well, a spirit starts in fright when it sees a mamu. The spirit can run in fright, to hide behind the back of the person. That's what spirits do, they hide and move from the front and will run to the back or to another part of the body. Or it might flee the body altogether.

After I swallowed that liver, I lay down and the mapanpa mamu came and gave me something shiny and said, 'This is for you.' After that I went to sleep. I left that place after swallowing that liver and taking that big mapanpa from that mamu. That's when I was still a child. And when I became a man I still kept going because I'd already been there to that mamu's place, in that spirit place when I was a child. I travelled in the sky and my father travelled under the ground and we arrived together at that place, the mamu's place, in the mamu world, where mamu have their meat that they cook. They cook the liver and they want to eat it but along we came and ate the liver instead, swallowed the liver. So from eating and swallowing that liver it's still strong and that's why I am so strong. I can go to that place any time. The father doesn't say anything when they take their children there. There's no talking going on when we travel there on a marali and things just happen. Something else may accompany us, which looks friendly, it may even look like a friendly and familiar person, but really it is that mamu, and that mamu will give us that liver to swallow.

We can heal people affected by mamu most of the time. Sometimes mamu kill people. The mamu can kill somebody from ear to ear, following that line under your chin and across your throat. The neck just below the ear is called the wilki-wilki, and a ngangkari can see all the mamu kill a person like that but they can't save the person that way.

My young brother was about eight years old when he was bitten by a mamu cat. I was about ten or eleven at the time and we were living at Kuru Ala. We were walking around the country and even though he had been bitten by a mamu cat we kept going, so we could visit our grandfathers, uncles, older brothers and grandmother. When we met up with them, everybody was crying for my young brother. I was sad. When the sun came out we climbed down a hill and when we looked up we saw something following our track. Someone said, 'Hey! Look over there at that hill at the tracks where you climbed down, look up! There's something sitting there, red, red, flashing red.' And we all looked up and it was that mamu sitting there flashing red in our tracks. We all got together and we just hid. It was kind of like a big camel and it was chasing me, to destroy me and it made such a huge dust storm, and dust with its feet. My father gave me all these spears, all lined up, and they made a line of people and they made a fire as it was running on our tracks, following our tracks and I think the camel thing was after me, it wanted to grab me. It was screaming like a cow and it was really big and fat and really frightening. All the ngangkari lined up and destroyed it when it got really close to us. They killed it, all the ngangkari killed it. They made a fire and everyone was happy.

The next day we went off and were collecting bush onions at Kuru Ala near Punuwara, near Warnkarnkingka. And then we went off to another place to another soak near Pipalyatjara, at a place called Pulalypulaly, and we were sitting at the base of the hill there. They said, 'Oh don't play there because of the mamu,' and they looked over towards a narrow opening where there was a big mamu dog.

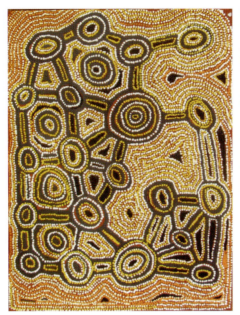
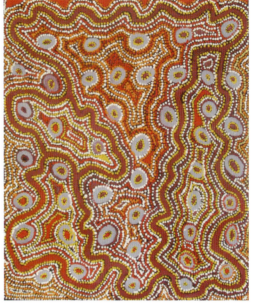

Top left: Sam Wimitja Watson, *Ngayuku Ngura (My Country)*, 2011. Acrylic on linen, 107 x 61cm.
PHOTOGRAPH VANESSA PATTERSON, © THE ARTIST, COURTESY NINUKU ARTS

Top right: Sam Wimitja Watson, *Ngayuku Ngura (My Country)*, 2011. Acrylic on linen, 91 x 61 cm.
PHOTOGRAPH VANESSA PATTERSON, © THE ARTIST, COURTESY NINUKU ARTS

Another man, a ngangka<u>r</u>i, killed it. We were only children then, and we were just playing, but I was ngangka<u>r</u>i too, and I was helping because I held a spear-like object, not a real spear but something else, along with my mapa<u>n</u>pa. All my family, grandfathers, uncles, older brothers, young brothers, and I joined together to help kill that mamu. My older brother didn't have ngangka<u>r</u>i powers then, and my younger brother didn't get to become a ngangka<u>r</u>i at all, because that mamu ate his kurunpa.

Another time, we were going to another place and we were collecting mai – collecting all these grains. The men were bringing kangaroos and kanya<u>l</u>a and all the kids were playing. They said, 'Sit down you kids! There are mamu around!' They said, 'Be quiet!' because it was getting dark. All that night, the whole night, nothing happened. It was a good night, we all got to sleep. And then we went off again.

The next day my father and my two brothers were separated from the other group. During the night, we had gone hunting possums at night – that's why we went. My father and others went to the one side and we went to another, walking by another route to join up while we were hunting possum. We saw dogs, they were biting something and we said, 'Grandfather, look, what are they biting?' And we saw two pythons, who were together. We burnt the tjanpi, the dry grass, so we could see, so as to kill the two pythons. Then we went off again, we kept going through the bush and we heard something, we heard a howling, and it was two possums up in the tree, in a hollow. My grandfather caught and hit those two possums, and then we kept on hunting, getting more possums. Next thing we looked up – 'Hey? Look at this! What is this? There are birds! There are lots of birds here.' The birds were going everywhere, they were all flying off and we were wondering, 'Well, what's going on here, then? There are too many...!'

Then the next minute we saw two lights, like car headlights, coming along, one coming first and another one coming after. They were mamu, that had put their two tails together – they were two mamu with their tails tied together that were coming along. My grandfather said to me, 'Sit down!' The lights were like a car but really it was those two mamu. It was like a light, like a car, but it was the Mamu Wipukarpilypa. This is referring to something which has its tail tied, and this was a mamu with its tail tied together with another one. The lights came and we heard those strange sounds, 'Woooooo', like the sound of dogs howling, which was probably the mamu. My father saw something in the front, and that is what kept us safe.

The next day we made camp at A<u>t</u>arangu, near Irruntju, and we cooked all the possums that we'd caught. The women saw lots of grains there, wakati, pig weed seed; they started collecting it all because there were grains everywhere. After that they went and they saw arngu<u>l</u>i, bush plums, near A<u>r</u>an and A<u>t</u>arangu. Then we all walked to another place, hunting as we went, and then we made camp. Again there was more food that they collected – this time all the women collected figs.

We were travelling during the winter. During the night people went hunting for possums. We set up our camp and went off hunting and came back. Everybody made windbreaks, and warm fires, behind the low walls. This was when we didn't have any clothes, we were living the traditional way in the bush, and so it was cold. The families – the fathers, mothers, grandparents and uncles – all used to camp close by because we were all afraid of mamu. We kept on going the next day. Another day we caught two kuniya pythons; we dug them up and killed them for meat. Then we kept on going and saw, 'Hey, there's a canyon there and all the kangaroos are going in through that narrow crevice.' So the men went and chased the kangaroos in through the narrow canyon in the hills and they were trapping them there. The kangaroos were probably going up to get water and so we were setting the dogs on them to help bring in our meat.

After that we set off towards a place called Manngu. Then after that we went to Walytjitjata, and from there we went to Lake Wilson. We stayed there for a while, going hunting at night and hunting during the day. We stayed there for a while and we were getting nganamara ngampu and wayanu – mallee fowl eggs and quandong. The women cooked the quandongs, roasted them quickly in the coals and made a paste with some water, they ground them into a lovely paste and we ate the paste. The quandong is a good quality fruit.

And then it started to rain, and we got completely soaked – soaked right through. We used to chase the kangaroos in the rain and the mud when it was wet. The ground was wet and all the dogs were chasing and killing our meat animals for us, such as kangaroos. We were still children then, and we would be playing, throwing toy spears at each other. And we saw a mamu come in! All the old men were using their mapanpa to get rid of the mamu that was coming towards us, getting the mamu. They were getting their mapanpa out from their arms and their abdomens and were throwing them at the mamu. The mamu got sick of all the mapanpa being thrown and it went away. I used to always throw my mapanpa at the mamu too.

I was a big boy, a teenager, when we saw a whitefella truck coming with food to give us. The whitefellas used to give us flour and sugar and tea; they used to pour it into our wooden bowls. We had never had flour like it before. They were giving us free flour and our grandfathers used to make something like porridge out of it. They used to put some food onto a spear thrower and give me some of it. Men used to use their spear thrower as a plate, they used to put their food and stuff on it. It was at Winpuly where I first saw white people. Whitefellas came there with food, giving it out to our families, at Winpuly near Irruntju.

We kept on going and the women were finding lots of kampurarpa and wangunu woolybutt grains growing everywhere. They would clean the grain, grind it up, make it into a paste and then pour the paste into the fire to make a big seed damper. Then we would get the damper and eat it like that, waru, hot! It was hot so you had to blow on it to eat it because you wanted to eat it really quickly. But you have to blow on it at the same time as you eat a wangunu damper. We used to eat nganamara ngampu in the pila – spinifex plain – and along the edges of the hills. We would eat emu eggs on the pila. Those nganamara lived in our country, in our area, in the Irruntju and Pipalyatjara area. I used to see all their eggs. When you found the nest you'd dig in it and you'd feel around inside it, and then you'd pull the eggs out. You'd feel the eggs that were in there and collect them. The mallee fowl always put their eggs in the earth, they'd make a mound and bury them. That's how they would lay their eggs and cover them and we'd come and find that mound and then collect the eggs. There'd be so many eggs! Sometimes we'd cover their mound back up and next time we'd come to that same spot and we'd find another lot of eggs and we'd dig them up again and collect the eggs and cover it up again.

Mallee fowl aren't around any more, they're all gone. Maybe they still live around near Watarru. Those mallee fowl have all been taken away to the cities, to Adelaide and that's where they live now. The mala, rufous hare-wallaby, and makura are also gone. Makura are like mice. They sit in the tjanpi or under the tjanpi, in the grass, or on the leaf litter, and you can feel them with your foot. They used to sit together, husband and wives, husband and wives. They'd live in the spinifex plain and in the sandhills.

Grandmothers used to dig a big hole to dig out all the kuniya pythons and they'd bring them out and put them on the ground and they'd just be lying there. Then they'd hit them on the head, then wind or coil them around and around, and cook them. Then they would pull the fat off the python. You couldn't really finish eating it because there was too much fat! It was too much to eat, too rich!

In the past we ngangkari were never allowed to talk about our power and the things we did. We have always kept it secret, but now we are talking about our work and explaining our methods.

My work is well known now, and all the things that I've taken out of people's bodies are there in the clinic. Some women might still say, 'Oh, don't risk looking at that man, because he's a ngangkari!' Once, a tourist took a photo of me when I was naked, and some people said, 'Oh, don't do that. Don't take photos of him, because he's a ngangkari'. Well, it is OK now for us to have our photo taken, because we've made our knowledge and skills known. We've made it known now, whereas in the old days we lived the naked way and we kept certain things hidden because of the way we lived. But now we live differently and some of our skills and knowledge are made known to the public.

We used to live at Ernabella Mission wearing clothes, when I married my wife, when I was still quite young. When we had a child, that's the time my photo was taken of me. I used to do housing work at Warakurna and Docker River a long time ago when I was a young married man. You can see a lot of my photos when I was working.

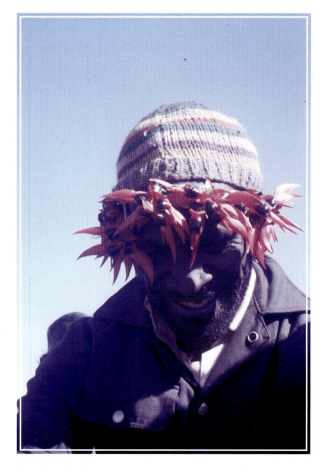

Sam Wimitja Watson wearing a malukurukuru (Sturt's Desert Pea) headdress, Amata, South Australia, 1966.
PHOTOGRAPH DAVID HEWITT, MARGARET & DAVID HEWITT COLLECTION, ARA IRITITJA AI-0000391

David Hewitt recalls, 'Sam was sitting on the back of a truck, probably returning from hunting, when this photo was taken. It must have been after rain as we did not often see Sturt's Desert Pea around Amata. All the men worked in those days and Sam Watson was the clinic gardener.'

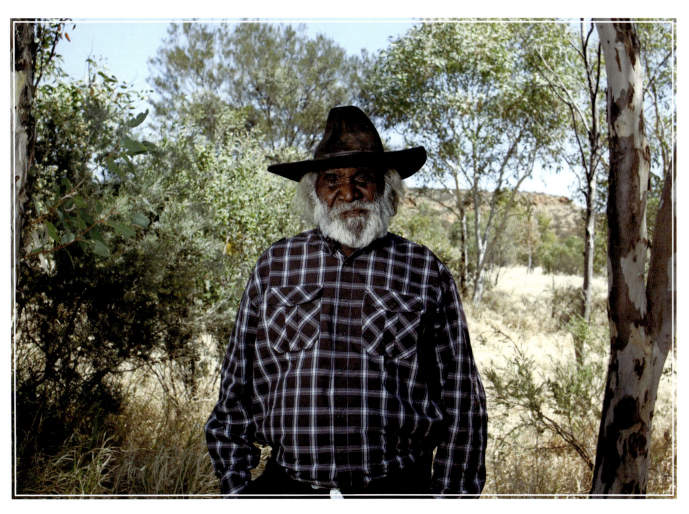

Sam Wimitja Watson, 2011. PHOTOGRAPH RHETT HAMMERTON

Once, two women linguists, Amee Glass and Dorothy Hackett, took a photo of me. When they saw me later they said, 'Ah, this is the man from Warburton', and they took the photo back to Warburton and showed it to people who said, 'Oh, he's the one who is a ngangkari. Well, he's there at Ernabella now'.

Women ngangkari and men ngangkari are level. I don't heal women. I mainly heal men and children. Women ngangkari usually heal women and children. They do lots of their own things. Many of the techniques the women use are unknown to me. We male ngangkari mainly just work with other men. But our powers are stronger, because we have been ngangkari long before the women, so we are more powerful than the women.

I'm still working as a healer even today in communities in the bush.

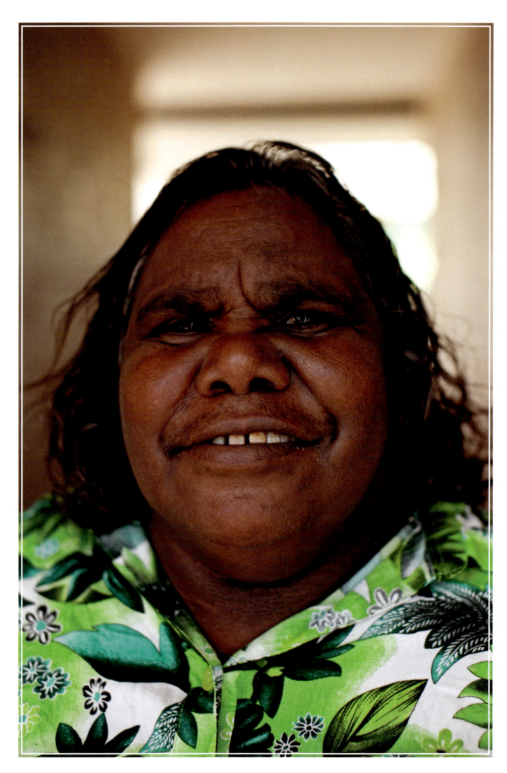

Josephine Watjari Mick, 2011. PHOTOGRAPH RHETT HAMMERTON

# Josephine Watjari Mick

At an earlier time, I wasn't a ngangka<u>r</u>i, but then in a dream I saw fire, a tongue of fire, just the bright light. I went towards it with my two hands and I was thinking, 'It's going to burn me!' That fire went into my hands, my two hands. After that I was thinking, 'Eh?' When I woke up, I was frightened and my hands were hot. I got up and my hands needed something, butter or water, and I was really worried about it. I asked my uncle, 'Why did that fire, the flame like a tongue, go into my hands?'

When I had that dream, I already had all my children by then. It was when my son Merlin was a little bit big by then, about five years old and starting school. After that is when I started working as a ngangka<u>r</u>i and I have always considered that it was important to help. I tried doing some work with my hands, working on children who were sick, and they got better. Then I worked on adults as well.

So I have a history doing this work. I went on a trip to Adelaide to work as a ngangka<u>r</u>i and as I travelled to different communities, people would spot me and bring children over. I did a lot of work at Ernabella clinic treating children with diarrhoea. These children would be at the clinic ready to be evacuated by plane and I would treat them and then they did not have to go away to hospital. I did this work in all the communities.

Today I still help to look after the children with stomach and gut problems. I'm still working with the healing ability that came through like fire entering my hands. I haven't handed it on to anyone else and so I am still working with the children. It's important work.

I can help with pain. I help people with pain in their heads. I use butter to do the kinds of healing work that we regard as women's 'separate' healing. I work on women with a number of techniques, using something like butter to work into the body. There is a blowing technique, used on the head. Openings can appear on the head and I am able to close these off.

Sometimes I go to the clinic to observe and help. I can see when a person's spirit is not sitting properly. This applies to children and adults. I don't say no to this work because I feel compassion for people.

Aboriginal people know me, mothers with children and people who have a sick relative at the clinic. They will ask me to go and see the person and I always go, I don't forget about it. A lot of women are too embarrassed to have men touching them. They really want to be treated by a woman ngangka<u>r</u>i. There are plenty of women ngangka<u>r</u>i on the Lands. Women can get embarrassed, you know, and I can help them, working on their bellies when they have symptoms like mental disorientation.

Just recently in town my daughter brought a girl to me who was yelling out and cranky and unable to listen to anyone. Her saliva was really flowing. I took hold of her to stop her writhing around and worked on her belly. I also removed things from her head. She is fine now, living back at home again. I've noticed that she is happy and well again. Before, her stomach and her head were seriously affected and she was crying out so much. This kind of thing is also my area of work. I don't ask people to pay me. I work on those young ones who suffer mental troubles. Yes, that kind of thing, I can work with mental problems.

I work on non-Aboriginal people as well. These days I also use bush medicines to help people to heal and to keep them strong. We travel a long way to get the plants. I tell people to use a preparation after their treatment. I helped a woman in Canberra, a top bureaucrat. She was getting severe headaches almost constantly and could hardly get out of bed. I gave her a treatment and three or four days later she told me she was feeling so much better and was so happy. She said she'd been hardly able to get up and now she was feeling well. Julia Burke can vouch for me. I worked on her at the NYP Women's Council office and fixed her headache, used the blowing technique and massage on her head with butter. This is how I work with children and women, removing headaches and also working on the belly where young women are affected and have become really off-centre. I can see it in them and do the work so that they can get on and do the things they need to do.

The way I'm thinking, our work as ngangka_ri is growing in importance again. It's good to be thinking about it. I think it's really important to look after family. There isn't another woman ngangka_ri beyond my home. Out east there are a number of women ngangka_ri, but in the west it is mostly male ngangka_ri.

I sometimes think back to that dream, and ask myself how I put my hands into the flame and how I gave myself such a jolt in my spirit, waking up in fright, holding up my hands. What a strange dream! And letting my hands recover. What a very strange dream!

I can feel a burning sensation inside my upper right arm, and I think, 'There must be someone sick somewhere.' It's telling me. It must be where my power is. It's as if it's burning inside and I rub it with butter and I think to myself that someone must be sick and that's why this is happening. The sick person might be thinking about me and I'm on the alert.

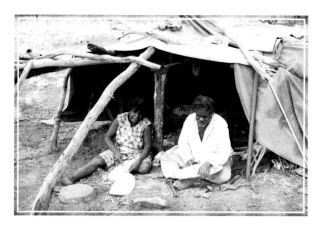

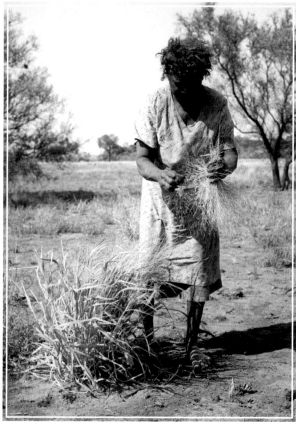

Top: Kunytjiriya Mick and Jacky Mick Mirankura (Josephine's parents) making piti (wooden bowl) beside their wiltja, Pipalyatjara, 1975.
PHOTOGRAPH PETER BROKENSHA, PETER BROKENSHA COLLECTION, A_RA IRITJTJA AI-0027891

Bottom: Josephine Mick's mother, Kunytjiriya Mick, collecting ka_ltu-ka_ltu (native millet) grass seed to make nyuma (seed cake), Pipalyatjara, South Australia, 1975.
PHOTOGRAPH PETER BROKENSHA, A_RA IRITJTJA AI-0027936

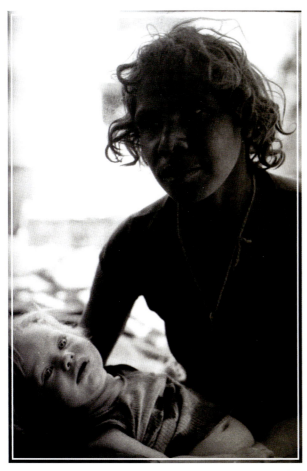

Someone might have a bad knee, and I will massage the tightness away, put butter on it. I treat babies too. I've been working on a baby and also my grandson, Aiden. I'm working on all the kids, massaging them and using butter. I was working on one baby to soften the tightness of his muscles and tendons to help him be more comfortable.

My mother was a ngangkari. She has left us now. She was healing people a long time ago and she helped people without taking any money, so that her family could be well and happy. I know her work well.

I remember her like this. She helped people and she would talk about what she was doing. I remember and I would watch her. She didn't pass it on to me. But she gave it to her granddaughter Palitja, Maxine's daughter. She is young, a teenager, so she isn't ready to do anything about what her grandmother gave her, it is not developed in her yet.

My mother used to work on Yaltjangki and she used bush medicines. I'm like her, I'm following her line, her Tjukurpa, using bush medicines as well. She would rub medicine all over the body and tell the person to sleep.

After a treatment I tell people to have a shower, 'Rub yourself all over with bush medicine and then sleep really well so you can heal.' This is what I tell to mothers with sick children or other people. If someone has a sore throat, so swollen that

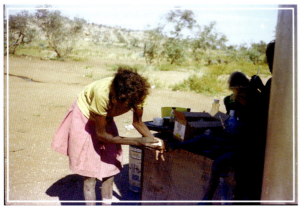

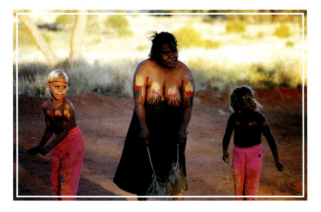

Top left: Josephine Watjari Mick with Suzanne Bryce's son Adji Rainow at the first NPY Women's Council General Meeting, Kanpi, 1980.
PHOTOGRAPH SUZANNE BRYCE. ARA IRITITJA AI-0036663

Centre left: Josephine Watjari Mick tending to a child with a sore toe outside the clinic, Pipalyatjara, South Australia, 1970–79.
PHOTOGRAPH SANDRA KEN, SANDRA KEN COLLECTION, ARA IRITITJA AI-0015432

Bottom left: Josephine Watjari Mick teaching girls Gina Tjitayi (left) and Geraldine Manyitjanu Curley the Waru Inma – black-footed rock wallaby ceremonial dance.
PHOTOGRAPH MAGGIE KAVANAGH, NPY WOMEN'S COUNCIL COLLECTION, ARA IRITITJA AI-0035364

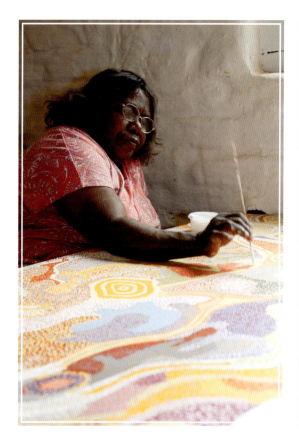
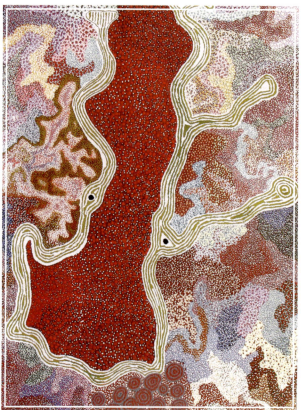

they can't swallow, I can fix that with rubbing on the medicine and giving a lot of water.

My mother made wangunu when Suzanne's son had mumps. For sore ulcers on the tongue, she burned the wangunu, pounded meat ants and mixed them all together with water so that it could be applied to the mouth. This was for pus-filled or weeping sores in the mouth. So the wangunu was scorched and turned into charcoal, the pounded meat ants mixed in and the mixture rubbed all over the throat, ulcerated mouth, and tongue to heal the problem. She used the base of the wangunu, a plant that had had its seed extracted. The grass could be thrown away, the root used, first burned in the fire.

Then there is another bush medicine, kalpari, rat-tail grass. The kalpari that is around about. It can be used everywhere, rubbed into the back, the stomach. It is pounded, and has a really strong scent and is good for blocked nose. Yes, that's kalpari.

Top left: Josephine Watjari Mick painting at Ninuku Arts, Kalka, South Australia, 2011. PHOTOGRAPH PAUL EXLINE

Top right: Josephine Watjari Mick, *Mamungari*, 2009. Acrylic on canvas, 130 x 94 cm.
PHOTOGRAPH CLAIRE ELTRINGHAM, © THE ARTIST AND NINUKU ARTS

Opposite page: Josephine Watjari Mick, *Mamungari*, 2011. Acrylic on canvas, 122 x 153 cm.
PHOTOGRAPH CLAIRE ELTRINGHAM, © THE ARTIST AND NINUKU ARTS

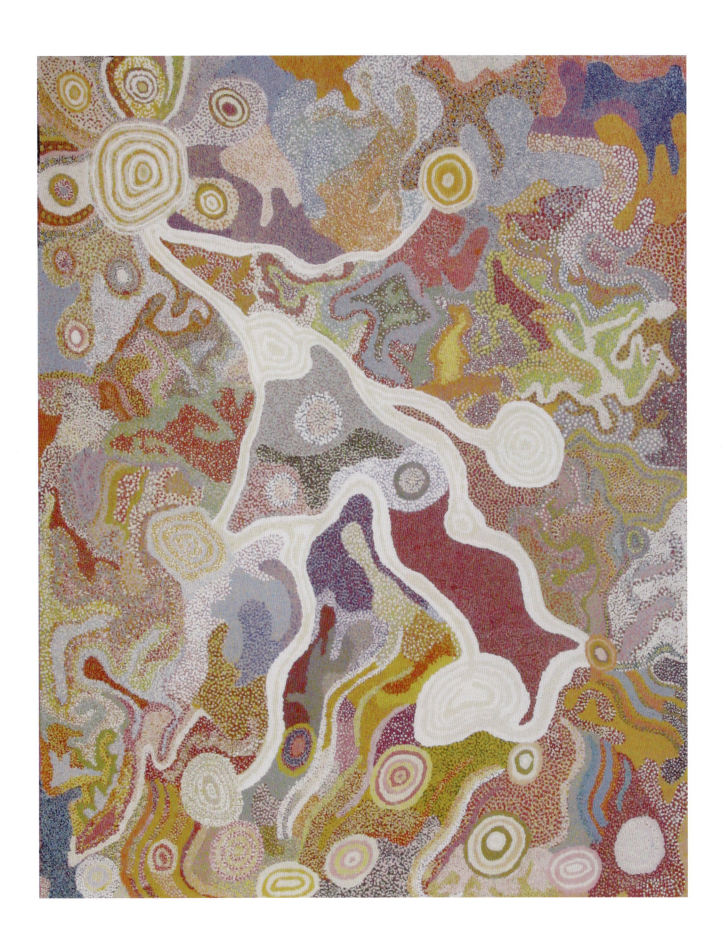

There is another one we cut to use and I have been asking a lot of people, 'What is this tree called?' No one seems to know, but one woman was going and getting it. They went to Kuru Ala, some women, and they collected it and started showing it to others. After that we all learned about it. It's a good bush medicine from a certain place but none of us knows its name. We just know the leaves, it's a bit like punti, cassia bushes, the leaves are bluish and inside dark green, they turn light green when they are burned and it has a good, strong smell. It's growing, not close, not on sand hills, not in the creek system, not in the hills, but a long way off, rirrangka ngaranyi – on a rocky, gravelly ridge. Rirrangka is a hill, a small gravelly hill – a bit like a sand hill, they have trees and different plants growing on them.

My mother made two bush medicines, the wangunu and the kalpari. Wangunu is the one for the sore ulcerated mouth in babies, used with meat ants mixed together with strong healing properties. Kalpari is good for the chest, for 'flu.

I'm happy to offer another story because people might want to know what it is like for a woman to be a ngangkari. I'm glad that my story is going to be seen, it's a story that is growing bigger. I'm happy to contribute to this book. I'm still an active ngangkari, working on women, children and senior women.

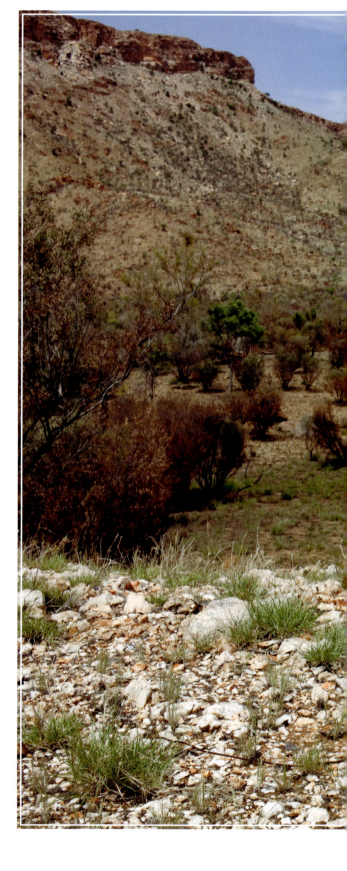

Josephine Watjari Mick, 2011.
PHOTOGRAPH RHETT HAMMERTON

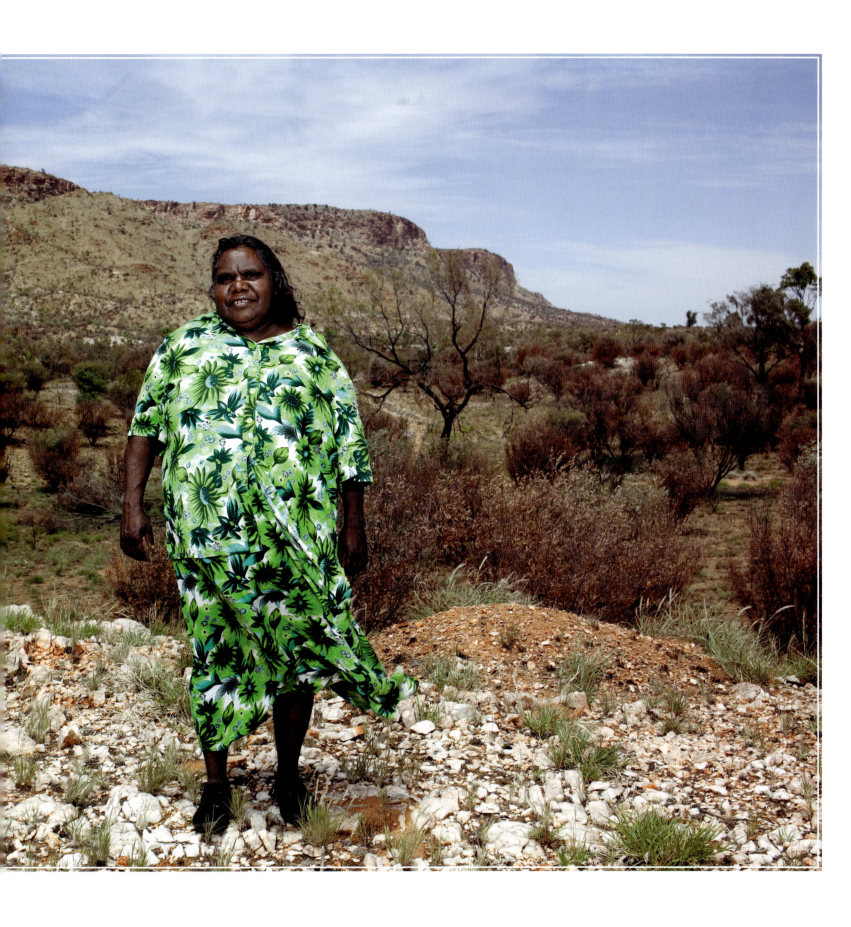

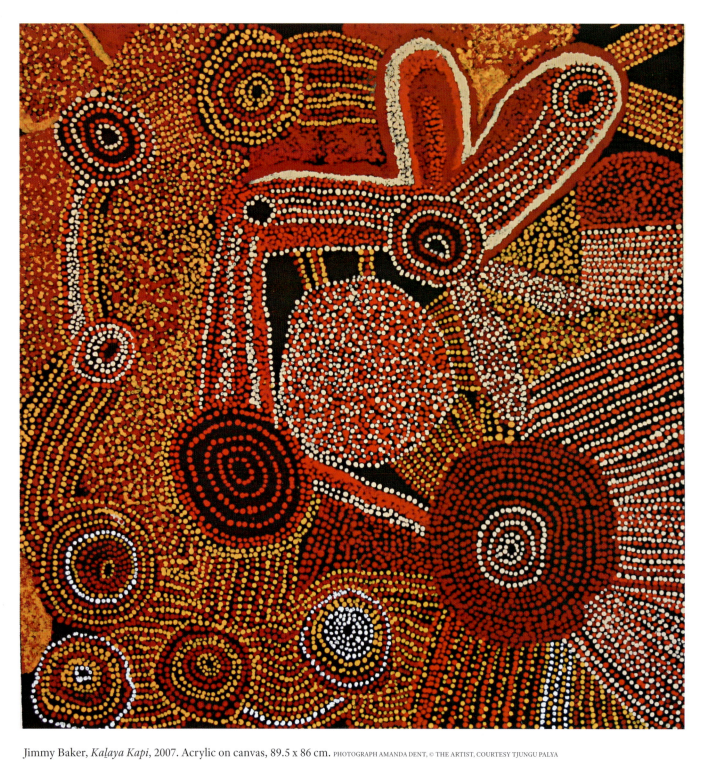

Jimmy Baker, *Kaḻaya Kapi*, 2007. Acrylic on canvas, 89.5 x 86 cm. PHOTOGRAPH AMANDA DENT, © THE ARTIST, COURTESY TJUNGU PALYA

*Kaḻaya Tjukurpa (Emu Creation). This is Kaṉpi. Ngayuku ngura (my home). These are all the rockholes around Kaṉpi and they all belong to the emu. The emu travelled all through this land, from one waterhole to another. This is my home and I am that emu.*

# Jimmy Baker

Let me tell you about the old days. I am not making any of it up. It is all true. We don't lie. Many years ago in the olden time, over in those ranges, there used to be many ngangkari. Most of those old ngangkari have now passed away. They didn't work for money. They didn't write down their work. They healed people and brought them back to health. That's what happened. In the olden times, all the old men used to do a lot of ngangkari work.

On the odd occasion when they couldn't help the sick person, they'd call in another ngangkari for additional help. They'd say, 'Hey! Can you come and take a look at this? I need help.' They wouldn't say out aloud what was going on because it would usually be because of something sacred. A sacred issue. 'Come and have a look at this. I can't seem to work it out. I've tried, but it isn't working.' So the other would come over and have a good look at the sick person and then they'd talk about what was going on. The other ngangkari would usually be able to fix the problem, and the sick person would soon be well again.

I was just a little child when I became a ngangkari. When I became a man I felt I was a fully fledged ngangkari. Ngangkari learn all the basics of ngangkari healing arts when they are children and we become more powerful ngangkari when we become adult men.

I am one of the leading ngangkari around here. Yet I have no money and no car. All I get is a little bit of pension. I am known far and wide. Sometimes I have to go to Port Augusta, Ceduna, Yalata, Tjunytjunytjarra and Kalgoorlie to do some healing work. I breathe the ngangkari healing breath on them to make them well again. I travel on the plane sometimes because I have no car.

When I was a young man, I used to heal people all over the country. This was for no money. I've never received money for my work, but these days we modern people have learnt about working for money. I have healed many people in my lifetime. I think that I would like to start getting paid regularly for my work, and put the money away until it has built up enough for me to buy a car. Because I am getting old and sick now, and I can't get around so much, a car would be good for me, poor old thing that I am. I can't move very fast at all and find it hard to see to the people like I used to.

When I do ngangkari work I don't get paid unless the health clinic calls me up and asks me to come in. I get paid for my clinic work, just a little bit. At the clinic they give sick people medicine, but I don't work with medicine. I work alongside doctors who use needles and medicine, there is often a lot of blood. The types of white man's medicines that are available to us are tablets, rubbing ointment, eye drops, needles and bandages for open wounds. We are all familiar with these things. Ngangkari don't use them, though. The ngangkari healing therapy that I use cannot be seen, nor can it be written down. It happens invisibly and usually quietly off to the side. Clinics need to remember to treat us ngangkari with respect, and to remember that we might have just come out of the bush. Our work is important.

We ngangka<u>r</u>i enter the skeleton by way of the spirit. We enter the body like that. We travel by spirit and enter the bones or the muscle. We heal from inside. We don't give injections and we don't spill healthy blood. Blood doesn't come out from the skin by our method. Doctors give a person who is having an operation another person's blood by transfusion into the veins under the skin. This can bring a person back to life, but the blood is still somebody else's blood. Sometimes the blood comes from a person who is now dead. We ngangka<u>r</u>i can see it. Other people's blood inside a sick person is a problem for us ngangka<u>r</u>i. We also believe that putting someone else's blood into a person can kill them. We worry about that dead person's blood being in a living person's body. We can see it and we can feel it. It can be the cause of that person dying during the operation. This is what we ngangka<u>r</u>i believe.

When somebody goes by plane to the Alice Springs Hospital, we worry for all these reasons. I have gone to see them there to help them. That's why I have to travel all over; Port Augusta, Alice Springs, Kalgoorlie, Papunya, Ceduna, everywhere! So when people are operated on, sometimes halfway through the operation they die. If that happens, it is probably because the blood they were given is from someone who is dead. The blood is old, and is not alive. Think about it. I am a ngangka<u>r</u>i. We know these things. We know if a dead person's blood is in somebody's body. We see it straight away. Poor things! When we see people's spirits, we see them as alive and moving. We see their blood, living and moving. Ngangka<u>r</u>i see people's spirits. It is easy for us. We see their spirits with our eyes and with our mind's eye too.

I have given ngangka<u>r</u>i healing therapy to people of all colours and ages. Old men too! I've been able to save them from having to have operations and injections they didn't want. Sometimes they have already had a series of injections, but have only got sicker and sicker. That is probably because they are being given dead people's blood during transfusions – at least, this is what I think. They have to swallow all sorts of substances, too, along with the dead blood. That's why so many people have died when they shouldn't have. We Aboriginal people don't really like the thought of operations.

I started work as a ngangka<u>r</u>i a very long time ago in Ernabella. Later I moved to Alice Springs and I worked there for a long time as well. I used to live at Kaltjiti. One day, someone came up to me and told me there was a sick person badly needing help. I asked, 'Where is the sick person?' I was told they were in Alice Springs. 'Can you go and see them?' 'Yes, why not? How am I to get there?' 'Well, you could catch a plane. Hang on, and I'll organise it for you.' 'OK. But what about my food?' 'Well, I'll organise that for you, too. I'll organise a purchase order.' 'Well, alright, then.' So I went to Alice Springs. Soon I was there. I went to see the sick person. Oh dear, the person was very sick. So I had a good look at the sick person. I did a good treatment on them. I spent the night nearby. The following morning I went back to see them. 'Hey! You seem good! Are you alright? You good?' 'Yes. I am good!' 'Hey good! That's great!' So that was that. Everything was

Opposite page: Jimmy Baker, *Pa<u>l</u>kapi<u>t</u>i*, 2007. Acrylic on canvas, 1190mm x 830mm.
PHOTOGRAPH AMANDA DENT, © THE ARTIST, COURTESY TJUNGU PALYA

*Pa<u>l</u>kapi<u>t</u>ila, Ka<u>n</u>pila kutu wa<u>n</u>ampi kutjara (the two mythical serpent brothers from Pilta<u>t</u>i headed towards Ka<u>n</u>pi, to a place called Pa<u>l</u>kapi<u>t</u>i). One brother was injured after his woman speared him with her wana (a wooden digging stick) in his back. He went past Ka<u>n</u>pi rockhole and kept travelling up into the hills. He was feeling sick from his injury and vomited. Apu pi<u>r</u>anpa tju<u>t</u>a (there are lots of white stones around here). Ngayuku ngura (this is my country).*

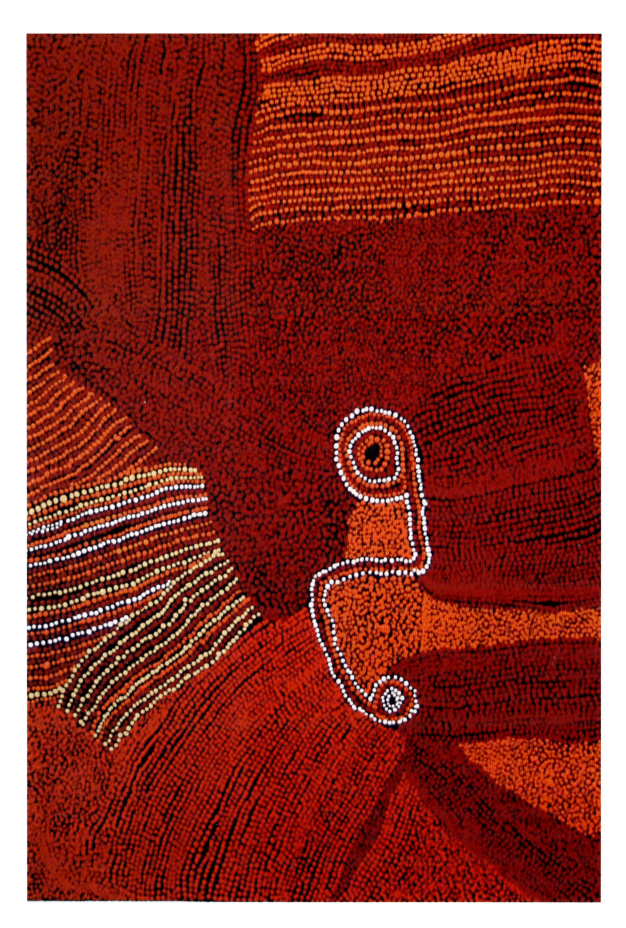

fine. I have come across many different ailments in my lifetime. I deal with the pain and the sickness so quickly that people sometimes say to me, 'What? Is that it? Is that all you are going to do?' So I say, 'Well? How do you feel? Better?' Then they say, 'Well, yes, as a matter of fact I do feel better! That was quick!' And I say, 'See. That's it!'

We call people who have mental health problems 'rama-rama' people. They can be rama-rama for a number of reasons and we can usually help them. If they have been touching too many wrong things, such as petrol inhalation and other substances like marijuana, they can ruin their brains. Ngangkari can't help them. Too many people are like this today. They might go from one ngangkari to another, but it won't work. We can't help with petrol sniffing and drug damage, no matter what you try to pay us! You know what I am talking about!

I was talking to Elsie Wanatjura about our money problems. She acknowledges how many years we old men have been working as ngangkari. She acknowledges that today we do not get enough money. Rupert Peter told me that he knew I had been a ngangkari for much longer than he has. This is true. Rupert Peter was still a child when I was doing ngangkari healing work all over the country.

Ngangkari don't use needles, tablets, pain tablets, eye medicine, ear drops or bandages. We weren't trained to use them. But doctors do. I'd like to ask, how much pay do white doctors get? Big salaries? Probably! I am sure you know how much they get! Well, look here. This is a ngangkari talking to you. We can talk. Put it in the book. I am one of the leading ngangkari of the Lands. I should be up front. I have been helping white men, black men, white women, black women, white children, black children – everybody!

Opposite page: Jimmy Baker, *Kalaya Tjukurpa*, 2008. Acrylic on canvas, 99 x 98 cm.
PHOTOGRAPH AMANDA DENT, © THE ARTIST, COURTESY TJUNGU PALYA

*Kalaya munu kiparaku Tjukurpa (this is the story about the emu and the bush turkey). The emu father had many chicks with him, but that poor old bush turkey only had one child. When the bush turkey came by he saw the emu sitting all alone and he asked, 'Where are all the children?' 'I didn't want all those children, they are too much trouble. They eat too much. So I killed them all!' The emu hadn't really killed his children, but hidden them in the bush. When the turkey's son heard this he said to his father, 'If you don't kill me I'll show you where all the tucker is'. But the turkey was thinking, 'I might kill my son.' He killed him, hit him on the head. While the turkey was sitting down at Kanpi he saw the emu come back with all his children. He realised he'd been tricked and was angry. He decided to kill that emu. He told the emu to grab his spear thrower and come with him. He hit him in the chest and killed him. When he got back to Kanpi rockhole all the emu kids were painted up for inma (sacred dancing). The kipara hid behind a tree and whistled at them. He was frightening them and they thought he was mamu (evil spirit). They ran off down towards Watarru. This is the true story for Kanpi.*

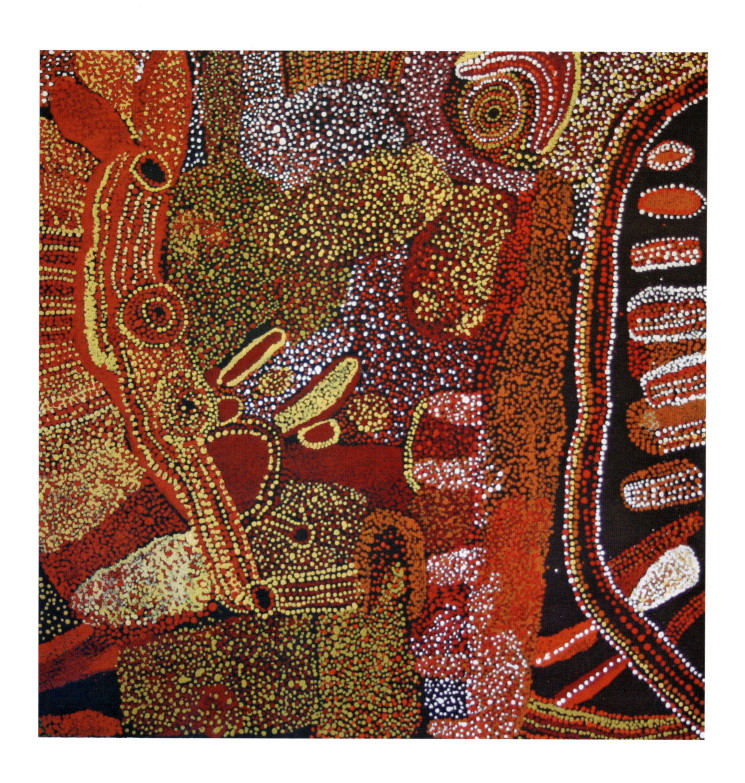

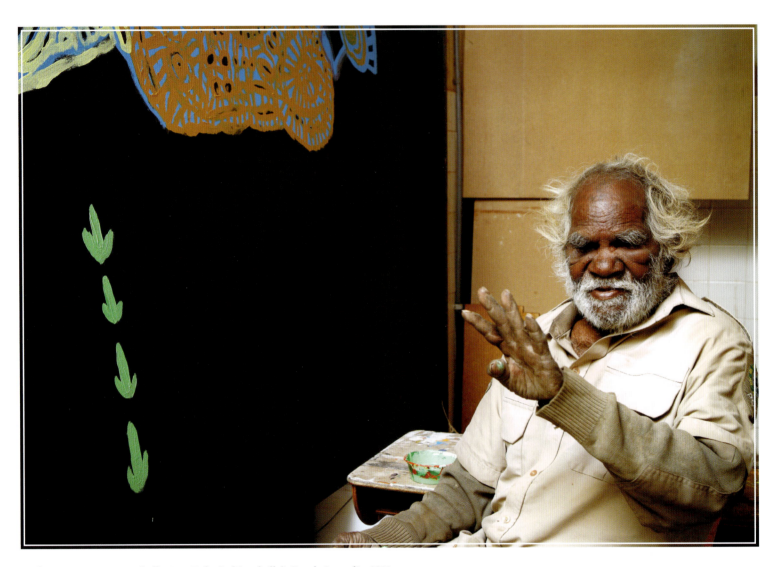
Dickie Minyintiri at Ernabella Arts, Pukatja (Ernabella), South Australia, 2011.
fPHOTOGRAPH ALEX CRAIG, COURTESY ERNABELLA ARTS

# Dickie Minyintiri

I was given only one name when I was born and that is Minyintiri and white people gave me the name Dickie. My real and only name is Minyintiri and I am a ngangkari. I was a ngangkari as a child and have been known as 'Minyintiri the ngangkari' all my life. But you can call me Dickie Minyintiri.

I learnt all my ngangkari skills from my grandfather and my older brother when I was a small child. They taught me how to touch in the healing way. They'd call me over when they were treating a sick person. The sick person would be saying, 'I am really ill.' I'd come running up and I'd watch and learn and listen carefully to what they were saying. They'd be saying, 'Here, check this out. This is what you've got to do.' They'd show me the sorts of objects I'd have to extract. 'Here, take a look at this. This is what you have got to extract from the sick person.' They'd wriggle the object out of the sick person's body.

So I'd work too, very, very carefully, with both hands. You have to be very careful because of the risk of actually spreading the sickness even more widely through the body. You must gently ease the sickness into a small, hard, round shape. Once it forms a kaputu, which is a small, hard, round ball, it can be extracted with two hands. I learnt how to do this when I was just a young child.

Grandfather and I used to sleep next to each other when we lived together at Tjintjulu. Grandfather was the man who gave me so much. He'd teach me and give me knowledge and power. He'd sometimes extract dangerous sicknesses from me. He'd then show me what he did with them and instruct me how to do it myself next time.

When I was still a child, I also learnt about mamu – evil, dangerous spirits. Mamu often arrive in clouds of dust. Some of these mamu are very dangerous. We'd know when they had come in close because there would be a lot of dust around. We'd get up and go looking for them. If we couldn't find them at first, we'd come back for our kulata and miru – our spears and spear throwers. Carrying them, we'd go off searching for the mamu. We'd say, 'Well, we know where they are. They are close by but they are hiding from us.' We would scare them with our power because they'd be shivering in their hiding places. They'd jump out and try to run away, but of course we'd spot them and we would take up the chase. 'Get them! Get them!' The mamu would get really wild when they knew that my grandfather was onto them. They knew that they would be beaten. They'd run off, stirring up dust and creating even more as they ran. We'd chase them and follow them, watching them until they disappeared, until we'd got rid of them from the area. Once they were gone, we'd go back to the camp to see if anybody had been affected. Mamu would sort of bite people and make them sick.

My grandfather would instruct me to work on someone who was ill. He would tell me that a mamu had bitten them and sucked out some of their blood. I'd go to see the person, who'd usually be hunched over, and extract the sickness that the mamu had given them. I'd bring back the object that I'd extracted to show him. I'd get the whole thing. I'd start by gently sucking out the sickness with my mouth. Then I'd carry the sickness away in my mouth and throw it away. I don't lose sight of what I dispose of from my mouth. I watch it closely until it disappears far off into the distance. I watch out for a puff of dust a long way off as it hits the ground.

Before I knew about these things I always used to think, 'How is it that ngangkari can extract these things from sick people? How do they do it? They can fix them up before they get seriously ill. All they have to do is touch them a bit and they get well really quickly!' I'd try to do it myself, by sucking with the mouth. When I was shown I could do it. I would be told, 'Here, give him a hand. He's really sick. A mamu has bitten him. He's going to remain sick until you heal him.' I'd do the treatment on the sick person with my mouth and my hands. I only use my mouth and my two hands. Grandfather always warned me, 'Go carefully. Carefully. Don't bruise them.' My big brother also taught me a lot. He'd say, 'Here, show me how you do it then. Come over here and show me.' He'd make me show him and he'd teach me what he knew.

I was only a child when I first started but soon I was treating men and women who were sick. They would ask me, 'Hey. Come here. What's the story? Can you tell us what's going on here?' I'd listen carefully. Something would be wrong. I'd say, 'Something is rattling around. Something is hanging around here. Crikey! Could it be a mamu? Watch out! The mamu will be biting people and eating their spirits up if we aren't careful! Quick grab your spears and come around quickly! Let's get him. Let's follow him and get him. You women, walk around very carefully, alright? Be careful while things are so dangerous for us. Watch out! Sit near the ngangkari to be safe! They'll be able to observe what's going on and let you know when it's safe to move around. We don't want any trouble!' We'd be very careful to look after all the extended family while dangers to our spiritual well-being were about. The ngangkari's job is to make sure everyone is safe. That is the work of ngangkari.

Ngangkari can capture negative energy inside the body and expel it, mostly by using the mouth, more often than using the hands. We can see clearly what is wrong with somebody. People

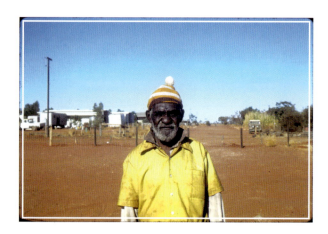

Dickie Minyintiri wearing a mukata (beanie) in Amata, South Australia, 1972.
PHOTOGRAPH NOEL WALLACE, NOEL AND PHYL WALLACE COLLECTION, ARA IRITITJA AI-0045916

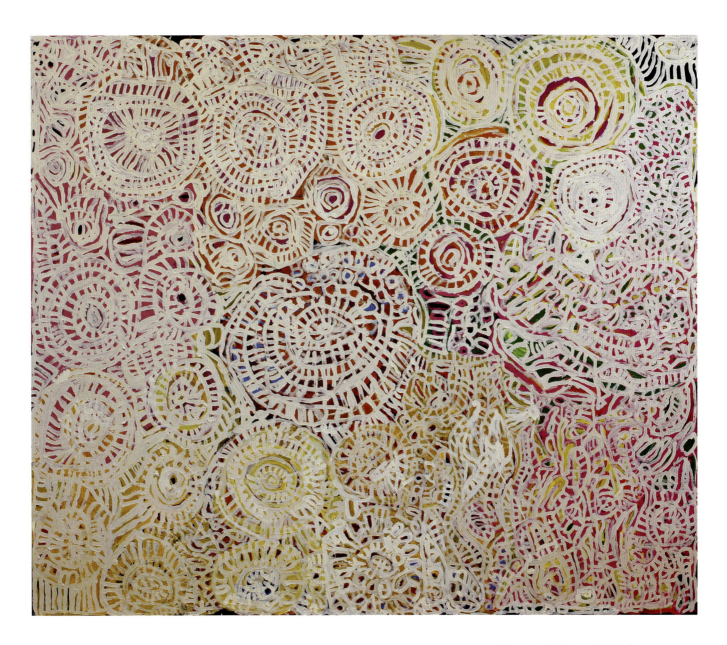

Dickie Minyintiri, *Wati Wiilu-ku Inma Tjukurpa*, 2011. Acrylic on canvas, 155 x 184 cm.
PHOTOGRAPH JULIAN GREEN, © THE ARTIST, COURTESY ERNABELLA ARTS

will complain about their eyes. They'll say, 'Oh, my eyes are dry and burning. Ouch!' We look at them for quite a long time, observing them. Then we'll look deeply into them until we find the object we are looking for. In these cases it is most often an object similar to a hot coal. 'So. Look at this. It's like a hot coal. This is why your eyes were burning up, see?' They'll say, 'Oh, right! So that's what's been scraping away at me, causing all that rough chafing and soreness.' If I extract a coal, or an ember, I'll get it out of my mouth, then show it to them so that they can see it. Then I will get rid of it. I'll destroy it.

I can throw some things away by using my miru – my spear thrower. A miru can help to throw things away much further. I'll throw away things like rocks and bits of bone. People's spirits suffer if we don't do this. Once we've got rid of things out of people's bodies they'll quickly feel much better. My grandfather told me, 'Be careful with the things you do. You've got to be careful because you can get sick yourself. Make sure you put it into your hand as soon as you extract it.' So I'd always hold onto these objects as soon as I got them, making sure they didn't do even more damage. It is to make sure that women and men live healthy lives.

I also go into the health clinic if people ask me. People will cry and cry if they are too sick. I don't really get paid money for any of this work. I am a bush ngangkari. I'm wati putjitja – a man of the bush. I work in the bush and I throw my spirit objects around in the bush. When I work as a ngangkari I get something from the people. I don't know anything about the health service. They don't call on me. They only employ health sisters and doctors in the clinic. They work inside the clinic buildings inside private rooms, so I can't say what they do. Their work is hidden. I talk to other doctors about how ngangkari work. I say, 'I work with my hands and my mouth. You work with a knife.' Doctors know I do this work. They know I help people to get better. Mostly, though, they don't know how I do it, because I work in the bush. They just know I do it, because I tell them. Most people don't understand this kind of work.

I sometimes get asked about my methods. I have to tell people that my work is dangerous. Ngangkari work with mamu. Mamu are dangerous, so you've got to be terribly careful. I don't want anybody saying bad things about the work that ngangkari do, because you can't underestimate our work. It is dangerous because of mamu. People do get sick. People get sick when it is windy too. I help them to get better by taking the sickness away from their body and throwing it away.

I am trying to tell as many of the young people about ngangkari work before I get too old. It is important that they know about bush doctors. I'd really like them to all know how important it is.

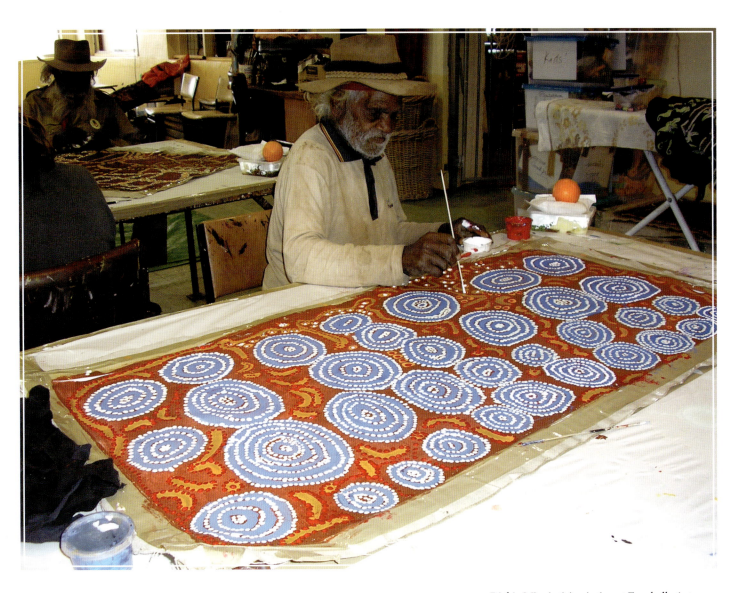

Dickie Minyintiri painting at Ernabella Arts, Pukatja (Ernabella), South Australia, 2005.
PHOTOGRAPH JOHN DALLWITZ, ARA IRITITJA AI-0051816

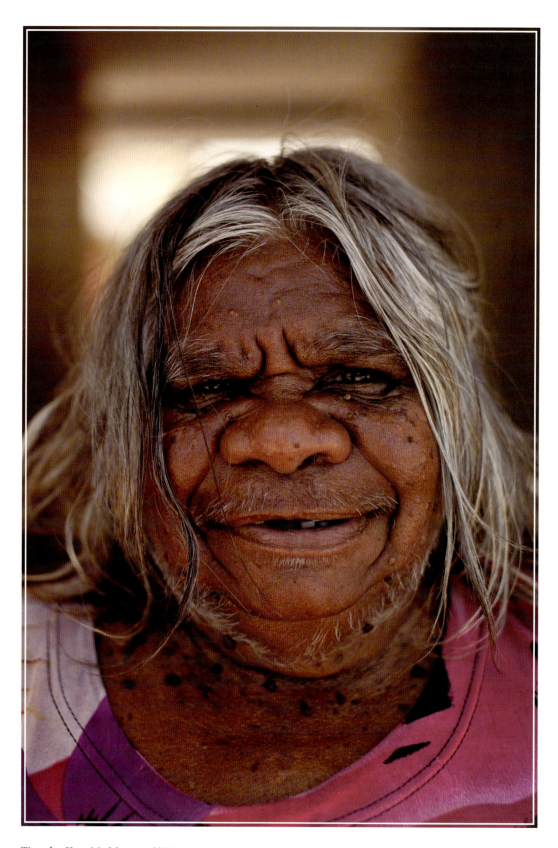

Tinpulya Kangitja Mervyn, 2011. PHOTOGRAPH RHETT HAMMERTON

# *Tinpulya Kangitja Mervyn*

When I was very little, I had no real idea of what a ngangkari does, but I used to watch the other ngangkari give healing treatments. I was always interested. I used to think, 'How does one actually do this? How can someone heal another?' While I was growing up I still wasn't fully aware that I had the power, but the strange thing was I used to have a certain power in the palms of my hands that enabled me to give healing to small children.

It wasn't until more recently, though, after we began to establish our community and we began building traditional shelters to make up the community, that I really started to question why the palms of my hands bother me so much. I used to think, 'Hey, what is it with my hands? They get so hot and sometimes they really bother me!' My palms were always getting hot and my arms would hurt sometimes.

In the end I talked to my sister, Nungalka, who is a ngangkari herself. So she gave me a healing treatment and felt my hands. Then she told me, 'Your hands are definitely hot. Oh, hang on! You are obviously a ngangkari too! That's what it is!' Evidently she must have felt my mapanpa in my hands and arms. She made me feel much better after she had given me the treatment. She then said, 'Alright then. Why don't you have a turn and try to heal this feverish child here?' But I told her, 'No. How can I? I don't know what to do.' But she told me to try and use my hands in the proper way. So I did try and the child cooled down.

Later on I went to Kaltjiti and Amata for a holiday and I found myself giving healing treatments to more sick children. This time it worked better. I found that if I went to the homes of the children and gave them a treatment, I could really help them. Doctor Kerry Gell once said to me, 'Why don't you see what you can do for these children, and afterwards I will take their temperature with a thermometer to see if their temperature has dropped.' So we did this and we found that after a ngangkari healing treatment, a child's body temperature drops to normal, in the case of a fever. Sometimes I will take a child back to its home to give it more treatments. Sometimes the child will have infant Panadol as well to help. We also found that if a child has got bad diarrhoea and is weakened, then a ngangkari healing treatment can help. A treatment can make things safer for the child, even at the point when the evacuation aircraft is ready and waiting to take the child to hospital.

As a ngangkari I focus mainly on sick children, healing them with my healing breath. I use the healing breath method to make them better, especially if they have problems with their stomach and digestion. I make them well again, and make sure they are balanced and happy, and have no fever. When I've finished with them I like to see them running off to play, better again.

Another thing I do is fix children if they've cut themselves or gashed their feet on a stake or a sharp piece of wood. I blow the healing breath on the cut and stem the flow of blood, and I heal up the wound with my breath. After that I might put a bandage on to help.

If someone's not paying proper attention while wielding a knife and cut themselves deeply, I can heal up the gash or cut by breathing my special breath on them and I will dab the cut with special saliva on my tongue and very quickly it will stop bleeding and close up. The cut closes up and seals together and heals.

If someone is weak and faint and feeling listless, I can make them feel perky again by blowing my special breath on their heads. That breath heals any problem they might have with their spirit. The same goes for headaches. I can take the pain right out of a headache in the same way. People get weak when they've got a headache or if they've got a fever and the breath will take away the pain and the fever very quickly and cool them down.

The breath works very well on painful joints. People in agonising pain in the joints or in the upper back will come to see me and tell me they're experiencing stabbing pain. Young women will come and see me for pain issues, as well as old people and young people.

Two of my grandsons were in a motorbike accident. One was evacuated in the Royal Flying Doctor plane. He was in a bad way and some of his bones ended up fused together, so he was in pain. I worked on him a lot, and loosened him up and took away the pain. His lower legs and feet were all swollen up and he couldn't walk at all. I saw him and worked hard on his tendons and strings and muscles, and I blew on his pain and really improved him to the point where he was able to walk again with a walking stick. So he's better now. His legs and knees are better and his back is flexible and working again. Two of my grandsons were in that accident and they are both better now.

I work on skin problems too, such as ringworm and skin eruptions. One mother brought her child to me to see. She was at her wit's end with the skin problems and asked me to help. I worked on the skin and I extracted all the eruptions and sores, took them away, and cleaned them up afterwards with the healing breath. I took out whatever germs were in there, extracted them and got rid of them and the child was better. The mother brought her child to me and showed me her child's skin to see, and it was perfect!

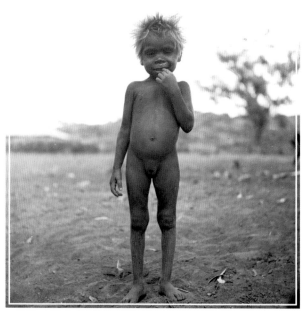

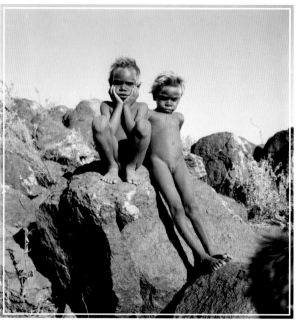

Above top: Tinpulya Kangitja Mervyn at Pukatja (Ernabella), South Australia, 1949.
PHOTOGRAPH RICHARD SEEGER, COURTESY MUSEUM VICTORIA (XP527)

Above bottom: Tinpulya Kangitja Mervyn (right) and Yipati Williams on rock, Pukatja (Ernabella), South Australia, 1951.
PHOTOGRAPH RICHARD SEEGER, COURTESY MUSEUM VICTORIA (XP 1127)

Opposite page, from left to right: Nungalka Stanley, Tinpulya Kangitja Mervyn and Malpiya Heffernan at Pukatja (Ernabella), South Australia, 1949. Nungalka, Tinpulya's sister, is also a ngangka_r_i.
PHOTOGRAPH RICHARD SEEGER, COURTESY MUSEUM VICTORIA (XP409)

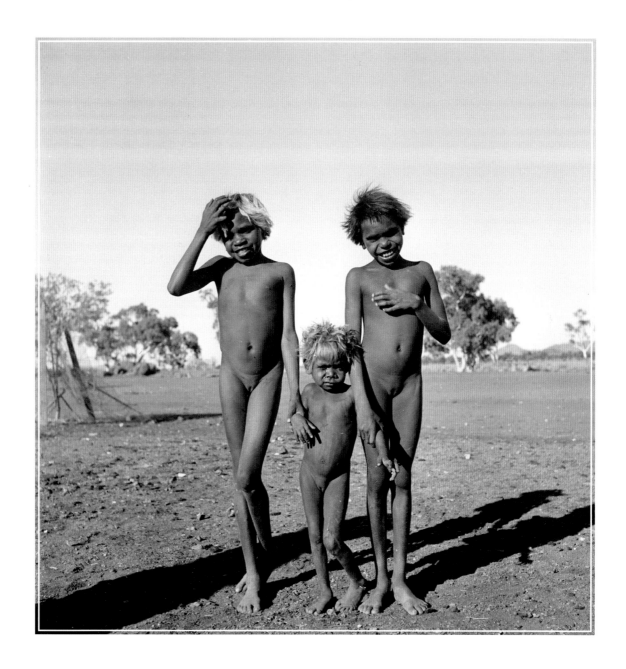

One woman from New Zealand brought her child to see me who had been lying in bed for five years. There was something terribly wrong with that child because she'd been bitten by a dangerous New Zealand spider. Though she was a white girl child, her skin was so bad that she looked black almost. I said, 'I'm not sure I can help here,' but I persisted and extracted the infection and blew a strong healing breath on her, and did the same again the next day, and, miraculously, the next day she was vastly improved. She got better and later, when she was visiting Kaltjiti to see one of her relatives, she showed me where the bite was, and it was almost gone. So that was success over a difficult case. Ngangkari can heal the bites from spiders and centipedes.

*Tinpulya Kangitja Mervyn*

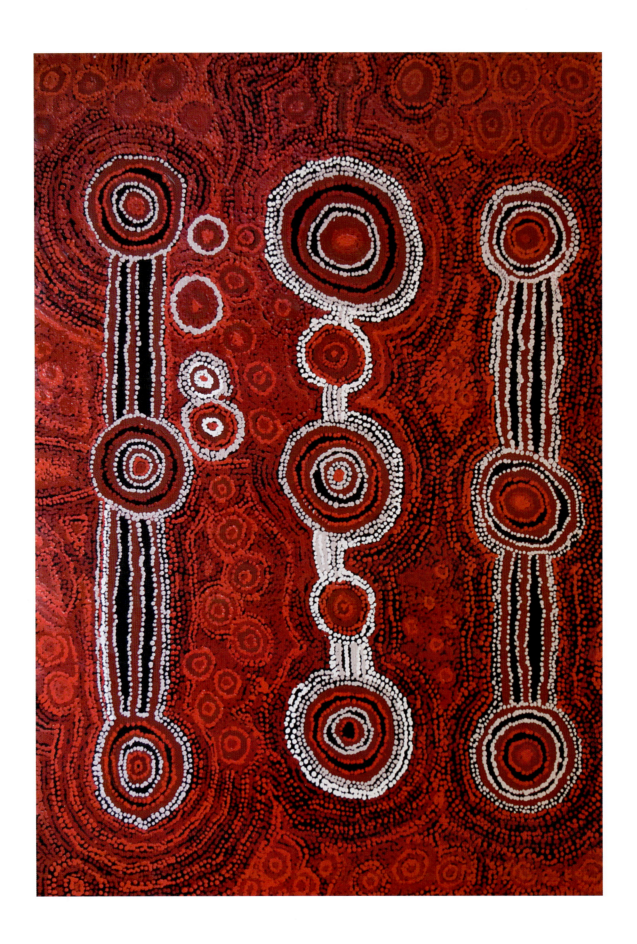

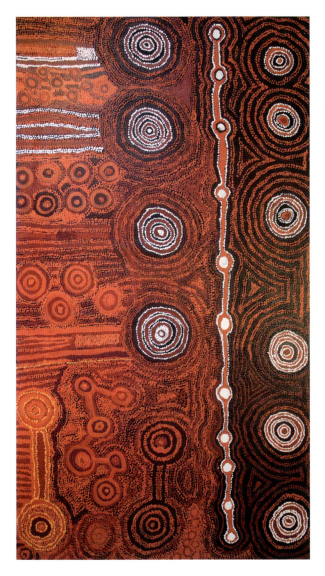

Above: *Panta*, Tinpulya Mervin, 2011. Acrylic on canvas, 111 x 200 cm. © THE ARTIST, COURTESY TJUNGU PALYA

*This is Watarru area. All the people travel from the main camping place along the travelling tracks to the smaller rockholes. They gather foods, bush foods, and stay for a while. For many generations our families have been doing this.*

Opposite page: *Panta* by Tinpulya Mervin, 2011. Acrylic on canvas 128 x 90 cm. © THE ARTIST, COURTESY TJUNGU PALYA

*This place is called Panta. There are large sand dunes here. All the children love to play in the sanddunes, while the mother and father go out for kuka. The women collect seeds of kunakanti, a type of grass, which are ground with water and baked into a cake. Tjiwa rungkani, grinding on a stone.*

Where I come from is Waru Tjukurpa, which means Fire Dreaming. Because of that Waru Tjukurpa I have certain healing powers. It is from there that I got my ngangkari powers to heal children. My healing powers take the form of special bones that look like bones in meat, but they are something different, that ngangkari from Watarru inherit and use. Some people are scared of ngangkari because of these things, but we are healers all the same. We healers hold these special tools within our bodies. We don't get them from other people. We get them from the special places that we live in. Sometimes we are not aware that these tools have entered our bodies until we feel the healing power stir within us, and then we realise we are ngangkari. After that we are able to heal. My sister has the same powers as me because she was born in the same Fire Tjukurpa place.

Ngangkari can heal many illnesses and problems, but not all. Some of the issues we cannot help with are problems associated with drug and alcohol abuse. Those physical and mental problems have to be treated by western medical methods and medication. There's nothing we can do with mental health problems associated with alcohol and drugs. Children born with Foetal Alcohol Syndrome are also unable to be treated by traditional ngangkari. They are modern problems that have to be treated by modern methods. Ngangkari have no problem helping with pain and fever and traditional problems.

Ngangkari can help people with sadness, loneliness and homesickness. Feelings like that can be eased and helped by ngangkari treatments too.

A long time ago, our people used to suffer a lot from wild cats that attacked people. We called those cats ngaya, and they used to be very dangerous. If they attacked someone, that person would die. Powerful ngangkari had to work on them very quickly with their most powerful mapanpa to get rid of the mamu that could kill people after these cat attacks. We would have to burn the country if there was a cat in it. These cats were very dangerous and have killed adult men and women, as well as children. They used to be around Pipalyatjara and Watarru back in the old days. There don't seem to be any around these days, thank goodness! But they are at their most dangerous when there is a drought. We've had good seasons lately, but if another drought comes then we expect those animals to get fierce and dangerous again. Of course, we are monitoring them with our Indigenous Protected Areas work, which is good. Watarru is our mother's country.

Our mother and father went over to Ernabella to become shepherds, and so I was born near Kunma Piti. That's how I came to be going to Ernabella School and learnt how to read and write in Pitjantjatjara. We used to read the Pitjantjatjara bible and sing hymns. It was good, and we can all read and write in Pitjantjatjara, whereas the younger people of today don't know how to.

In recent years people moved back from Ernabella to Kaltjiti, and then they moved back to Watarru. These changes happened around the same times as changes of government. Now we are living back on our own traditional country and quite a few of us are working for Land Management, cleaning out rockholes, monitoring rare and endangered species such as brush-tailed possums and black-footed rock wallabies, mallee fowls and great desert skinks and marsupial moles.

We are cleaning out the same rockholes that our strong and healthy grandfathers and grandmothers would clean out and drink from. We are caring for the land that they cared for and which gave them fruits and seeds and berries with which to raise strong and healthy children. I was raised differently to those early-days children, because I was raised in a modern way. But my healing is as strong and as ancient as the old ways, because the healing doesn't change. It is still as strong as the strong, old days and the strong, old ways.

There are many new young ngangkari coming up. I am passing my ngangkari knowledge on to two of my granddaughters, Loretta and Rosemary, who have been given their healing tools by Langkatjukur. They are confident and sure of their skills and they will be strong ngangkari when they are older. Nowadays I am working on behalf of the NPY Women's Council, doing healing treatments as part of their ngangkari program. I hope that the ngangkari healers of the future have the same sorts of opportunities as I have.

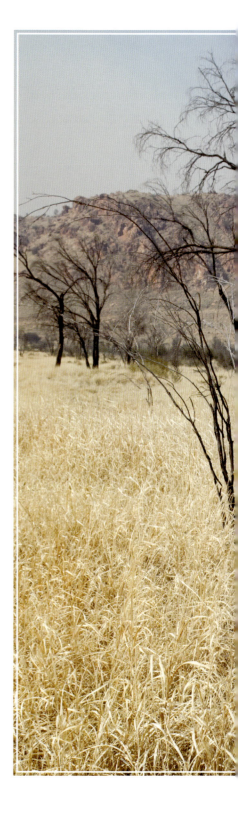

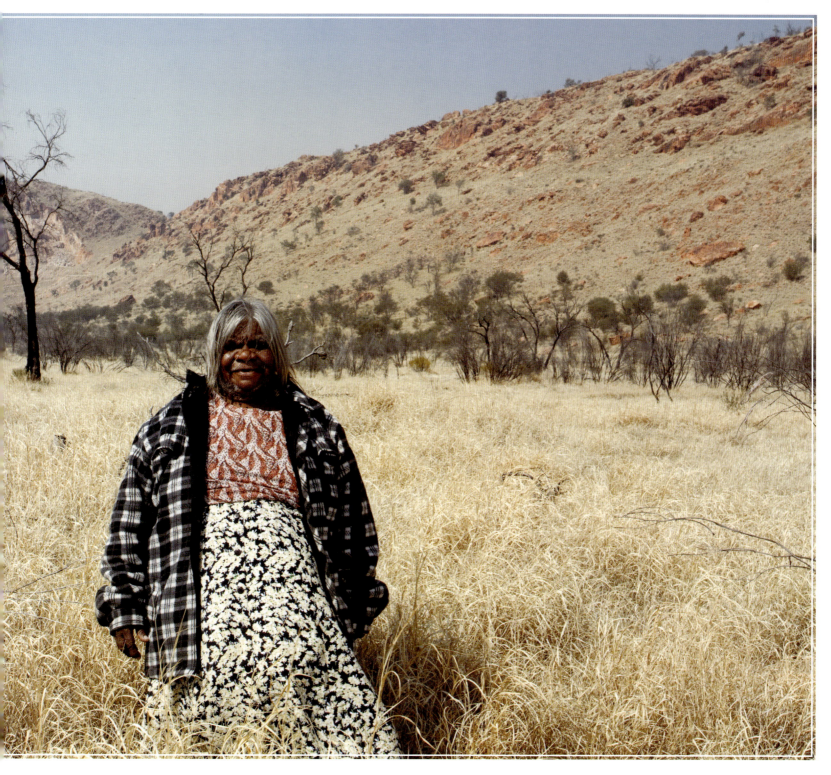

Tinpulya Kangitja Mervyn, 2011.
PHOTOGRAPH RHETT HAMMERTON

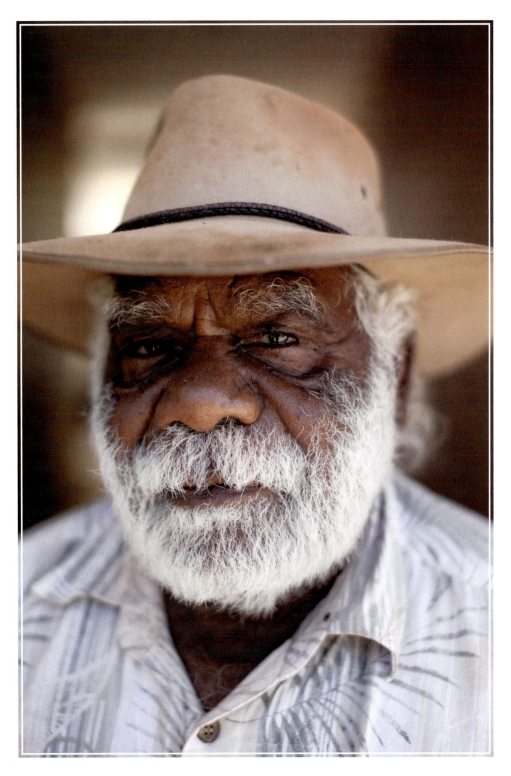

Bernard Tjalkuriny, 2011. PHOTOGRAPH RHETT HAMMERTON

# Bernard Tjalkuriny

I was born near Waltja, near Kunamata. Not far, but in the bush, you understand. Waltja is a kapi piti – a big waterhole deep into the ground, by the name of Waltja. It is close to Kunamata, just to the south of it. It is a waterhole in the ground and I look after that waterhole. We travel down from Nyapari and go that way in to Waltja waterhole. We look around and make sure everything is doing well around the area, and then we go back home again.

My mother's country is Watarru. My mother is a Watarru woman, but she lived in the Kunamata area. My father ordered her to leave Kunamata when she was expecting me, telling her, 'You are a southern woman. Walk back towards the south to have your baby. You can't give birth around here'. So my mother left and walked in a southerly direction to Waltja. Not only my father, but all the men were saying this. So she obeyed, headed off south and so that is how I was born at Waltja. She walked away from Kunamata and she went south because she was told to.

My mother's father was from Watarru. He was an emu man from Kalaya Piti. My mother's father was born at Kalaya Piti. My father's side is elsewhere, at Aparatjara, near Amata, near Nyapari. Not far from Nyapari.

I was born in the bush, as I said, but I grew up in my early years around Watarru and Malara. I lived around Malara a lot. Malara is near Kalka, and that is where I lived and grew up. I also spent a lot of time out in the west. That is when a lot of outside people arrived for the first time, with camels. They were whitefellas, arriving with their camels. None of us had ever seen a camel and we were all amazed to see them. We saw them that time not far from Malara. We saw this strange animal and we didn't know what it was. We called it an auru. Emus stare intently at things and that is what we did too!

We also noted these strange people with white skins arriving and walking around. They had really white skins compared to our dark skins. We were frightened of them. We touched them to see if they were real. The men and the very old men were much more confident and they went up very close to these people, very bravely. My father was among them. They acted like children and they played with us children.

Another mob arrived at Kirpiny, which is a sacred place. They went into our sacred place, those whitefellas. My father followed them to see what they would do. Fortunately they left. My father followed them all the way to Ernabella Mission because they'd told him about the food that was available there. The whitefellas were wandering at will around our country. They did not ask permission or request to go anywhere. They just went where they liked and departed and went to another place, depending upon their whim, with their camels. The men returned with the whitefellas to Ernabella Mission. Only the men went. The white people had made themselves understood enough for the men to realise that they were saying that there was a lot of food available at Ernabella. I went along as well because I was a big boy. My older brother, Ingkatji, and I both went. He was a big boy and so was I; Ingkatji was born before I was, so he's a bit older than me, but we played together.

We arrived at Ernabella and we stayed on. Reverend Love said, 'Do you want to go out hunting for dingo scalps?' White people wanted us to get dingo scalps, dingo skin. Reverend Love was a white man who lived there, he was a missionary. Mr Young was there. Mr Young was a well-digger and he organised for quite a number of wells to be dug. After that, another man arrived to take care of all of us children; whose name was Ron Trudinger. He kept us children after that.

Large groups of us would go hunting dingo scalps. Everyone went, and I went as well. We all went together, walking around the country hunting dingo scalps. A large group of us went south towards Fregon and we got many from there. Another large group of people went east towards Kenmore and got dingoes from there. Others got them from closer to Ernabella and another group went to Makiri. So we got our dingo skins from many, many places. We walked, everyone walked in those days. We all walked together in a large group. Mother and father and all of us, everyone. There were a lot of people, with a lot of senior men. We took blankets with us, bundled up on our heads.

When Ron Trudinger arrived he told us, 'Right, first of all you children must all go on holiday. When you come back from holiday you must start school'. Holiday time for us was when it was cool, not too hot, still cool but warm enough for us to need wiltja for the shade. We'd leave for holidays then, in order to be away for when the dingo pups were big enough. We'd go when there was the maximum number of dingoes around. We'd be told, 'Now you all need to leave and go hunting dingoes'. This is the time when the dingo pups are starting to come out. Just like this time of year. We'd get so many dingoes then. I went away, for

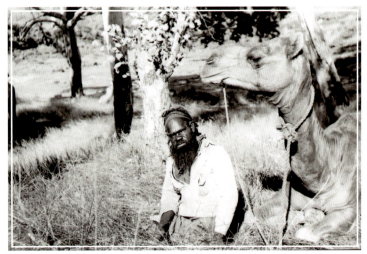

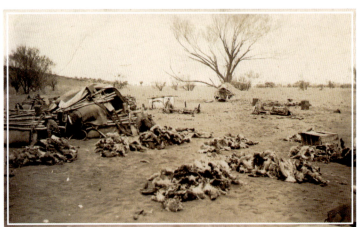

Top: Andy Tjilari's uncle, Jimmy Yaka, who was 'kamuḻaku ninti' (experienced with and knowledgeable about camels), Aparina, 1934.
HH FINLAYSON COLLECTION, AṞA IRITITJA AI-0057671

*None of us had ever seen a camel and we were all amazed to see them. We saw them that time not far from Malaṟa. We saw this strange animal and we didn't know what it was. We called it an auru.*

Bottom: Piles of dingo scalps at a dogger's camp, Musgrave Ranges, South Australia, 1927–31.
PHOTOGRAPH ALAN BRUMBY, RAMON BROWN COLLECTION, AṞA IRITITJA AI-0035182

Opposite page: Bernard Tjalkuriny, *Kaḻaya Tjukurpa*, 2011. Acrylic on linen, 120 x 200 cm. PHOTOGRAPH AMANDA DENT, ©THE ARTIST, COURTESY TJUNGU PALYA

*All the emus from the creation time were travelling from Kanpi heading south. They came to a stop and half decided to travel west while the others continued on to Wataṟṟu. They were running, the emus. Tjuṯa mulapa (really many many emus). On the western side they stopped at the line of deep rockholes. They created this country. Tjukurpa mulapa, Tjukurpa puḻkanya (this is Law strong and true!).*

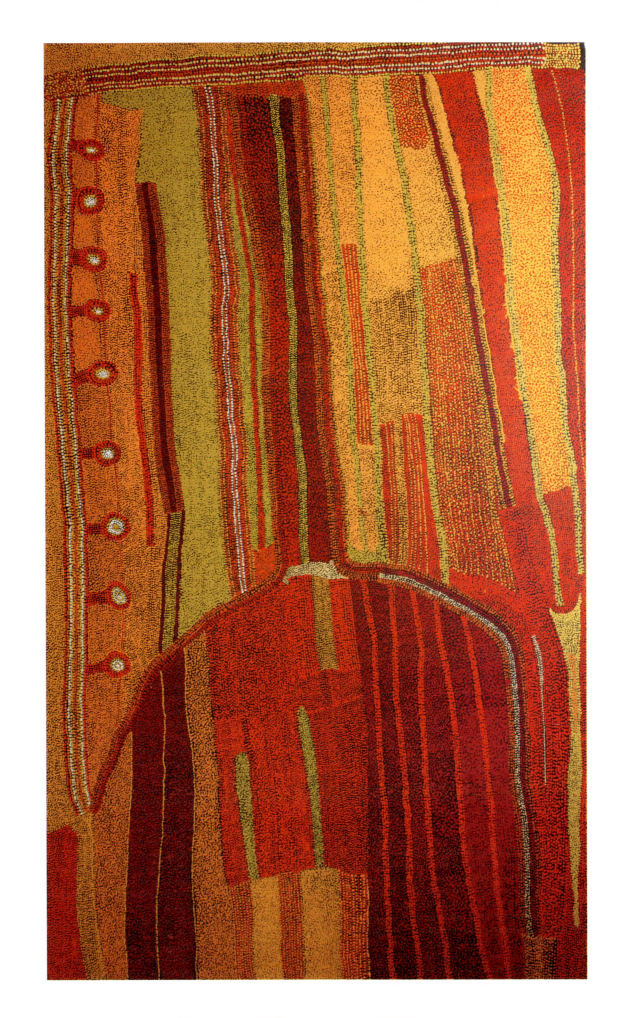

a big holiday, and we were living at Anpin, which is not far from Aliwanyuwanyu, a large and important waterhole.

My first experience of the ngangkari world was when I saw something very unusual. Even though my eyes were shut, I saw something out of the ordinary. My cousins, Ingkatji and Tjilari, were there. 'What was that?' Ingkatji and I had to have a good look. It was some sort of opening. We figured out it was where a mamu had entered the ground. There were hordes of mamu about in that country then. My father had a surprise: 'See how observant these two children are! They saw a mamu!' And we had indeed seen a mamu. We warned everyone and we blocked up the entrance hole. We told everyone, 'Watch out! A mamu is inside that hole'. The three of us saw it at the same time, but I saw it first.

Our ngangkari talent was born at that moment. From that moment on we went into proper ngangkari training. That's the moment when I became a ngangkari. I am now a senior ngangkari. I had seen the mamu and warned everyone. My father knew it was true and he backed me up. After it was under the ground we never saw it again. Ingkatji had seen it. We stomped on it and compressed it down. We blocked up any chance for it to escape, and made sure it stayed down inside. Mamu can still move around underground so I am sure it eventually burrowed its way out elsewhere. The mamu left the vicinity. Mamu go into the trunks of trees. After I had seen that mamu, Tjilari stamped on it and squashed it down completely. Tjilari became a ngangkari too.

Connelly was a very clever ngangkari. My older brother was there when Ingkatji stomped on it. By midday we were seeing dozens of new mamu. The senior men had to get rid of lots of them, they were put inside or buried on a regular basis. I saw them before I was awake, when I was lying down with my eyes shut, and I saw the mamu with my special other vision – then I opened my eyes and saw it with my ordinary eyes. Children have good, clear vision. This happened at Anpin, then after that we went elsewhere.

Putting a mamu into the forehead makes one a ngangkari. It gives the ngangkari powers. That's what we do. We were only children, we were just starting out and we had a lot to learn. The senior

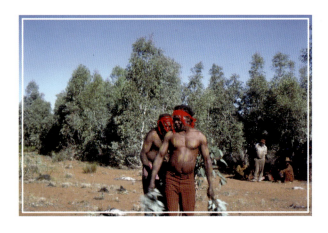

Above: Bernard Tjalkuriny (front) with Ray Ken performing inma during the Edwards' farewell, Amata, South Australia, 1980.
PHOTOGRAPH BILL EDWARDS, BILL EDWARDS COLLECTION, ARA IRITITJA AI-0014571

Opposite page: Bernard Tjalkuriny, *Kaliwani*, 2011. Acrylic on linen, 200 x 120 cm.
PHOTOGRAPH AMANDA DENT, © THE ARTIST, COURTESY TJUNGU PALYA

*This country is this side of Watarru (north). The boomerang went all around and came back. The hunter picked up the boomerang and got going, travelling along and leaving a track behind him. This is a special place from the Tjukurpa, the creation time, a place called Kaliwani.*

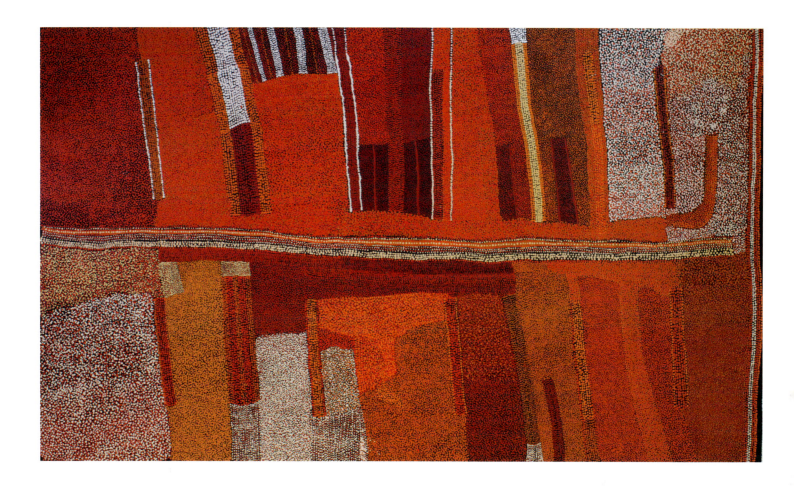

men had told us that's what they did, so we already knew it was the done thing. Ingkatji and I already knew how to do it, in theory.

I had no idea that this would happen. I had no idea! That old man selected me to have the mamu put into my forehead! He said to me, 'Come here, child!' I went over to him. He immediately inserted it into me, making a hole, while I was going, 'No, no, no, don't, don't, don't!' I was a big boy then – but he still shoved that mamu bone right into me! That mamu bone went into me and became my mapanpa. That old man put that bone into me, in the sight of all the other men, and the men commented on how it wriggled when it entered me. I was only a boy. The bone went in and wriggled around. The men saw it and everyone knows what happened to me. That bone became an important mapanpa for me.

That mamu left completely because all the other ngangkari chased it away and it just disappeared in fear of them. We two saw the mamu, we two children. We could see things like that now we were ngangkari, and we had become quite fierce. We pushed them into the ground and murdered them. We made sure mamu couldn't get back up out again. We'd block them in and they'd never resurface. This happened all around that same area. Later on I became a man in my own right and an experienced ngangkari. Other new ngangkari were starting work also, new women ngangkari and new men ngangkari and child ngangkari.

So I gave treatments to anybody: men, women and children. I was still young but I gave everybody treatments. There were no other options. We didn't have a modern medical service like we do today, back then it was just us ngangkari handling all the medical situations. We were the only healers, children healers and all.

I saw camels long before we went to Ernabella, but the previous senior ngangkari were still operating then, and they were really busy with mamu and wild cat mamu. We children had already seen camel mamu before, and we started to see them a lot more often after that. We saw white people travelling through our country. They were giving the old men food.

After I became a nyiinka I kept the same mapanpa. I was still learning. Ingkatji was learning faster than me, I was coming along behind him. I was still blocking mamu holes up though, stomping on them with my feet. But I didn't understand everything. Then my older brother died, he took some stories with him.

I saw mamu. Only ngangkari can see mamu. The old wati tjilpi ngangkari – senior elder male ngangkari – can see them really clearly. I see them when they are close. The ngangkari see mamu and grab them and take them far away from people. We put them into holes and fill them in and block them in and tell them to go away. We don't want them to come out and bother people.

There are other mamu that live in the bark of trees. Another one looks like an emu and he is called Karpirinypa. He looks just like an emu. He even has feathers like an emu – wipiya feathers. He's still a mamu. Mamu Karpirinypa is his name. There is another mamu that lives inside the ground. There are many, many Mamu Karpirinypa – too many! Like a great flock of emu. But of course we ngangkari are numerous also. The men hit mamu and knock them over. I did not see a Karpirinypa Mamu when I was a child but I could still easily hit mamu and kill them.

That Mamu Karpirinypa is a giver of special things though. Kanti and kuuti and the like. He gives them as gifts. Bones and special things. That Mamu Karpirinypa gives children and ngangkari gifts. He gives feathers and so on. Mamu Karpirinypa gives gifts to ngangkari. He looks just like an emu. I have personally been given dozens of special things by Mamu Karpirinypa. The things he gives me I do not put in my pocket but I store inside my hands. My older brother, Mr Miller's grandfather, also had a lot of things and he gave a lot to me. He was full up of them! We keep what we are given by Karpirinypa, we keep them inside our kurunpa.

Karpirinypa gives the mapanpa so we can keep our children in strong, good health. We look after our children well despite the dangers from these powerful mamu. There are so many dangers but there are so many ways to look after them. We are powerful healers. We give our children healing to make them strong to withstand these external forces.

The reason a mamu gives ngangkari things is because he is scared of people and wants to keep them on his side. Senior men are very fierce and can easily frighten him, so he gives them gifts. He gives gifts to ngangkari and his gifts make ngangkari strong. We keep them and use them. We see him coming when we are asleep, when we go on our marali journeys. On those journeys we take the children along with us. Ngangkari travel all through the middle of night. We hear the mamu going, 'Oh, Oh, Oh!' He is dangerous and will kill little children if they are sick. Children hear that noise and they cry in fear. We rush to their aid. Women do also. And men. That mamu is travelling towards that child underneath the ground. It will be sent off by the ngangkari. The ngangkari take their children away for safety straight away.

The eastern people are very experienced in this. They will take the child over to the east. The men capture that mamu under the ground and bury him and leave him there. That particular kind of mamu is very nasty and dangerous. The ngangkari job is to settle him down, to make sure he doesn't hurt our little children.

When I was still a child I lost my ngangkari powers. My old grandfather died. My forehead had closed up. It was closed up. The body of my grandfather was lying in the ground and I was given something from him. But my forehead remained closed up. This man here, Andy Tjilari, re-opened it again, but unfortunately I hadn't had it re-opened for so long and I hadn't worked for a long time or said anything and I hadn't worked much as a ngangkari.

I was a child still. There were still lots of dangerous mamu around. Rupert knew me then. He would be saying, 'Look out! Look out! There's a mamu around!' He was always working. He taught me a lot and he got my confidence back up again. From then on things improved for me as a ngangkari.

As a child I lost my ngangkari powers from lack of use, but when old Mr Miller's grandfather died, everything in me that was closed up was re-opened. I had treatments to make me clear. I was given the blowing breath. Everything became clear. My ears were open. My hands were blown upon and they became active again. My head was blown upon and my intellect sprang into life.

I was able to do the same treatments to children and I would work on children, using the blowing breath. Children have been given the blowing breath treatment by me and they all benefit. I have treated men and women and children ever since. We ngangkari bring with us over the course of our lives many varied treatment styles. We have songs to gain more mapanpa. We sing those songs, which are important to us. We are always finetuning our methods. This is the work of a ngangkari. We sing a song about getting more mapanpa. We watch out for the health of children. Make sure their feet and eyes are good. A treatment is very simple really. The healing breath is the main treatment, and it is very effective.

We always use the blowing breath, and it works very well on children. We blow onto women's abdomens, and on their heads. But men ngangkari do not touch women on the abdomen, though we do use the blowing breath treatment on their abdomens. We don't risk touching women below the abdomen in our culture. Though the women sometimes say, 'Please work on my stomach area. My digestion is not good. Please just straighten me out again'. We may do that but we men do not touch a woman's lower abdomen. We are too nervous to do that. We are always warned by the senior men to never work below a woman's abdomen. I certainly never do. We have to be really careful about what we do. We have standards and there are also deep cultural reasons why we can't, it is ngangkari business.

We never lose the Mapanpa Inma. That song is about getting mapanpa back. We remember that song and always keep it in our minds. Some of our songs are sacred. Many of our inma are extremely sacred and secret.

We have told Tjukurpa wirunya, a good story. There are so many stories. We have been painting some of our stories. I have been painting a story about emus walking to Watarru. I've also painted a picture of children dancing at a place called Waru Piti. It is a children's song. Ngangkari are good painters because we have such amazing stories so our imaginations are very alive. We know many wonderful things.

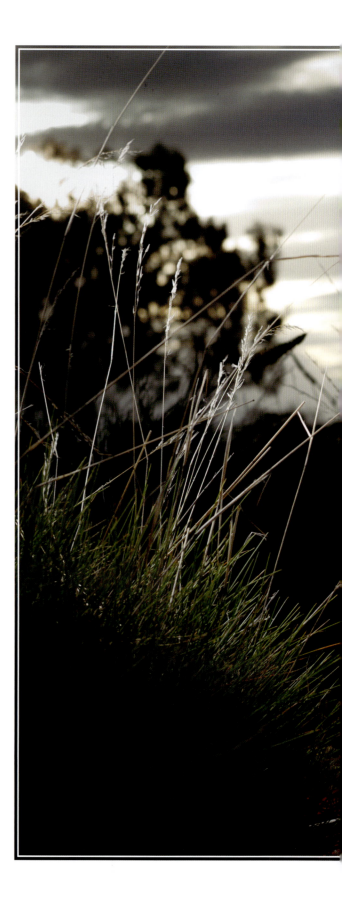

Opposite page: Bernard Tjalkuriny, Yulara, Northern Territory, 2010.
PHOTOGRAPH STEPHEN OXENBURY

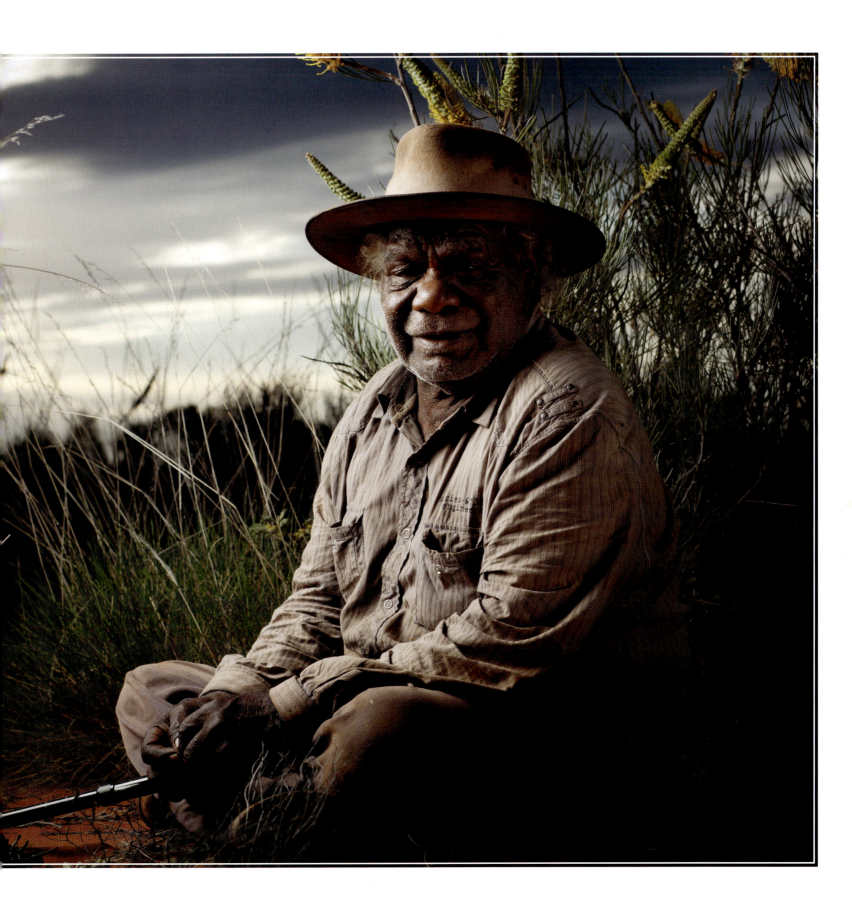

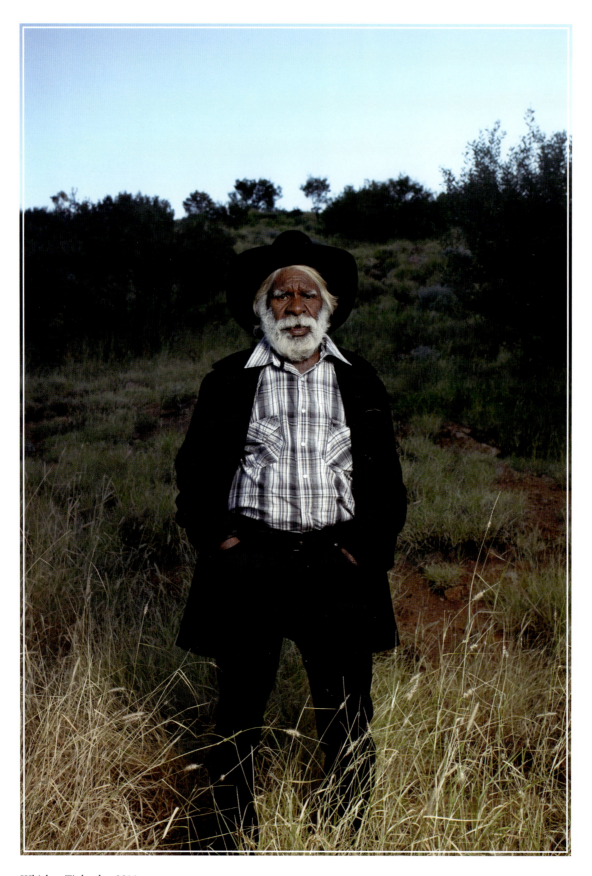

Whiskey Tjukanku, 2011. PHOTOGRAPH RHETT HAMMERTON

# Whiskey Tjuka*n*ku

When I was little, my own grandfather gave me the power of working as a ngangkari. I was still a child, mind you! Yet from that early age, I was able to heal men and women and I healed problems experienced by young women as well. This was in the early days when we were still living in the bush.

People come to my home to see me because they know I am a ngangkari. When people come to see me they ask me for a treatment. We don't talk about money. We just get down to work straight away. Money doesn't come into it really. This is because I believe in the importance of healing, and I love it. It is my skill and I am proud of it and I want to help people.

Well, we were still walking around that area then, all those years ago, we were walking around the Maralinga area. We didn't know anything about that poison, that contamination, then. I was travelling around in my marali – spirit body – quite often at the time.

I gained more skills when I was travelling around in my spirit body because when ngangkari do that, they get to see and hear sick people calling out for help. People, children and adults, ask for help in their dreams. Their spirit calls out for help, and our spirit bodies hear them and go to them.

My mother helped me greatly to do my work when I was a junior ngangkari. I started my life as a child ngangkari, healing people, and now, as an old man, I am still healing people. So I have come full circle.

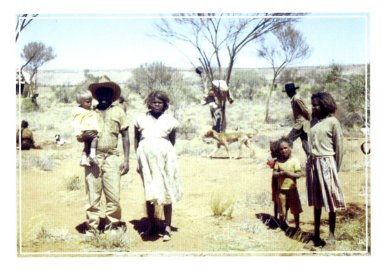

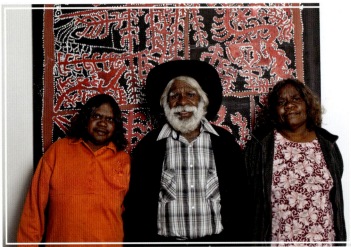

Top: Whiskey Tjuka<u>n</u>ku with his family on camp. From left (foreground only) Whiskey Tjuka<u>n</u>ku holding Mona Whiskey (his daughter), Emily Nyuniwa Whiskey (his wife) and to the right Frankie Wangka (Whiskey's nephew) and Puna Mary (his niece, Frankie's sister), Indulkana, South Australia, 1966. PHOTOGRAPH DON BUSBRIDGE / BETTY CULHANE, A<u>R</u>A IRITITJA AI-0022680

Bottom: Whiskey Tjuka<u>n</u>ku with daughters Lippsie Whiskey and Mona Whiskey at his solo exhibition, RAFT Artspace, Alice Springs, April 2011. PHOTOGRAPH RHETT HAMMERTON

Opposite page: Whiskey Tjuka<u>n</u>ku, *Arrernte Country*, 2011. Acrylic on canvas, 153 x 153 cm. PHOTOGRAPH HELEN JOHNSON, © THE ARTIST, COURTESY IWANTJA ARTS AND CRAFTS

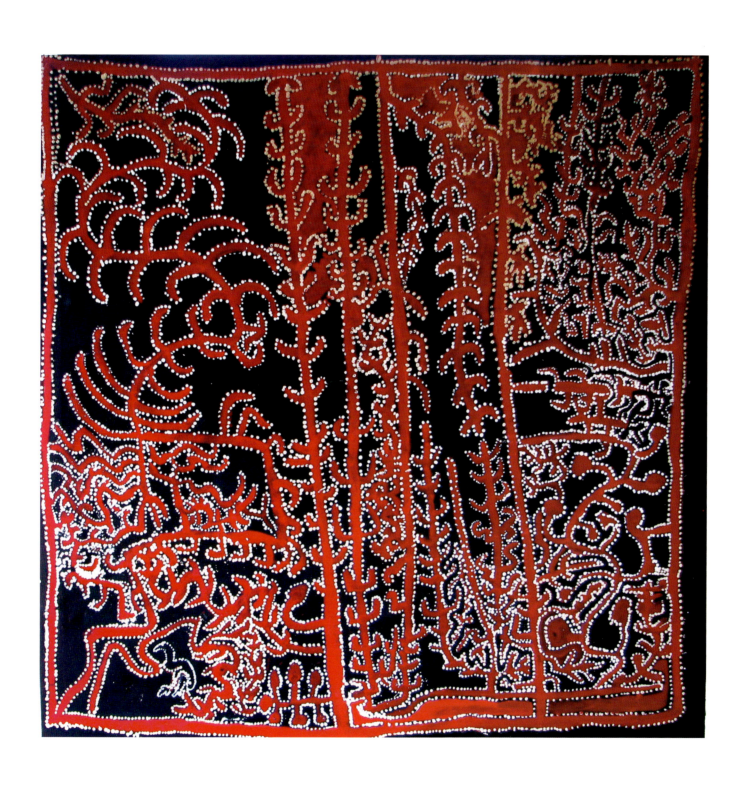

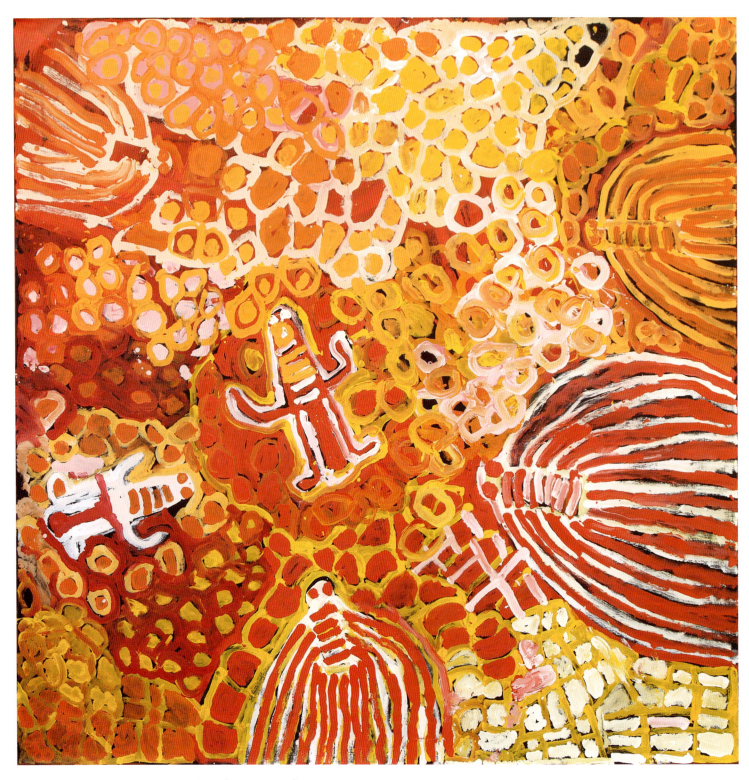

Harry Tjutjuna, *Wati Nyiru munu Wati Wanka*, 2011. Acrylic on linen, 183 x 183 cm. PHOTOGRAPH PAUL EXLINE, © THE ARTIST AND NINUKU ARTS

# Harry Tjutjuna

I am a ngangkari and I am just going to say a few words.

Sometimes we ngangkari hear of bad things going on in our society. Swearing and fighting by our people is not approved of. We older men and women do not like it. It is very bad. We older people remember the more peaceful, healthier times of the past. People were happier in the past. People felt happier in the past. They felt happier in their bodies, in their stomachs. But today, we see so many Anangu who are not happy. Their gut feeling is not happy. The feeling people have in their gut plays a big part in their lives.

We are sad that so many babies are born in hospitals today, who come home to start their lives, but who never get smoked like they used to be. Smoking babies is strong Law and I'm sad to see that the practice seems to be dying out. The old strong women's Law with child rearing practices seems to be getting weaker now. It is a shame for the new younger generations being born not to get the benefit of our old healthy ways. Babies used to be born without any medicines. Of course, I can't talk any more about this because it is women's Law. With our traditional health practices, the women have one road to follow, and the men have another.

Sometimes I hear of young girls saying things they shouldn't. Girls shouldn't talk like that. It is not right for young girls to swear or utter sacred words. I can't tell you what those words are, because obviously I can't say them out aloud. We must never utter sacred words, as it is dangerous. Sacred words and sacred ways must remain secret to us.

We men have sacred and secret stories, traditions and words. Women must never say secret sacred words, which belong to men.

Women have their own culture, which is secret and sacred to them. If young women wrongfully get hold of sacred information they might easily pass it on, especially if they are intoxicated. This is wrong and very dangerous. The uttered word can be dangerous. Many words should either be spoken very carefully, or not uttered at all. Wrong knowledge or inappropriate knowledge is very bad for the spirit of the person who may have heard it. Do you understand me?

Young children should never be exposed to bad language or information not intended for young people. Children should only ever hear playful language. Children should only be playing and having fun, such as splashing in water – I'm not referring to deep rivers, but just in little pools or rockholes that children can play in safely.

We should remember that our old culture is very respectful and also safe for children to grow up in. We need to remember the old Laws of life, and to live by them. If we do, we will have a better life.

We Anangu love each other very much. We like our people to be healthy and happy.

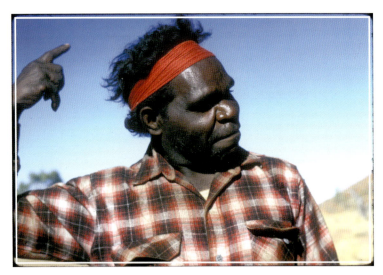

Left: Harry Tjutjuna, demonstrating the hand sign for 'wati' (man) in 1972.
PHOTOGRAPH NOEL WALLACE, NOEL AND PHYL WALLACE COLLECTION, ARA IRITITJA AI-0046176

Below left: Harry Tjutjuna, work in progress.
PHOTOGRAPH CLAIRE ELTRINGHAM, COURTESY NINUKU ARTS

Below: Harry Tjutjuna at the Arts Centre, Pukatja (Ernabella), South Australia, 2006.
PHOTOGRAPH BETH SOMETIMES, SOMETIMES AND FREEDMAN COLLECTION, ARA IRITITJA AI-0061837

Opposite page: Harry Tjutjuna, *Kungka Tjuta*, 2011. Acrylic on linen, 167 x 183 cm.
PHOTOGRAPH PAUL EXLINE © THE ARTIST AND NINUKU ARTS

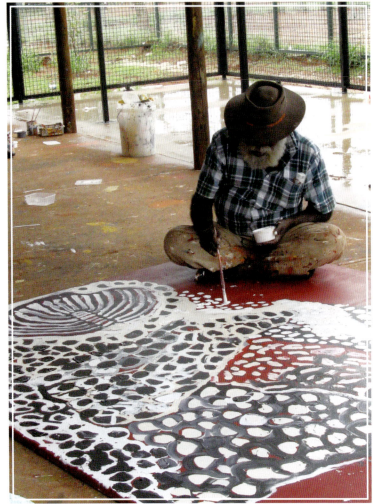

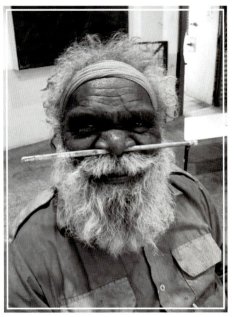

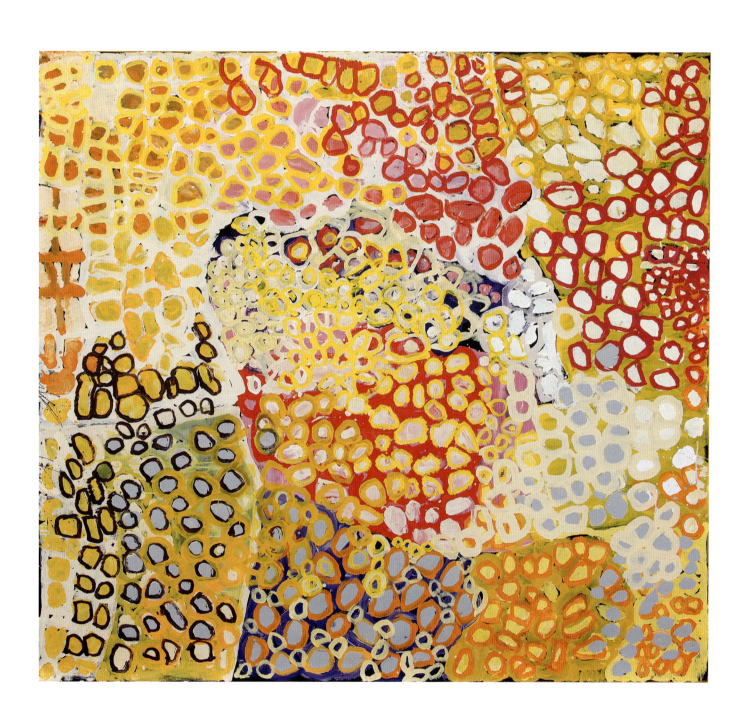

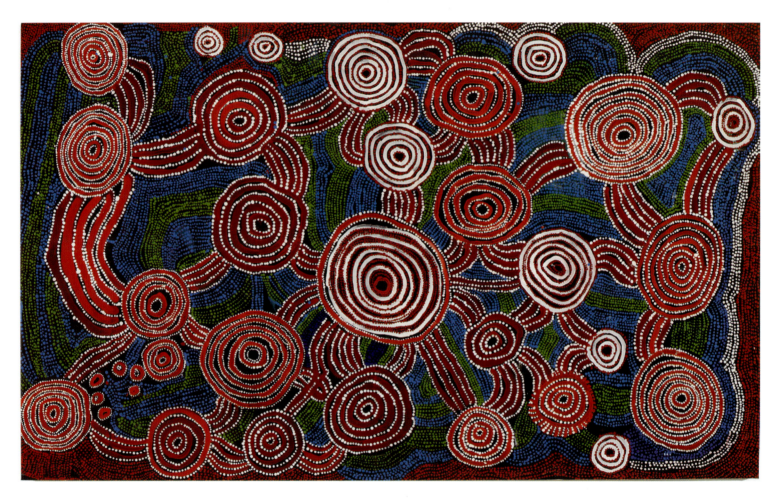

Nyakul (Nakul) Dawson (*c.* 1935–2007), *Irrana*, 2002. Synthetic polymer paint on canvas, 120.2 x 201.5 cm.
Gift of Dr Milton Roxannas 2011, donated through the Australian Government's Cultural Gifts Program.

PHOTOGRAPH CHRISTOPHER SNEE, COURTESY ART GALLERY OF NEW SOUTH WALES [302.2011]

# Nakul Dawson

My name is Nakul. I was given this name a long time ago when I was a baby.

I was taught to be a ngangkari when I was just a little child by my grandfather. I trained at being a ngangkari by giving people practice ngangkari healing treatments. In this way I got a lot of practice, because, after all, I was a tjitji ngangkari – a child ngangkari. Since childhood I have learnt how to give full and proper treatments, and I have been working as a ngangkari ever since.

Once I had grown up, I saw white people moving into this area, and I watched them establish health clinics. I started going to these clinics and working in them from time to time. I have been shown many things by white people and I, in my turn, have taught them many things. White clinic staff come up to me from time to time and ask me, 'Please come up and see someone in the clinic.' I go up there and I check someone out. All they want is to be healed and then declared to be well. So I give them a ngangkari healing treatment. I have even given a healing treatment to walypala, white men, and to walupara, white women.

I have heard some wrong stories about me, for instance, 'Oh, I have only just heard about you. So are you new to this then? So you weren't around before?' But it isn't true. I have been a ngangkari all my life and I'm an old man now! That walupara made me quite upset, considering I have been healing people all my life, white people included! I am still working and I will keep on working despite how I feel at times.

I sometimes tell doctors to go slow when they say some Anangu should have an operation where they can expect to be sliced open and have their blood pouring out. That should never happen. Anangu should never have their abdomens cut open like that. It's not good. We are Anangu. We should not have that kind of thing happen to our bodies. Despite what is said, we do not believe that it is clean or safe. That's all I am saying on the subject for now. I can't change my mind, because I have lived all my life working hard, healing hundreds of people, and banishing their illnesses in the ngangkari way. I heal sick people: children, children with upset stomachs, sick women and sick men. I specialise in problems with the head. If a woman with a bad head problem needs help, I can heal her. It is one of my specialities. I heal them in the clinic too, inside that very clinic just over there.

I don't know how to take a person's temperature with a thermometer. I only know about mapanpa or special sacred tools. Mapanpa can look like small pieces of bone. They are kept in water or inside the hand. They are kept inside the hand and help to locate punu, or little pieces of wood, that get lodged in people's bodies. I find these pieces of punu in people's bodies, drifting in the blood flowing along the inside of their veins. I feel them floating inside and I can grab them and extract them from the vein. Once I have got them out I take a good look at them, in order to identify them. I sometimes get a surprise with what comes out.

I can usually determine if a person has been sick for a long time or only a short time. I can tell if they have something rotten inside of them. I look at the object closely and I blow on it – this is called puulpai. I blow on it from above. This can sometimes neutralise the sickness. My spirit gets a strong feeling about what to do. Next, I usually have to grab it and throw it back to where it came from.

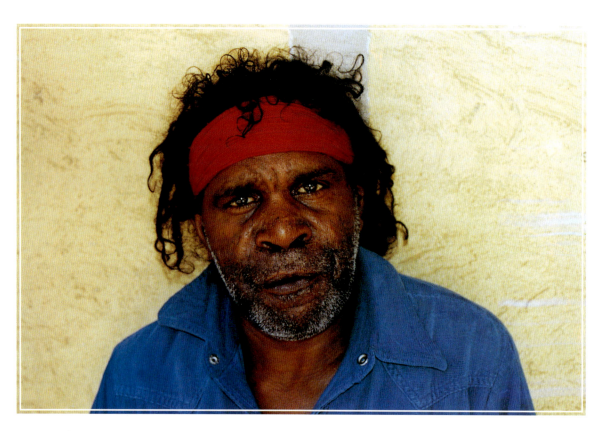

Arnie Frank, 2000. PHOTOGRAPH ANGELA LYNCH

# Arnie Frank

Ngangkari work with the spirit. Our work is to touch and heal people, to bring their spirits back and make people so much happier than they were. Our traditional way has always included many ngangkari in the community. We hold strong Tjukurpa and all ngangkari have to look after this Law. We always want to have ngangkari around. We always need to have ngangkari. They are good for us. We never want to lose our ngangkari. We want to have ngangkari with us for all time. Always.

Ngangkari sit down with people and then give them a healing treatment with the healing touch. It seems simple, but don't forget that what we do is special and sacred and nobody else can do what we do, except Anangu, who have been given this sacred skill and power. The knowledge of what we do remains with us Anangu and nobody can take it away from us. Remember that.

Ngangkari live on the earth but they travel to the skies. We ngangkari, including myself, oversee Anangu life, from up above in the sky. Up there are many beautiful and wonderful things that have been taken there by our ancestors. It is a good place. When we look up into the sky we have a lot to think about. We are reminded of many things, even budgets and the money line. Yet the sky is really a place of Tjukurpa and spirit. Really, we shouldn't be thinking about money when we look up at the sky. We don't like the way money has got into our minds. It has caused us a lot of problems.

The earth is beautiful too. It is a beautiful place with lovely wildflowers blooming everywhere. When we see these beautiful places, we feel happy and proud that it is our Tjukurpa that has made these places come into being. We own the Law surrounding such beauty and wonder, and we know that it has been like this for countless eons. We know that the land was beautiful even before there were humans on the earth. We know that the earth had an idea to put people onto this lovely land, and so we were created, in ancient times gone by – according to the Tjukurpa – and all without hospitals.

We were born in the days before hospitals. As babies we were bathed in smoke and it made us strong. But today, we are seeing the tragedy of these ancient times coming to a close. We don't want to see these ways come to an end. Never. There are so many issues that are important to Anangu which we must never allow to pass us by. Because of this, we have had great struggles, and we need to solve a lot of problems. We can't see any other way.

Today, we are learning so many new ways. We are learning about money, budgets and motorcars. We think about Toyotas now. Ngangkari want cars too. Our spirits never knew what they were before, but now that cars are among us, we see them and we want what we see. We Anangu have always loved the beautiful environment in which we live, and all the things around us, and this hasn't changed. We have always lived with papa, dogs. Dogs have always lived with us. They can warn us that something is not right. Dogs can warn us if children are sick and are having problems with their spirits, and if they are getting seriously ill. This is an ancient tradition with us. They are important to us.

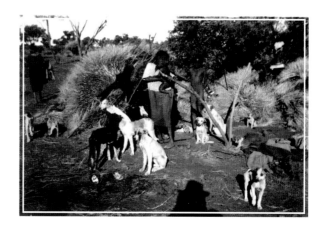

Rupert Langkatjukur Peter (standing right) and his mother (who is also Tinpulya Mervin's mother's younger sister), with many dogs, Mimili, South Australia, 1951.

PHOTOGRAPH BILL ELLIOTT, BILL & ALLISON ELLIOTT COLLECTION, ARA IRITITJA AI-0019372

*We have always lived with papa – dogs. Dogs have always lived with us.*

Anangu own a lot of information and Law, from healing to gathering bush tucker and wild foods. We have always had this knowledge and it has been taught to others by example. We have spent our lives following in the footsteps of our elders and they taught us by example until we became proficient ourselves.

Ngangkari learn from other ngangkari. We are taught from a long heritage of traditional healing. There are ngangkari men, women and children. All ages can be a ngangkari. Ngangkari speak many different languages and dialects. Ngangkari become ngangkari because somebody else has given them the power. Ngangkari teach by example. A person will inform a ngangkari about a certain person's sickness, and that ngangkari will then go about healing the problem.

We support families with our work. We prevent even more sadness from entering families' lives by preventing the death of a family member. Sometimes people can become so sick that their very lives are threatened. For instance, they can suffer great internal pain, as well as feel great sadness and distress. They are desperate for help. Ngangkari can help. We ask the sick person to lie down or to sit down, and then we begin the healing process by touch. After we arrive we sometimes consult with the spirit ngangkari in the heavenly skies for help. By doing so we are given even more strength to do our work. Only ngangkari can do this. Families really value this level of communication, as it brings a special power to the ngangkari and a special level of healing to their sick loved one.

What a very special gift we have, don't you think, when we can get in touch with the spirit ngangkari who reside in the skies? I don't know anyone else who has such an intimate relationship with the stars. What are stars? Lumps of stone? Not really! They are kililpi – stars – and they are made of special substances, and they are very, very ancient. Kililpi have their own spirit. The spirit descends from the stars down to us on the earth just like a waterfall. They are also teachers. Our own fathers told us, 'Never forget about the spirit of the stars. Watch them all the time. They can teach you.' So we keep this Tjukurpa alive, because it is so important.

Ngangkari can heal people, because of all this power and old Law. Ngangkari are called Wati Tjukurtjara – men with ancient power. Men who can heal people inside without cutting open their stomach.

It's always been like this. Nothing's changed. We were born as babies into this world and this is the world in which we live. We live here on this land in the bodies we've been given in this life. That includes nyumpu

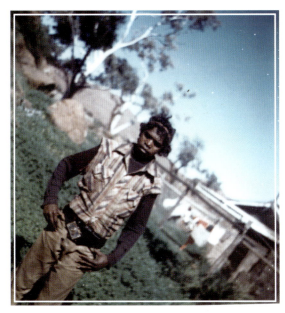

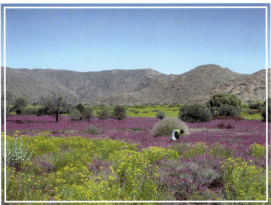

Top: Arnie Frank as a nyiinka (young man) in Pukatja (Ernabella), South Australia, 1980.
PHOTOGRAPH ANNIS BENNETT, AṞA IRITITJA AI-0030402

Bottom: Minyma (woman) picking wildflowers north of Pukatja (Ernabella), South Australia, 1979.
PHOTOGRAPH BILL EDWARDS, BILL EDWARDS COLLECTION, AṞA IRITITJA ARCHIVES AI-0014248

tjutaku, people with disabilities. Some people are kuṟu pati, blind. We'd like to help the people with disabilities to walk and the blind to see. We want to help all people to live a good life with good health. It is important to be healthy.

We live and work on our land and we have been given strong Tjukurpa from this land. We have been taught the stories of the land, which we now inherit. It is our duty to keep on working, so as to be able to pass down the Law that we know. We do not want to die without properly passing it down to the right people. We are not much use to the living if we are dead. It is a pity that some of us have given up on life and died. It's as if they have split off onto their own path and gone off to die, leaving us bereft. We need to be as strong as we can so that the culture we have can be held really strongly by living, healthy people.

Yet, in truth, we gravitate towards people who need our help, towards sick people. Sick people call for us. We go to those sick people and we ngangkaṟi give true spiritual and physical healing. This is called wiṟunymankupai. Wiṟunymankupai means for a ngangkaṟi to give true spiritual and physical healing. People ask for us to come. We see them, give them healing, and, later, we see them walking around well. That's because of the skill of the ngangkaṟi. We can heal people. All we have to do is see someone and we know straight away that they are ill, and what is wrong with them, and how to put them to rights. We go to them, ask them how they are, talk to them, and heal them successfully.

So what is it we want? Well, we want all the good things in life like everybody else does and the means to look after our sons well. We wish to be more respected for our skills and to get better work conditions and pay. Some ngangkaṟi say that the work they do is very sacred and important. So they really need more support such as an income to help them to continue their important work. So we are trying to make it plain and obvious, by speaking out truthfully and clearly, about who we are and what we do, so that you will believe us. We don't want to keep on talking about it, only to be forgotten. That wouldn't be fair. How can you remember us? I think a good thing would be if every time you looked up and saw the stars shining and glittering in the night sky you could think of us.

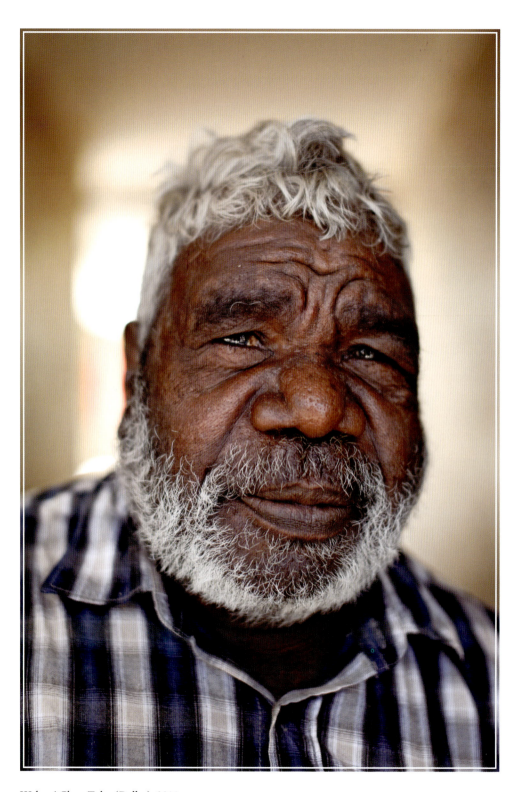

Wakupi Clem Toby (Dalby), 2011. PHOTOGRAPH RHETT HAMMERTON

# *Wakupi Clem Toby (Dalby)*

My grandfather gave the name Wakupi to me when I was just a little baby. I was born at Ernabella and my grandfather gave me his name there. I was born during the mission times, a long time ago, and my mother gave birth to me in the bush. There were no hospitals back when I was born.

My mother's father was from Irruntju, and my mother was born there and lived there during her earlier years, and then she came to Ernabella, where my father was already living.

My father's name was Witjiti Toby. My father is a Yankunytjatjara man, who was born at Imanpa. That is our country there, Imanpa and Waltanta (Erldunda). He was a stockman, and he had been working at Waltanta. Later, he went to Ernabella to look for his wife, my mother. They met at a well near Amata, and decided to get married and to go back to Ernabella, which is where I was born.

My grandfather gave me the ngangkari powers. That grandfather died a long time ago, my old grandfather, Old Mr Jimmy Brumby. He was Jimmy and Harry Brumby's father, my own grandfather's brother. My grandmother was also his cousin. They were like sister and brother. My old grandmother's name was Murika. A long time ago grandmother Murika used to live at Irapuwa and at Imanpa. When my father was born she left Imanpa and went to Mutitjulu and Aniri, near Atila. She lived at Aniri then, as well as Tjukaltjara. Aniri and Tjukaltjara are connected. There were some white people there, but they had no business being there. That is our country. Our people were working for the white people. My uncle, Punch Thompson (Kawaki), was born there too.

So Harry Brumby's father gave me the powers, my old grandfather gave me the ngangkari powers. He opened up my body and bestowed upon me his mapanpa. This means he loaded his mapanpa into me, to give me the power to heal. He told me to leave them for a while, to settle down and to give the powers a chance to build up. 'Wait,' he said, 'just in case those mapanpa disappear!' He told me to wait for a while, and then came the time when he said, 'OK, you must now touch this sick person.' That's what they say to us apprentices. They give us the permission to work on a person at a later date. 'OK, you can work on them now. Go ahead,' they will say.

My grandfather took me on my very first marali and showed me the ropes. We journeyed to many places that night. Another night, he took me, and we travelled to many more places, and it was from those journeys that I became experienced in the skills and tasks required. He said to me all those years ago, 'We are going to take you under our wing and teach you and we will make you into a good ngangkari, and we are never going to forsake you. You will never get lost, and you will learn how to heal men and women using ngangkari techniques.'

After that my grandfather didn't work as a ngangkari himself for ages, but he was busy teaching a number of apprentices about the ngangkari work. There were a lot of mamu around at the time, and he asked me to spend one or two months seeking out mamu around the place. Ngangkari work with mamu. We are mamu experts.

I would dream about mamu and ngangka<u>r</u>i all the time, but I was safe in the company of all the other ngangka<u>r</u>i. We dealt with the mamu ourselves. Soon I was a graduate ngangka<u>r</u>i, able to work on people then with my mapa<u>n</u>pa tools. I would send my own kurunpa to see other people and let my kurunpa do the work. I once stopped a serious case of vomiting and made the sick person well. 'Hey, this kid is well again!' I gained a lot of confidence from those early days, and yet I was confident always and I got more confident after that first success. So then I began working in earnest, and by the time I was a big kid I had had a lot of experience.

My father took me back to Erldunda, and I started working with the horses, but I was also a practising ngangka<u>r</u>i, right from the start. I became a stockman on Erldunda Station. I was a tall boy, still a teenager and not yet an initiated man, working as a stockman. I gave the stockmen ngangka<u>r</u>i treatments if they became unwell. I used to give other stockmen treatments deep in the bush while working as a stockman myself. That was a lot of extra work, treating a mob of stockmen in the bush. But they were all in good health because of me. I never stopped being a ngangka<u>r</u>i when I was a stockman. I was giving healing treatments on Erldunda and Kenmore Park Stations. Rupert Peter and I were working together then. Many of us worked at Kenmore around that time.

A long time ago when there were no doctors our ngangka<u>r</u>i were our sole health practitioners. They took care of the health of all our people. My grandfather's generation were our only doctors. They lived beside warming fires, inside sheltering windbreaks that looked like small yards. The yards were for safety, and inside would be good fires burning. Ngangka<u>r</u>i lived inside these homes with their families. Ngangka<u>r</u>i make their own fires.

We were living at Mount Cavenagh at the time of the Maralinga bomb blasts. There were a lot of children living at Mount Cavenagh at the time. Three times they exploded those bombs, maybe four. Many A<u>n</u>angu lost their sight from that. Everyone was crying out from sore eyes. They were badly affected by the puyu smoke, the puyu was blown out from the blasts and entered people's eyes. Everyone had eye problems from Maralinga. The ngangka<u>r</u>i had a difficult time of it during those terrible days.

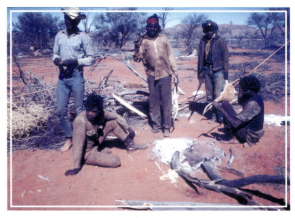

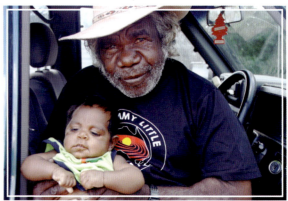

Top, left to right: Ronnie Norris, Wakupi Clem Toby (Dalby) (sitting), Sandy Mutju, Rapa Mervin and Jacob Puntaru sitting around the ashes of a fire with hunted kangaroo and joey, Amata, South Australia, 1970.
PHOTOGRAPH FAY BLACKMAN, FAY BLACKMAN COLLECTION, A<u>R</u>A IRITITJA AI-0007478

Bottom: Wakupi Clem Toby (Dalby) with his grandson, 2007.
PHOTOGRAPH ANGELA LYNCH

Dickie Minyintiri was working flat out then. He helped many children along the road. Dickie helped many of the children that were living at Mount Cavenagh. All those children had serious eye problems. We all had infected eyes. Dickie was busy helping everyone with treatments; in fact, he was the only ngangkari around the Mount Cavenagh area at the time, apart from my grandfather, old Jimmy Brumby.

A lot of people got sick, mostly the young children. The children suffered most from eye infections. Yami Lester was one of them. He got a serious eye infection at that time and was blinded. We all used to play together. Rupert Peter's grandfather passed away. Toby Baker got really sick too. This is a true story. Many people were struck down by unknown illnesses because of that bomb. Every single person at Ernabella was seriously affected from that puyu.

I give treatments to women, anywhere on their bodies that is needed – in the abdominal area and so on, as necessary. I heal children, women and men. However, pregnancy is in the realm that we generally do not go. A female ngangkari can work on a pregnant woman, they have always done so. Josephine Mick is one of those. Josephine is a true expert! She is a strong ngangkari.

I generally enjoy very good health myself, and keep myself in balance, so I have good health. This is because I have special powers. I have a special power in the form of a dog, or papa. He lives within me and the two of us travel together, and he looks after me, and also helps me with my work. He's smart and direct. He's a real-looking dog but he stays well hidden. Well, he's not a person, not Anangu, he's not visible like that. He's papa mapanpa. Hidden papa mapanpa, kurunpa ngangkari. I keep him hidden away. We travel around together at night. We travel on a marali. He comes with me and points the way, 'Someone's sick over here!' Once, down in Mutitjulu, my little baby grandson became sick and so in the middle of the night the two of us went over to see the baby and give him a treatment and balance him back up again. Next morning I was told, 'His health has been restored!' I did that! We travel around at night. My body lies sleeping but in fact we are travelling around. We go out travelling and all it takes is one day, not many days, one day is all it takes. We return home very quickly. This takes place while I am asleep. That's a marali. That's what I am referring to. That's what a marali is. It is a night time spirit journey that ngangkari take. The kurunpa takes the journey. Our journey resembles the flight of an eagle. We soar. We fly, similar to an eagle.

That particular time I went to see my baby grandson, I travelled there marali and gave him the treatment he needed and soared back home again, during the night. The next morning he was already cured! I often give healing treatments like this. Rupert and I often go together. Sometimes we go huge distances to see people who are calling out to us. Even though this occurs within one day, we do travel massive distances. These are marali spirit journeys. I am deeply asleep and not seeing anything. I am travelling marali. I return at dawn. I may have only been gone two or three minutes. Marali can be quick, regardless of distance.

Papa is my own spirit dog. His name is Papa. He's mine. He resides in me, inside my body. He's got his own body. He lives back at my camp. Nobody can see him. I can see him. Some of my grandsons can see him. He's like a white dingo. We work together as a team. He sees things and lets me know. He travels ahead of me. When my other grandfather, my mother's father, had his own papa, he would travel marali.

He gave that papa to me, and told me I could now travel marali as well, and after that, he died. My old grandfather died.

My father's mother was a Yankunytjatjara woman. She was from this Northern Territory side. My grandfather was an Irruntju man. My mother was an Irruntju woman. That's far away in Western Australia. My father and my uncle Windlass, and my grandfather and my grandmother. My father (Witjiti Toby) was number one, the eldest. Number two was old Nellie Armunta, old Dickie Minyintiri's wife (poor old thing has passed away now, bless her), Windlass was next and Stanley was the youngest. There were four of them, three brothers and one sister. My father died. Armunta died. Windlass is in an old people's home. Stanley died.

From them I became a traditional owner of Uluru. That's my grandfather's place. Mantarur and Mutitjulu. That's Yankunytjatjara country. That's why I worked in the eastern area, because it is my father's country, Imanpa area and so on.

We work our whole lives to banish sickness, our work is endless, and our treatments are successful. We hear the words, 'I'm OK now!' a lot.

If someone has been playing football and has broken their leg, a bone fracture requires a different approach altogether.

When a snake has bitten somebody, a ngangkari will be called. We'll bind up the place which has been bitten, to prevent the contaminated blood from moving around. We will hunt around and find the snake and hit it and hit it until it is dead. We'll block off the blood flow, and kill the snake, too, and the person will survive. I know because this happened to me when I was involved in a snake bite near Alice Springs once. A snake had bitten David Ingkamala's daughter. I quickly bound her up tightly at the site of the bite and then we went and killed the snake. We always kill the snake because snakes are poisonous. They have mamu, and their mamu can sneak around. Snakes are mamu. They are really bad. Snake poison becomes mamu also. Mamu with sharp teeth. They have dangerous teeth, so we have to kill them and bury them and stamp all over the surface of the ground. We hurl the poison away for safety's sake. We throw it away onto the ground. Snake mamu is big and bad and long and dangerous. It's poison goes into the body very quickly, so we have to work fast, but it is very hard to do. We do what we can and quickly.

My mother's father gave me my first mapanpa, and my father's father gave me some others, but the main ones came from my grandfather, my mother's father, he was the main one. He died a long time ago at Mutitjulu. My mother's father was Nugget Dawson's father. My mother was the eldest, number one, and Nugget was number two.

Ngangkari mapanpa are otherworldly. Lights … like the little lights you see glinting in the bush as you travel around, lights like that, live at a special ngangkari place. They are special mapanpa. Children are never allowed near a place like that. Mapanpa come and go. They have their own place, where they go and rest. A place a bit like where a spider might live. Ngangkari mapanpa have many special hiding places where they enter. But we can't put our hands inside to find them because spiders live in there too, and you'd always get bitten. Mamu take many forms like spiders living in the trees. Lightning can also be mamu. It sets fire to things. It sets fire to the trees and burns them down. Lightning can kill things. Sometimes mamu live in trees, but not if lightning strikes it. If that happens they get killed. Lightning strikes hard, because there is a mamu spider living inside the tree bark, a bad mamu more than likely. The lightning sees it and kills it. It gets hit by lightning. Mapanpa live inside tree bark as well, where there are biting spiders living sometimes.

Mapanpa cannot die. Mapanpa are eternal. But if our grandfather dies with his mapanpa inside him, then they are forever trapped inside and then they do die.

Something comes during the night and takes people's teeth. It is a wanampi, a rainbow serpent. Wanampi come in and see them, they come around and they think they'll steal teeth. People never see them of course, only ngangkari. Ngangkari know when they've been around, and, actually, ngangkari get happy to know there are wanampi around or if they see one. They'll think, 'Ah, it's gone off with a tooth!' It will come around at night and it will take out a tooth and sneak away with it! The wanampi will use mapanpa to hit it, it will rise up above the mouth, waving its tail and it will go upright into the sky, and then it will go straight back down again into a hole. Its head will enter the hole and its tail will follow quickly behind. Ngangkari witness this, and they try to grab the tail before it disappears, and then it gets dragged inside too! I've been dragged into a well myself. I'm telling you a Tjukurpa here. Where there is a wanampi there is plentiful good water where green vegetation grows.

They take the teeth because the teeth drop out. They can put mapanpa inside the head after that. The wanampi is right up above, looking down, not moving. Dead straight. A ngangkari will know what is going on and when a tooth drops out the ngangkari heals the spot quickly. When the wanampi gets close to its hole it starts to go inside. It has a long tail. People are scared of it. It lives inside the hole, that's his home – water is there and springs bubble up. Wanampi live in springs, they always have done, from a very long time ago. Wanampi look after people because wanampi look after the water, which is life-giving to the people. Most wanampi are gentle and kind, but some are fierce and dangerous. The ones that live underneath salt lakes are the most dangerous because the water they care for is unpleasant and undrinkable usually. They live inside these salty waters. So ngangkari are busy all the time caring for people who have had visits from wanampi. It is hard work for them, but, still, wanampi do a good service for people, caring for their water sources inside the ground. Wanampi come up to the surface, bringing water up with them, and when it all bubbles up again and the water level rises, they go back down inside. They do this because other ngangkari may steal someone else's wanampi.

Wanampi move around and they make the groundwater level rise up. At Uluru, the traditional owners call out to the wanampi there and cause the waterfall to flow, at Mutitjulu waterhole. All my old grandfathers call out at Uluru.

In the past, if someone has got an agonising toothache it means the string holding their tooth in is infected, and causes great pain inside the tooth. So what we can do for that is to jiggle it around with a stick, which further breaks the connections holding the tooth in and out it comes. The string inside the tooth is obviously infected and is dissolving inside. But ngangkari find it hard to fix that string. He will just pull the tooth out. There's just the one string. String is an English word, but we say pulyku. Pulyku. Yes.

Strings inside the body are called pulyku or malypanypa. Malypanypa or pulyku. I guess pulyku is an easier word to say! Malypanypa, pulyku. String is what white people say. We just feel around until we feel it, and then we push everything else aside, but if we can't do that, then the energy running down the pulyku doesn't work properly. Only half goes. So ngangkari have to keep on trying until we properly locate it and then, there you go! It is all sorted and brought back to proper working order. Think of it as a blockage in a tap, which you fix and then all of a sudden the water starts flowing again. Energy flows along it, but if there is a blockage of any sort, the ngangkari has to find that blockage and get it shifted. They might have to search all over the whole body from head to foot. It will be inside somewhere. This is my work. It affects the kurunpa. The spirit is affected. There are many strings in the head, coming down to the forehead and down the neck.

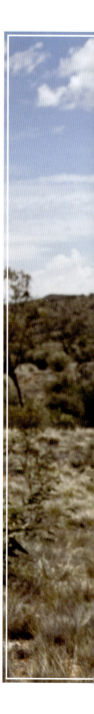

Sometimes, if we have a difficult case, we might decide to call in a second ngangkari to help us. Malparara. That's called malparara, or working with a companion. We all work like that from time to time. In the past, one ngangkari at a time will work on somebody, while any other ngangkari might sit on the person's back and massage it back and forth, while the other ngangkari straightens the person up and does any extraction needed. Even four might work together on one person, malparara way. Two ngangkari could work together while another two will work together, in that way, nothing is missed. Ngangkari know how much hard work it is hunting and carrying a kangaroo on the head a long way back home with a bundle of spears, and lots of aches and pains will come from that. Of course they'll get a good feed out of a kangaroo, but the person carrying it home with all those spears and spear thrower will sometimes need to see a ngangkari when he gets home, poor thing! He will need to go out hunting again tomorrow so he needs to be up to the task. That's how we work. All ngangkari are the same. We are no different.

There are new young ones coming up. We ngangkari will be passing on our mapanpa to the younger generation later on in the future. We are not old enough yet. My old grandfather used to take me around, old Clem. I'm 'young' Clem. He used to take me around and he told me one day, 'When you are old enough and I'm old enough, I shall be giving you my powers. I will then slow down, and after that I will go to my eternal rest'. Then it became my time and, as he said, 'I will bequeath unto you my powers. They will become yours, and after that I can die.' So when I hand mine over, the whole lot in its entirety is bequeathed. None is kept. Other items are bequeathed at the same time. Spirit items. I can't tell you everything.

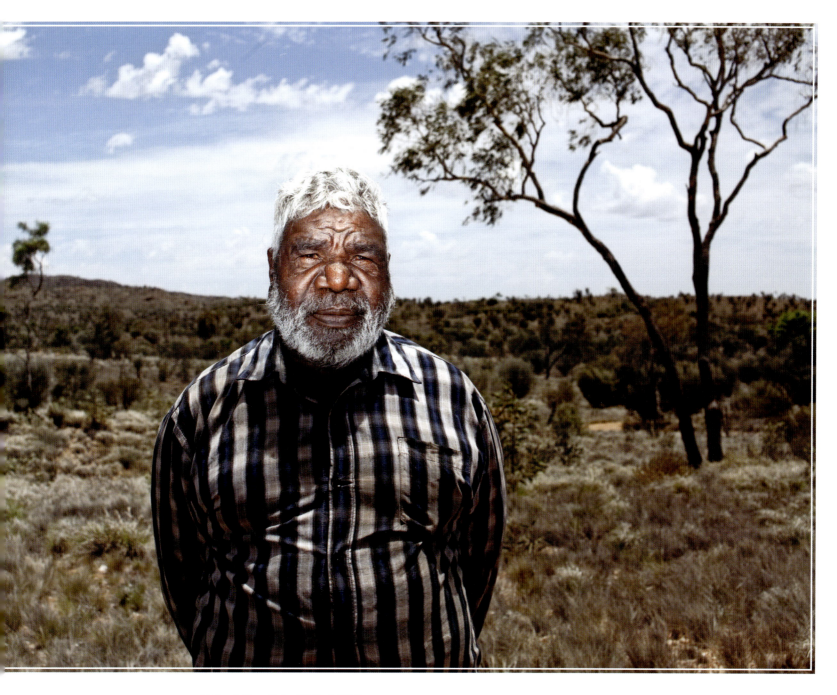

Wakupi Clem Toby (Dalby), 2011.
PHOTOGRAPH RHETT HAMMERTON

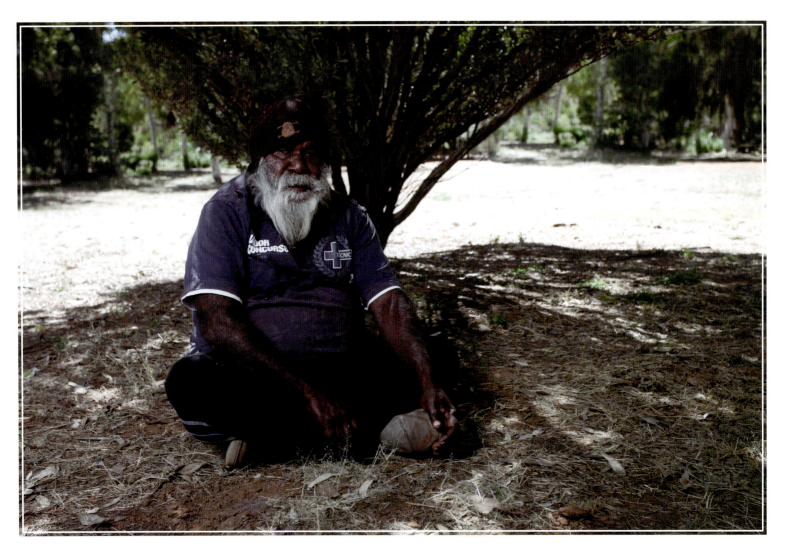

Martin Wintjin Thompson, 2011. PHOTOGRAPH RHETT HAMMERTON

# Martin Wintjin Thompson

I am a Pitjantjatjara man. My real name is Wintjin, which is an old name given to me when I was a baby. I was born at Kunatjara, which is not far from Pipalyatjara, just a little south of Pipalyatjara.

When I was still a child but hadn't become a ngangkari yet one day, I heard a ngangkari song. Upon hearing a song, I grabbed onto it and held it tightly. I grabbed the song. They were singing a ngangkari inma in preparation for going on a marali. Upon hearing it and holding onto it, I went on that marali too. It was that song that made me become a ngangkari. I was given the power at that time. This happened at Kunatjara. I was still a child. One of our ancestors, a very powerful old ngangkari, passed his powers down to me. His powers were very old. I became a ngangkari because he handed his power down to me. He'd died a long time ago and so had no name that can be spoken. He was an ancestor by then. After I became a ngangkari I inherited his name and his mapanpa.

Ngangkari have mapanpa, which sometimes look like bones. My mapanpa were inserted into my body. I was given many mapanpa, perhaps five, and the power of them spread right through my body.

After that, if someone was lying down very sick, and one of the men would come up to me and ask me to give them the healing touch, I would do so. A man might say to me, 'Please touch him here, because you have been on a marali and you carry the mapanpa now. You have been flying like an eagle with the ngangkari and you now have the power'.

We travel on marali travels. We travel to the special ngangkari place and then we come back. People know this and they ask ngangkari like me to help out, if they know of someone who is kurunpa ultu. Kurunpa ultu means they are spiritless or empty of spirit. Our job is to find their spirit and put it back into their bodies, which quickly heals them. Even children do this if they've got the ngangkari power in them. I gained a lot of confidence in myself after I became a new young ngangkari. I was fearless when travelling on marali and when dealing with spirits and illnesses.

I remember someone at Pipalyatjara who became ill and lost his spirit, and I was responsible for regaining his spirit and repositioning it back in his body, where he quickly regained his health. After he'd lost his spirit he was very weak. A ngangkari like me will seek out his lost spirit, find it and bring it back to him, and will make sure it is put back where it belongs.

When one becomes a ngangkari, be they a child or whatever, they'll have the ability to see clearly and will easily see a lost spirit lurking in the bushes. We can easily go and get it. That is Ngangkari Law.

As a new young ngangkari, I began working around my area and as I got older and travelled further afield, I began giving treatments to people further away. There were no white people around, back in those days. We Anangu were responsible for our own health and treatments, and ngangkari were our only doctors.

Our extended family walked around our own country for as long as we could remember, until white people established Ernabella. After Ernabella was established most people walked there to see it, and then everybody else went there to go and see their relatives and to try out the new food on offer.

Before then, we lived on our own lands and we centred our lives around our own waterholes in the Kunatjara, Pipalyatjara, Anumara Piti, Atjal, Amuntari and Pukara area. When there was drought, and no water anywhere, we only had a few places where there was dependable water. Sometimes we had to go to Kunytjanu for our water.

Our people lived like that, all basing themselves around their own areas and own waters. We did the same in our own area, basing ourselves on the life-giving waters between Kunytjanu and Irruntju. In the days before white flour, this is how we lived.

When I was still a child, but taller, we heard about this place Ernabella Mission, and we walked there to go and have a look. I was a fully practising ngangkari then. We went to Ernabella for the flour and the food we'd heard about. Our people know the entire landscape from near and far and so the news came to us that there was this place, and food was being given out, and then white people started making forays into the land on camels, and would be handing out flour, so news travelled fast.

I walked to Ernabella with my mother and father and Toby Baker and his family. He's my nephew-son, he's my father's grandson.

My father was named Itimini and my mother was called Kunypiri. The Pipalyatjara area is my father's country and my mother comes from Makura Piti, that's her country. He married her and they lived in the Kunatjara and Pipalyatjara area, which is where I was born. We moved to Ernabella, and there we stayed, until the Maralinga bombs. My parents died as a result of the smoke and the fallout from the bombs.

I continued working as a ngangkari at Ernabella and I gained expertise in dealing with kurunpa and spirits. There were more people and more displaced spirits and more complex

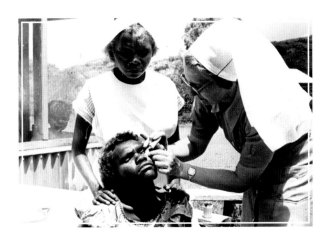

Sister Natalie Graham and hospital assistant Mayawara Minutjukur tending to their patient Tjukupati outdoors beside the hospital, Pukatja (Ernabella), 1952.
PHOTOGRAPH HAMILTON AIKIN, UNITING CHURCH (NSW) COLLECTION, ARA IRITITJA AI-0005344

*When we were living at Ernabella a new way of healing was established when the white people built a hospital, and doctors and nurses started working inside.*

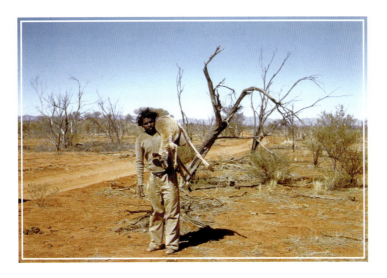

Martin Wintjin Thompson carrying a red kangaroo, Ernabella region, 1961.
PHOTOGRAPH SHIRLEY GUDGEON (HILL), ARA IRITITJA
AI-0006276

problems. I used my special tools, especially my kuuti. Ngangkari keep kuuti, which we use as powerful tools. We use them as visible tools of healing power, which we can put into people's bodies and get back after they've done their healing work.

We have power in our hands. You can't see it but it's there. Once the power goes into our hands and arms, it lives there and comes and goes as needed. You can't see it, it looks like we've got closed skin on the palms of our hands, but that power can come and go through the hands nevertheless.

Ngangkari travel into other worlds in the same way that a bird flies. We soar and glide the same way that an eagle soars and glides high up in the skies. This is not my own special activity – all ngangkari do this. We travel and fly together to a special ngangkari place, where mapanpa are stored.

When we were living at Ernabella a new way of healing was established when the white people built a hospital, and doctors and nurses started working inside. Meanwhile, we ngangkari continued our work, but we stayed hidden from the white people. People would go and see sisters and doctors in the hospital and get medicines from them, which they liked, and the medicines were good. But we ngangkari were just as busy working outside. Our work was outside, whereas the doctors worked inside. Some of the Anangu who were working in the hospital were ngangkari too, and they worked two ways!

Ngangkari will never stop working because we are in great demand and always available on call throughout the bush. We give our healing treatments at people's homes.

Jacky Kurlturnyintja Giles Tjapaltjarri (b. 1944, d. 2010), *Kaliangku*, 2005. Synthetic polymer paint on canvas, 101.6 x 152.6 cm.

MOLLIE GOWING ACQUISITION FUND FOR CONTEMPORARY ABORIGINAL ART 2005, PHOTOGRAPH JENNI CARTER, COLLECTION ART GALLERY OF NEW SOUTH WALES [338.2005]

# Jacky Tjapaltjarri Giles

While living here in Karylwarra I called the two ngangka<u>r</u>i, Andy Tjilari and Rupert Langkatjukur Peter, to come and visit me, which they did. We three sat down and talked together and I told my story for the book. You are welcome to listen to what I have to say.

I am a maparntjarra, or ngangka<u>r</u>i. I work in Tjirrkarli, Karylwarra, and Warburton, where Yarnangu people know me. When sick people go to the health clinic they call me and I walk to their house and I see them afterwards.

When people are in pain, I give them a treatment and they get better. They say they have got bad pain and nothing will stop the pain. So I pull out the pain from them and I show them what I pulled out, so they can see what caused their suffering. Ngangka<u>r</u>i use the mouth for sucking out sickness. This cleans out any sickness or pain. Our style of healing brings children in particular right back to health very quickly.

I help young children by giving them healing treatments. Their parents are grateful. I give the children treatments openly, so that the parents can see what I remove from their bodies. It makes it better if the parents know what is going on with their children's health.

There is a lot of demand on us ngangka<u>r</u>i to give healing treatments. People demand treatments from us at all hours of the day and night. We are happy to help, of course, but we are frustrated that though we are doing more than a full-time job, we just cannot match it with the kind of income that we are worth. Where do ngangka<u>r</u>i get their income from? The health clinic? No, from Yarnangu people who receive the treatments.

Not many of us ngangka<u>r</u>i have cars, so it is hard for us to see all the people that want us to give them treatments, particularly if they are a long way away in the bush. I would like to travel further afield.

There are some very powerful ngangka<u>r</u>i in Western Australia. The Wiluna ngangka<u>r</u>i are particularly powerful and have strong, important Law. I worry about the new young apprentice ngangka<u>r</u>i these days. They are not getting the same bush upbringing that we old men did. I worry about them. Ngangka<u>r</u>i business is too important to lose.

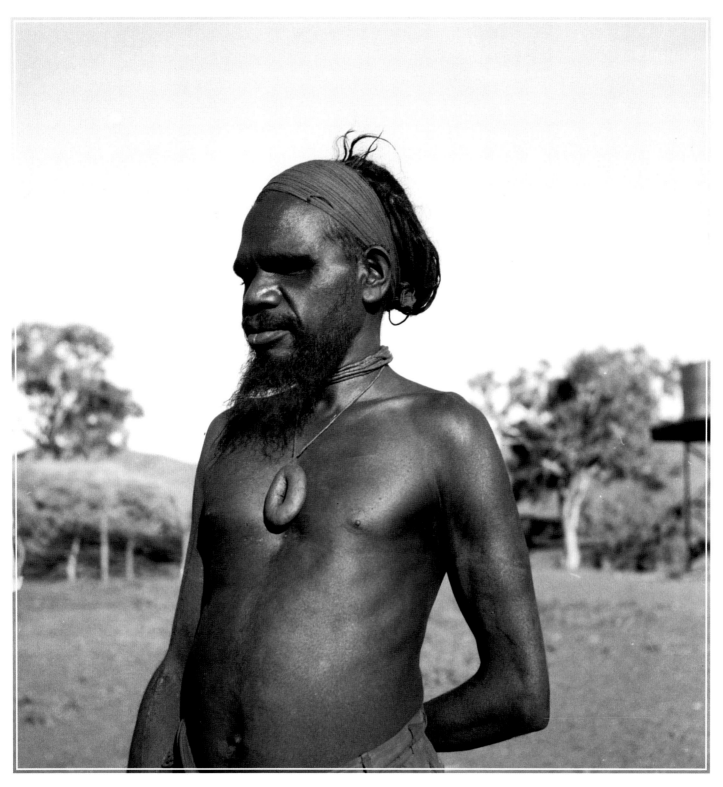

Ngulitjara, also known as Palingka, an important and powerful blind ngangkari at Pukatja (Ernabella), South Australia, 1948.
PHOTOGRAPH RICHARD SEEGER, COURTESY MUSEUM VICTORIA (XP87)

# Ngulitjara

Ngulitjara passed away a long time ago, but his legendary healing abilities are still talked about today. These stories about him are included to honour the warm memories many of us hold of Ngulitjara.

## Ngulitjara was my own loving mama too

There were once two brothers; Pilpira was the eldest, Number One, and Pilpira Number Two came next. They came from very sacred men's country out towards the Pipalyatjara area. They were kangaroo men, Wati Malu, from Aparatjara, Putaputa, Tjangi, Ilitjata, Punuliri and Nyira, which are such important places that nobody is allowed to go to them without permission.

These two men were the fathers to a large group of children, and Ngulitjara and my own father were two of those children. The first son was Nura Ward and Kawaki's father (Punch Thompson), who was also one of my own fathers (uncle). Then came my auntie Ada Imala, then my auntie Maringka. Then came my uncle, mama Ngulitjara. After that came my auntie Nyingkalya, followed by my own father, Bossy Pungkayi. After my father came my auntie Nyuniwa Alison, followed by my youngest father, Barney Wangin.

All of these brothers and sisters had many children, who are in turn all my brothers and sisters. Nura Ward, Kawaki, Maggie Mumu, Atipalku Lewis, Amuntari, Tana and I are all brothers and sisters. Pilpira Number One and Pilpira Number Two are our grandfathers. We are all kangaroo people, from those two men. Pilpira Number One is the father of Ngulitjara, who was a very famous, blind ngangkari.

I am my father's daughter and I am carrying his blood. The same blood ran through his father, to his son, to me. Ngulitjara was my own loving mama too. We come from the same family line. He loved me very much, and that is why, when I first saw that photograph of Ngulitjara, my father, I knew that our family blood had been flowing through his veins, and it made me sad, so at first I wanted to keep his memory hidden. I wanted to just forget about him, because it made me too sad to be reminded of him. Not just me but all of us, it makes us all sad. But so many people have wanted to hear about him and to see his picture that I have relented, and I am now reconciled about his photograph being in the ngangkari book and am happy to talk about him.

My father was born on that men's country area near Putaputa, near Tjangi, in that sacred area. I was born at Areyonga. My father, Pungkayi Bossy, died there and is buried there at Areyonga. I went to live in my mother's country at Docker River and around the Western Australia/Northern Territory border and it was there, a long time ago, that I heard the news on the bush radio that Ngulitjara had died at Pukatja.

He was buried at Pukatja, along with his own father, my grandfather. Those two brothers Pilpira Number One and Pilpira Number Two are both buried at Pukatja in a family group. My aunties have died as well. In Mutitjulu there is a line of graves: Ada, Maringka and Nyingkalya are laid there, those three sisters. We are a very big family group.

Ngulitjara was born blind because he was born on that very sacred country. He was blind but he was very powerful, the power coming from the powerful land. Not only the land made him strong, he also grew up on bush tucker, which made him strong and healthy in his body. He grew up and lived his life on incredibly sacred and powerful lands and he only drank sacred water and ate meat and food growing on sacred earth. This gave him extraordinary powers. His eyes may have been blind but he still had the ability of vision from his forehead, and also from behind his head. It was as if he had a torchlight beaming from the front and the back of his head. While he slept he could see things and would warn the people. He could kill dangerous things such as serpents that came in the night. He was very precise and never missed his targets. His family benefitted from his spiritual protection and in return he was provided with delicious food from the surrounding land, good clean water, fresh fruits and meats. Not tea.

He did not get his mapanpa from his grandfather. He got them from the land and from the sacred places. He could see the landscape in his mind's eye even though he couldn't see it through his actual eyes. He was only blind in one sense of the word. In the other sense, he was like a superman who could see things nobody else could.

He was born blind. Some people say his mother made a mistake by giving birth where she did, and causing him to be born on such a sacred place. But it happened, and he was born blind, but he was very talented. His mother was Graham's aunt, Kulyuru and Nyinguta's father's older sister.

My other father, Barney Wangin, would look after Ngulitjara during men's business time. Sometimes Ngulitjara would ask to help with the spearing of meat, and so Barney would load up a spear into his spear thrower for him to try, but he just couldn't do it, and this would make the men laugh hilariously. They would laugh, 'Hey, we are going to lose our meat if you are the hunter!' and they would laugh some more. Sometimes this made Ngulitjara sad, because he couldn't help with the hunting. His brothers would go hunting on his behalf, and they'd bring the fresh meat back to camp. Ngulitjara would be there, and sometimes they would find him feeling sad and sorry for himself. They'd say, 'Hey, don't be sad!' and his brother would make him laugh about something, and so he'd cheer up. They'd tell him funny stories about the hunt and sometimes make up stories about Ngulitjara helping to hunt the meat animals. At least he could see the funny side of it.

When we were all living together in Pukatja, my younger brother Tana and I used to be his helpers. We would take him fresh water to drink and food to eat. We would help him make up his bed and we would tell him, 'Lie down and rest now. Have a sleep, and we'll come back to you later' – but he would say, 'No, don't leave me. Take me with you. Take my hand and lead me to where the other men are. Leave me there and then play close enough to me so I can hear your voices.' So we'd play near him in his immediate area and we'd shout out to him from time to time. Then when he was ready to go home he'd call out to us, 'Come back and get me!' We'd take him by the hand and lead him back to our home camp. Tana and I looked after him well. At night we'd all lie down to sleep and he would tell us wonderful stories before we slept.

I always remember him as my own loving and caring father. He would refer to us as his own children. He never married or had his own children, but he was still father to his brothers' and sisters' children. He used to ride around everywhere on the back of a donkey, and his sons would lead the donkey. His sons would look after him – and that included Andy Tjilari. Ernabella missionaries would come to see him and would give him things. But we are the ones who cared for him.

Ngulitjara became the most important ngangkari on the land. He gave hundreds of treatments, using his own specialised skills. One of his specialities was by using his mouth, blowing and spitting. He also used his hands, drawing out the sickness. I would watch him work. It was fascinating to see him heal people so quickly and effectively. People would come to him and ask him for healing and he gave superb treatments and was recognised as having very special powers. He had a god-given power of unusual strength. He was an especially gifted man, who had a sacred body, who was born on sacred ground. So you can imagine what a high level he was working at, and how revered he was.

Even his grave is a sacred place to us. He was a tjilpi when he died. He was an older man, but not an elderly man. It always makes me sad to think that I was such a long way away from him when he died. I still miss him.

Kunbry Peipai

## *I can remember Ngulitjara clearly, he was a lovely man*

I remember Ngulitjara as a young man. He would wear trousers but no shirt. He never wore shirts, because he didn't like them. The people used to look after him. His older sister would kill rabbits with stones, and bring the meat back for him. He was a good man, and always gave treatments to the small children. He and I would give treatments together. He used to say to me sometimes, 'I'm a bit tired, could you do the treatments for me? You can see those white people, but I can't, and I am scared of them'. So I would give some treatments on behalf of him, if any white people were about. There were a lot of men in those days who lived their lives hidden and privately, and others who lived their lives openly and publicly. This lovely man lived openly, in view of everyone.

Mr Trudinger (the superintendent at Ernabella in the forties and fifties) came along, and Ngulitjara said, 'Who is that there? I am going to kill you!' Ngulitjara was scared of him, that's why. Trudinger replied, 'It's only me, and I'm not going to hurt you. Don't hurt me!' But Ngulitjara was scared of him, poor thing. We said, 'Mr Trudinger is a good man, so don't hurt him.' Trudinger asked him what he was doing, 'Are you sucking blood, or what?' He'd been watching him work on a patient, 'Are you biting him?' he asked. Ngulitjara was a great ngangkari, but he was really frightened of white people, and he would never, ever knowingly give anybody a treatment in front of a white person. He would say, 'No, not now, wait until they are gone.'

Ngulitjara and I both had mapanpa from that creature that looks like an emu. I was given some and I still have them. He had some too. That creature would walk around, and he would look and walk just like an emu, but he wasn't an emu. His name was Karpirinypa, and he would walk around in the rain. I have some mapanpa from him. Karpirinypa would walk around amongst our ancestors and the old men who are now passed away. Anyway, we both have some mapanpa from him and that is something we two share, something we have in common. Oh yes, I can remember Ngulitjara clearly, he was a lovely man.

We would spend a lot of time together – bless him! He would ride a donkey, clicking his tongue to make it go, I think he called it Tika-Taka. One time he was taken with our group a long way away, on his donkey, and I remember accompanying him on parts of that journey, where our objective was to get dingo scalps for the bounty. We travelled into Yankunytjatjara country and he would ask me, 'Son! Where are we now?' I'd tell him where we were. This was in the days when the first money came in, the government bounty for the dingo scalps.

Andy Tjilari

## *He was a very powerful ngangkari*

Kurutjara (Ngulitjara) was a ngangkari. He did not have sight but he had a great number of mapanpa. He kept his mapanpa in an emu tail. He was a very powerful ngangkari. He was my uncle. He was Martin's brother and Rama's cousin brother as well, from one country, one family, near Pipalyatjara. I used to spend a lot of time with him. He once gave me half of his mapanpa – but he took them back again! Kurutjara had so many! He had many more inside of him, like little lights, they were. Like lights, like sparks. Lights. Tili. Tili mapanpa. Ngangkariku mapanpa, not made by the hands of men.

Wakupi Clem Toby (Dalby)

## *When I was a little girl, he made me better again*

There was a ngangkari in Ernabella who was blind, that was Mike Mulayangu's old uncle. That old, blind ngangkari was his old uncle. He was a very good ngangkari and he would give us children very good treatments when we were sick. He healed many children. Once, when I had bad eyes, when I was a little girl, he made me better again. He lived at Pukatja in mission times. He lived in the bush in the early days and came into the mission when the missionaries arrived.

One of his relatives led him along, leading him along with a stick. He had a stick of his own that he would poke about, feeling things. He was a powerful ngangkari. He was Kunbry Mankutja's uncle. His name was Palingka. He was her father's older brother. Old Palingka was Kunbry Mankutja's father's older brother. He used to ride a donkey. He used to get around on a donkey. He'd go straight to where he wanted to go on a donkey. Kunbry used to walk and take him with her on a donkey. He would be able to travel easily and directly riding on his donkey. He'd meet someone halfway and they'd tell him where to go, and he'd be off, going down the right road. He'd find out where he was all along the road. This was during Dr Duguid's time. There were a lot of people around in those days.

Pantjiti McKenzie

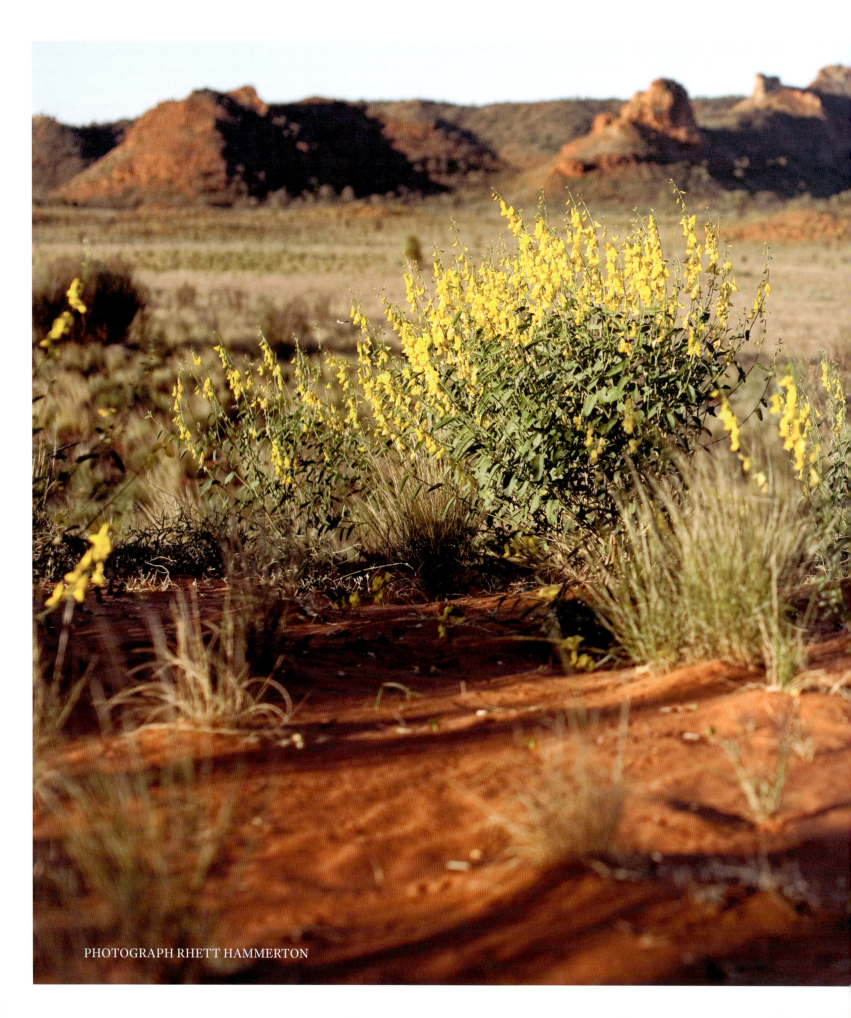
PHOTOGRAPH RHETT HAMMERTON

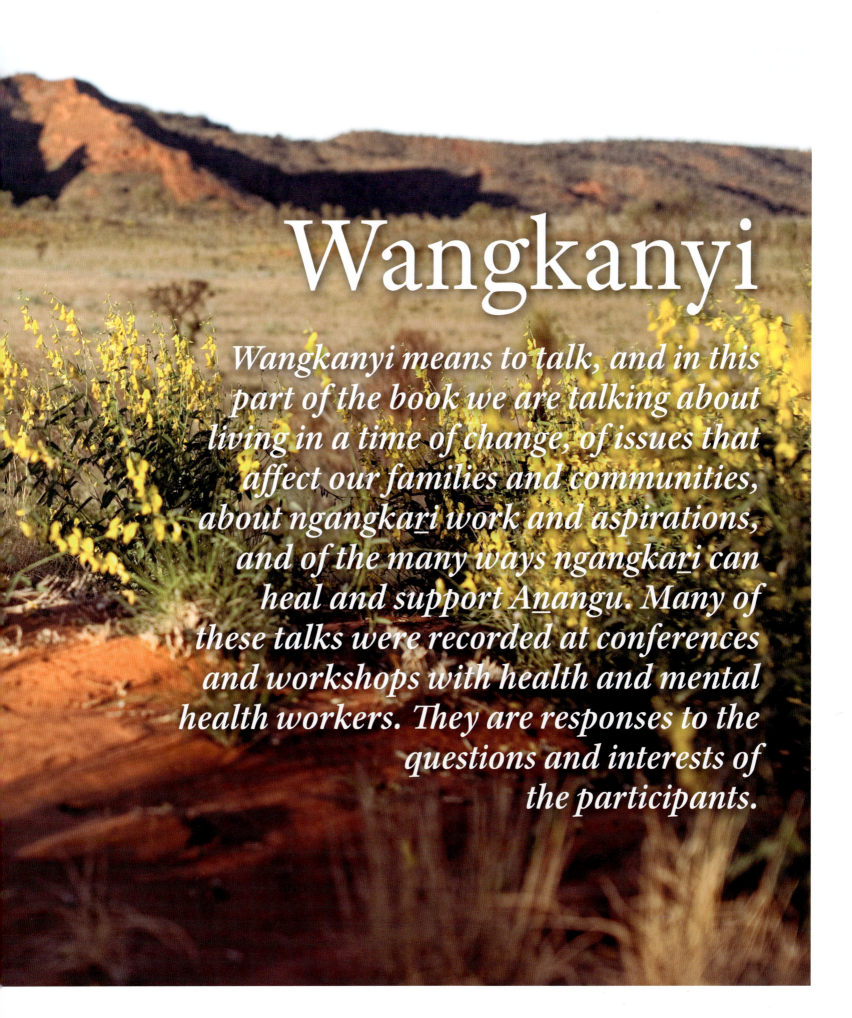

# Wangkanyi

*Wangkanyi means to talk, and in this part of the book we are talking about living in a time of change, of issues that affect our families and communities, about ngangkari work and aspirations, and of the many ways ngangkari can heal and support Anangu. Many of these talks were recorded at conferences and workshops with health and mental health workers. They are responses to the questions and interests of the participants.*

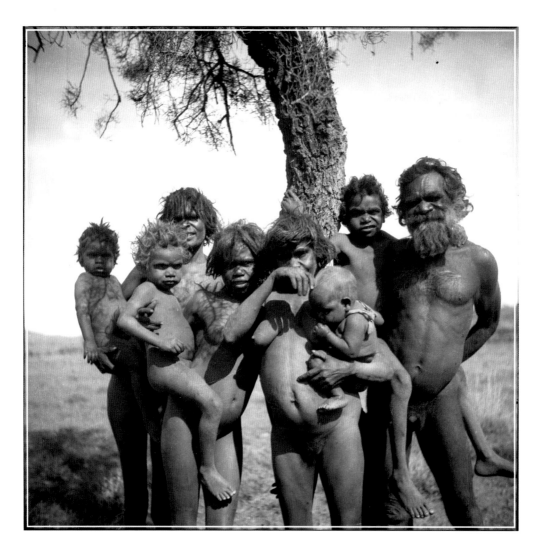

Tinpulya Mervyn's family in 1946, from left: Amanyi Young holding her son Yirwinti Young, Sandy Tjulkiwa Mutju holding Intjintjin, Tinpulya's mother, Wintirangu, holding Tinpulya (the baby) and Tinpulya's father, Ram, holding her sister Muwitja Wipana Jimmy.
PHOTOGRAPH DR CHARLES DUGUID, DUGUID FAMILY COLLECTION, AṞA IRITITJA AI-0030489

*Once upon a time Aṉangu were fit, healthy and happy. They spent their lives hunting and gathering and eating traditional foods.* Tinpulya Kangitja Mervyn

# Changing World

### *Once upon a time A̱nangu were fit, healthy and happy*

Once upon a time A̱nangu were fit, healthy and happy. They spent their lives hunting and gathering and eating traditional foods. There were no mental health problems. It is only since white people came on our lands that mental health problems have started, and people have become alcoholics and drug addicts and cigarette smokers.

Before, our people only ever died of old age. Old men and old women only died of old age, that is, unless they died of other things like perishing in the heat and sun without water. People lived with very little water, and had to dig for their water deep in the ground. Waterholes would dry up very quickly but soakages deep in the ground hold water a lot longer. People would dig out the holes and get the water out, using grasses to sieve out the bits. The water would be cool and fresh and people lived on it.

Nobody had diabetes back then. Renal failure and dialysis were unheard of. Nobody had high blood pressure because everyone was so active and busy hunting and foraging every day. Our fathers, grandfathers and all the young men were occupied entirely with hunting for meat. They hunted all their lives and were very strong because of it. Nobody had scabies or skin problems. Everyone carried firesticks and started their fires when they made their new camps.

Ngangka̱ri would be needed for all sorts of simple injuries such as burns. If someone was burnt we had a special caterpillar's nest we would use as a burns sheet. For a snake bite we would cut open the skin at the site of the bite very quickly, to make the poison pour out. Then we'd seal up the wound with a hot coal, which sealed the cut up and prevented infection.

Tinpulya Kangitja Mervyn

### *It was a time of great change*

In the old days in the time when the measles really hit us hard, it was an epidemic and many people became sick. That was a big time of change when things started to go wrong and it was harder to teach the Law. Many people passed away. My father told me about it. It was a really difficult time, a time of change. Many people survived to go to places and learn Tjukurpa and keep things even and balanced again.

But it still hit really hard and as many as half our people passed away at that time. The time of the measles epidemic (1948) was a time of great change, and the way of life that we once had was changed forever. We had this one clear path, one clear line, Tjukurpa, but since the epidemic many other things came in that made life confusing and less clear. Things started to change and there were more and more mental health problems within our world and people's thinking became spoilt. Up until that time it had been a clear path to follow.

Many people passed away during the measles epidemic. Its effect was very harmful to us, similar to the way marijuana and petrol have been really harmful. It was a time when things really hurt us and when things started to go wrong.

Rupert Langkatjukur Peter

## *In the old days*

In the old days when people walked very long distances, there was always great concern about when they would be able to come back. It was more difficult to communicate then, and sometimes you wouldn't know how long people would be away for. When they did come back again, there was great relief and happiness.

In the old days when people walked the country they had to make long and difficult journeys by themselves. For example, if a man went to get mingkulpa, he may need to go a long way for it. He'd get the bush tobacco but then, in the distance, he might see smoke on the horizon. He might then decide to go to the source of the smoke to spend time with other family members for a period of time. Meanwhile, family back at the original camp would be concerned about their man. They might pick up his tracks and follow them to where the tobacco was, determine that he'd safely got there, and then they'd see that he'd headed off in a new direction.

They'd follow the tracks up, and arrive in the camp to see their family member there with a number of people they'd never met before. The man would say, 'Look, I'll introduce you to your family here! This is your brother, these are your sons, this is your uncle, this is your grandfather.' They were being introduced to people that they hadn't met before, yet who were part of their family. And in turn you might say, 'Oh, that's my grandfather over there,' and go to live with him for a few months, and travel with that family then. Over time you'd get to know your whole extended family in this way.

A man might arrive in a new camp, of, say, one or two wiltja, shade shelters, having travelled from afar. He will walk towards that camp and then sit down, at a distance. He would be carrying meat, having come from hunting to join that camp, but the people in the camp may not be sure who he is, where he's come from, how they're related to him. It's only later on in the evening when their own hunting party returns that they'll recognise him and see that he's part of their family.

He is shy and a bit embarrassed, so he'll sit waiting at a distance from the camp rather than go into it, until he's formally welcomed in. They might say 'Oh good, my son's arrived!' and then go and give him some water and invite him in. Everyone's really happy and they laugh together and it's a good feeling. They talk together, all sitting together, happy to be together after their travels.

In the old days, when people were walking the land in the height of summer, they were forced to travel during extremely hot times because of drought and lack of food and water. They couldn't just shelter all day in a shady wiltja on account of starvation and had to travel during the middle of the day risking

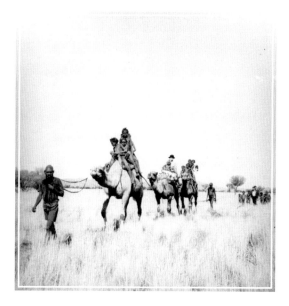

'Harry' leading string of camels to Itjinpiri for a picnic; the party included Andy Tjilari's Grandfather Yapayapa Tjapaya (walking behind camels) and teacher Ron Trudinger. Andy Tjilari says he used to travel with these people but 'I was too scared to ride camels, I'd be told "Come here and climb up." No Way! I would not!" Titu, near Apara and Pukatja (Ernabella) 1940.

PHOTOGRAPH CHARLES MOUNTFORD. COURTESY OF THE STATE LIBRARY OF SOUTH AUSTRALIA, PRG 1218/34/1255C

sunstroke. By the end of a long day searching for food the sun would be really striking them hard.

The sun beating down enters the body and head and causes considerable harm. It really affects people's thinking to the point that they would return home almost dead. Often these poor people would become disorientated and collapse under an old tree and may not even know where their home camp lay. The sun can cause great harm; people's thinking gets confused, they can lose their sight, become disorientated, they get extremely hot and burnt.

As a young ngangkari who has lived through drought, I worked on those poor hunters who staggered back into camp, collapsing under an old, dried tree and sat there staring.

Ngangkari have a really important role helping people who are struck by the sun. We quickly remove the effects of the sun and the heat from people by cooling them down and giving them water to drink. Mothers and fathers and other family members would help cool the person, cooling their head and giving them a little bit of water.

Andy Tjilari

## *The ngangkari had the sole responsibility of caring for everyone*

There is a really long tradition of ngangkari in the Anangu world. Well before my time, the old men and women ngangkari were responsible for looking after, and the healing of, their people. And that is what they did – in the bush, in an environment where there were no hospitals. The ngangkari had the sole responsibility of caring for everyone and making sure they were OK. This was before my time. Today we work really confidently and together in the hospitals – it's a new way of working. So we have seen that time of not having hospitals in that world and ngangkari having the sole responsibility, to coming closer and closer, until today where we see ourselves working really quite closely with people in hospitals. We do that through the NPY Women's Council work, a lot of meetings and talks, getting to know each other's style and skills. This is something that has grown over time and we work really closely today.

Rupert Langkatjukur Peter

*Changing World* • 175

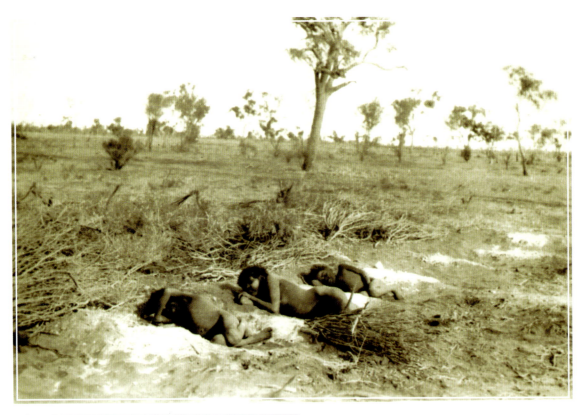

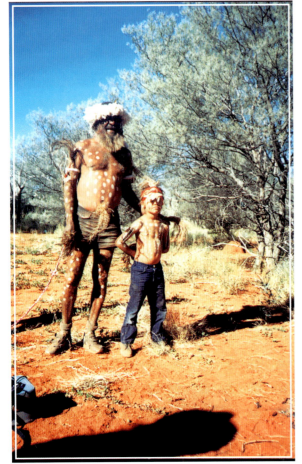

Above: Aboriginal children sleeping in trenches behind bush windbreak [undated].
PHOTOGRAPH DR CHARLES DUGUID, DUGUID COLLECTION, COURTESY SOUTH AUSTRALIAN MUSEUM, AA 79-1-1593

*As a child I remember how they warmed the earth. They put coals on the ground and warmed a beautiful bed for me and then cleared it all off and smoothed it out and lay me on it to warm me when I was getting cold. Everyone had ways of looking after each other.* Toby Minyintiri Baker

Left: Andy Tjilari and Pirpantji Rive-Nelson dance Inma Ngintaka at Atal, South Australia, 1990.
PHOTOGRAPH LINDA RIVE

*In the past grandparents, parents, uncles, brothers and sisters cared for and really looked after young children as they grew up in a way which gave them a really clear understanding of the proper way to do things ... We really want to hold on to that proper way.* Andy Tjilari

## *Everyone had ways of looking after each other*

As Rupert said, my father and his father and those generations grew up in the bush. Ngangka<u>r</u>i were responsible for the spiritual well-being and health of the whole community – all the family. They had many ways of doing that – they did a really good job.

As a child I remember how my parents warmed the earth. They put coals on the ground and warmed a beautiful bed for me and then cleared it all off and smoothed it out and lay me on it to warm me when I was getting cold. Everyone had ways of looking after each other. There were ngangka<u>r</u>i right across the Lands – as there are now – and everyone had them. In this case I was describing a situation where, in winter, when it got really cold and we didn't have blankets, that was a way of keeping warm. Without being warm and being looked after, if you had a cold and it was raining, you would get hypothermia. That was the way I was kept warm as a child and, if I got a cold, I would quickly recover. Our parents made sure we didn't get sick in those really cold or wet times.

Toby Minyintiri Baker


## *We want to hold on to that proper way*

The whole family – grandparents, parents, uncles, aunts, and brothers and sisters – play a role in growing up young children. The children grow with a really clear understanding of the proper way to do things. Children know what is right and what is wrong when they grow up in strong families with clear minds.

In the days before the aged pension we lived to a great old age and though we may have a good, clear head we may have become physically disabled. But we were cared for in our camps, by the young people, and we lived a long life.

We want to hold on to that proper way. We want to continue to help our young people learn the dangers of the world. We want our people to be able to think well and live long and healthy lives.

It's from their kurunpa, their spirit, that they learn. When young people are strong in their kurunpa and they are clear in the head, they have the strength to be able to reject negative influences and harmful habits. They can say, 'No! I want to live properly and learn well.' So it's really important that we keep helping young people to have happy and healthy spirits and a clear mind.

Andy Tjilari

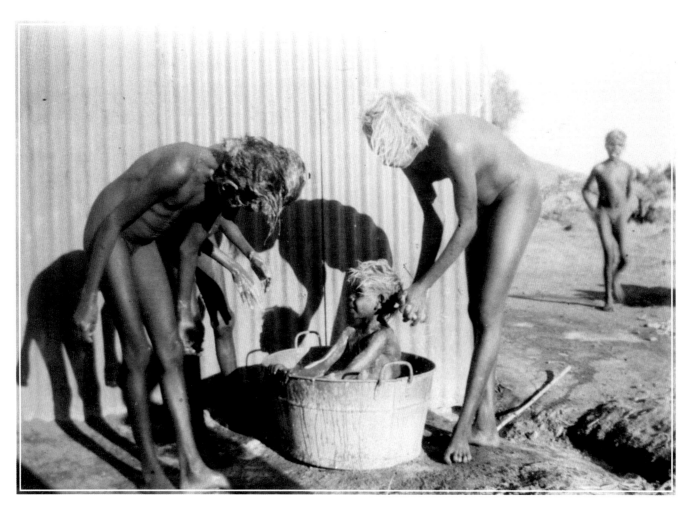

Students washing outside the shower block to catch the sun's warmth, prior to entering school, Pukatja (Ernabella), 1951. From left: Purki Edwards, Tinpulya Kangitja Mervyn (in the tub) and Tjariya Nungalka Stanley.
PHOTOGRAPH BILL ELLIOTT, ARA IRITITJA AI-0019345

*It was one Law that everyone followed*

Our way of thinking used to be really clear. It was a life that revolved around using mingkulpa, the bush tobacco, eating meat, drinking water – these were what we lived on. The whole family shared a clear understanding – all the grandparents, uncles, fathers, mothers, sons, daughters – on the proper way to look after each other. People would go and talk with each other about things, uncles would talk with their brothers and people would say, 'Great! That's what they're saying and we understand the same.' It was about the proper way of looking after each other. It was one Law that everyone followed.

Whereas now you see people a lot more isolated – living one by one – by themselves, on their own and not sharing the same understanding of what's going on. And this has come about with marijuana and drinking and petrol sniffing. So now things are a lot more mixed up. Those people that are using those substances aren't joining in and are not learning about things in the proper way. We can see that – we can see people becoming more isolated. We can see the value of the knowledge of our grandparents and of that Law and people learning it over time. It's important that people do get to learn it – and people do learn it – but some people, especially those who abuse those substances, are not joining in and not being part of that learning process.

A lot of bad things have come with the marijuana and the drinking and the sniffing. We really need to break the cycle of substance abuse in the communities. We need to get rid of those things so that people can begin to learn again the proper way of living together and being together and following a Law in the same way as their parents, grandparents learnt in the past. It's really important they get back to that and slowly learn to understand, learn about culture and the proper way of doing things and of looking after each other.

Substance abuse is causing a lot of problems. It's the wrong path to go down and people that do are really mistaken in their thinking, often very confused – it's like a rope that has frayed. Their understandings are all over the place, they are not following one Law properly.

You see with the whitefellas how parents teach their sons and daughters about work and about the proper way to live and they grow up learning about those things. In the same way, our understanding has come by way of our grandparents and parents, who have been taught the proper way and have given us a good understanding of how to live our lives. Those who are abusing those substances are not getting what has been given to us. They are not listening and understanding about that Law in the proper ways. They are using these things, the alcohol, petrol and marijuana that have come with the white people, and their understanding of things is really frayed.

Rupert Langkatjukur Peter

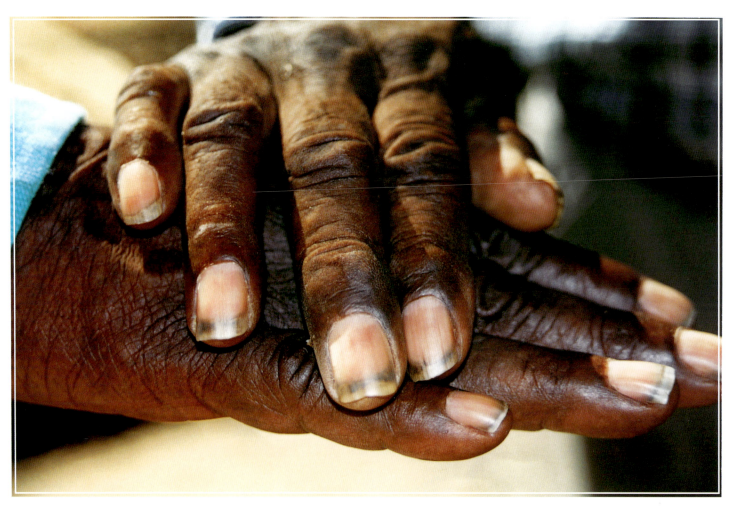

PHOTOGRAPH ANGELA LYNCH

# Ngangka<u>r</u>i Work

### *Mapa<u>n</u>pa – the force that allows us to do our work*

Our ability to heal people comes from our grandparents and they got it from their grandparents. That tradition has been passed down over a really long period of time. The powers that we have, the things that are given to us to do our healing, are the same – they are the same powers given to us through those lines.

The reasons we use them changes all the time though – the reasons people are suffering grief, the things that have actually happened, and all the new circumstances change. However, our ability to look after people and our powers have remained the same.

Those powers that are given to us are called mapa<u>n</u>pa – they can't change. They are the force that allows us to do our work. They are things that allow us to find someone's spirit and place it back within them. The reasons why they have lost their spirit change all the time. But that power to find it and place it back comes from the mapa<u>n</u>pa – they are given things. We can't change those.

Toby Minyintiri Baker


### *Mapa<u>n</u>pa or mapa<u>n</u> are 'healing tools'*

Our powers have many names: mapa<u>n</u>pa or mapa<u>n</u>, which means 'healing tools', or else it can be described as a<u>n</u>angitja or puntutja, which means 'residing in the body' or 'of the body'. Those are the words we use.

Maringka Burton

## *Kuuti are mapanpa*

Some of my kuuti come from the west. Once I travelled in a westerly direction on a marali, a Ngangkari spirit journey, and I was given some kuuti from there. Kuuti are mapanpa. That's what they are, mapanpa. Mapanpa can be made of bone. They are all mapanpa. Kanti mapanpa. Kuuti mapanpa. Puunkuninypa mapanpa. Puunkuninypa are the same, but they are black. They are the same and black. Kuuti are black also. There are thousands of kuuti available. Ngangkari go west all the time. We go there on journeys and we get meat and food from there also. We travel there and sit down there and we hear that call, 'Paaaaai!' And we have to watch out for mamu – harmful spirit beings, dangerous spirit force or energy – while we are there. We travel together for companionship and safety.

I had some wipiya, emu feathers, that my grandfather Pangkalangu gave me. The mamu that has wipiya is known as Karpirinypa. That is his name and he gives us presents freely. I am given the presents, too. We carried them around in wipiya bundles because in our days of being naked, we didn't have pockets. The presents that Karpirinypa gave us we carried around in emu-feather bundles. We never had pockets, we were naked. We couldn't carry anything unless it was in a large bundle of wipiya. We couldn't carry the bundle in our hands because we needed our hands to be free. So we would tie our bundles onto our heads with our puturu – our headbands. We'd also carry mingkulpa, wild bush tobacco, inside our feather bundles, along with extra mapanpa. In that way we could easily carry things around.

Andy Tjilari


## *Oh my goodness, he's left his mapanpa behind!*

A grandmother will give mapanpa to a granddaughter, and a grandfather will give them to a grandson. Men can give women things. The woman will give it back to her husband later. It is a husband and wife thing. Husbands and wives share things. A woman can keep a man's mapanpa for a while. A man might hide his mapanpa inside his windbreak, mapanpa ngangkari. He might put them inside for his wife to look after while he goes off hunting kangaroo. The wife will go, 'Oh my goodness, he's left his mapanpa behind!' and she'll take care of them for him while he's gone. She'll put them inside his windbreak, perhaps inside a bundle of emu feathers. A woman can help look after them while the husband is off hunting meat. She'll keep them somewhere she can keep an eye on them, to make sure they are safe, while he's gone. She'll say to herself, 'Oh look, that man has gone hunting and left his mapanpa here for me to keep an eye on! That's risky – the kids could throw them away!'

Wakupi Clem Toby (Dalby)

## It is a kind of physio work

Anangitja – that's something that belongs to you. If you say the word anangitja you are referring to your mapanpa. Wirulymankupai – that's with the hands – when you touch the body, you are massaging it. This is wirulymankupai, or making smooth. It is a kind of physio work, using oil and using irmangka-irmangka oil. We use irmangka-irmangka oil – a powerful bush medicine – when we are utilising our blowing technique, or puuni. When ngangkari use the puuni that means we are blowing air onto the head.

We make bush medicines and we use the bush medicines such as irmangka-irmangka. A lot of people use that irmangka-irmangka medicine, because it is so good for skin infections. Tiwilpa is a word meaning stiff, so if someone is tiwilarinyi and tired in the muscle, that's when we rub the muscles to make them flexible again. When we make the muscles soft we refer to that as tjulani, or to 'make soft'.

Ilawanti Ungkutjuru Ken

## Pampuni is the healing touch

Pampuni is the word we use, meaning 'touch', referring to the 'healing touch' that ngangkari gives when giving a treatment. Pampura ngangkarinanyi. It isn't *that sort* of 'touching' – it is the *healing* touch! So the first time I gave someone the healing touch, ngayulu kurunpa pampunu – this means, 'I touched their soul', or 'I touched their spirit' – what I am saying is, I touched their spirit and I did something to them, similar to synchronising everything inside them, and then I replaced their spirit. So I was a practising ngangkari then, yet I was still only a boy! After that experience I had to have a lie down to regain my own equilibrium!

Kurunpa is easy for us ngangkari. Kurunpa is visible to our eyes. Kurunpa is visible and therefore easy to treat. Kurunpa is easy to care for. Things easily get lodged in the kurunpa, though, but are easy to remove too. Things like bits of splintered stick and wood. So we give the healing touch and work on that area directly, and draw the sticks out. The kurunpa will instantly feel better and health will improve. Vomiting will cease. Some people have problems with their heads, and so we give them the healing touch on their heads and foreheads and pull the problem out of their foreheads. We pull the problems – in the form of objects – out of their foreheads and have a good look at them, and then we dispose of them.

Wakupi Clem Toby (Dalby)

## Things that cause harm and sickness

There are a range of things – sticks, bones, small stones – that are causing harm to people. These things cause people to become sick. Ngangkari have the ability to get hold of those harmful things and take them out. We can draw them from a person's body with our hands. Ngangkari can get these – but only ngangkari. We can get those harmful things out there in the bush, in the country, in the world, that cause people to get sick when others can't. If they can't be got out, then a person remains sick. These are the things that cause harm and sickness within people. In ngangkari hands they're not dangerous but they are very harmful when other people have them or if it's within someone.

Andy Tjilari

## We have equally sophisticated ways of drawing out illness

Western techniques like x-rays allow people to see into a person's body, see where an illness is, see where there are blockages that are affecting their blood flowing. Ngangkari have the same ability to see within a person, can see where something has caused the blood to stop flowing. It might be in someone's forehead in a vein, the blood has turned like a black stone. We can see that and actually draw it out, draw it out, get hold of it and take it out – without any outward signs of the operation – and get that stone that's causing the illness and show the person.

When a person's blood has stopped flowing in that way and there are blockages causing harm, you can feel their head getting really, really hot, and you can see where the blood's stopped flowing and it's dried out. They're the things that we can remove and see within people – in the same way that doctors use x-rays to assess the situation.

With Western techniques and sophisticated ways to help people by operating on them, you can see a scar that's left behind. In our case we have equally sophisticated ways of drawing out illness without leaving a sign of it. As ngangkari we have the ability to see inside someone. We are able to use our hands to get out those things that are causing the harm and help people be well again.

Western doctors have a great ability to help people with kidney disease by transplanting another good working kidney. They're very clever at that. You can see how they replace a person's kidney and connect up all the things that need to be connected so the blood flows well. That's a great ability to be able to perform transplants, operating on a person and placing another kidney within them.

As ngangkari we too can help people with kidney problems. We can feel the heat build up around the kidneys where the blood flows. I've given treatments to my family where I can draw out that heat and help them. In my granddaughter's case she had problems with her kidneys. With my hands I could feel the heat build up around the kidneys and remove that heat without operating in the way that Western doctors do. I could just draw that heat out to help her.

Rupert Langkatjukur Peter

## *Things that cause people harm ... can be removed in this way*

We work in the same way that Western doctors do. They too work with people with mental health problems whose thinking has been harmed. Western doctors work with people and have a range of techniques including operations and so on, and we work in the same way. We can see into a place where the blood has stopped flowing because the bones and arteries have joined together. We like to straighten those out, get things flowing again, and remove any bad blood which is causing those blockages, so that good blood can flow again to the person's head.

We treat a number of young people with mental health issues. Where we see that harmful things have caused blockages in their arteries in their neck, we try and open this up to get the blood flowing again. When veins have joined together we work to straighten them out and get them flowing again.

The blood can become blocked in the arteries in the neck and stop the flow of blood to the brain. This causes harm to the way people think. These harmful things can turn the blood to stone and those black stones can be removed. We can do this to help people get better and help their thinking. When the blood turns to stone and the flow gets blocked to the head, you can feel the person's head becoming really hot and the brain is damaged. When harmful things are causing the blood to be blocked, it gradually dries in this place and then becomes like stone.

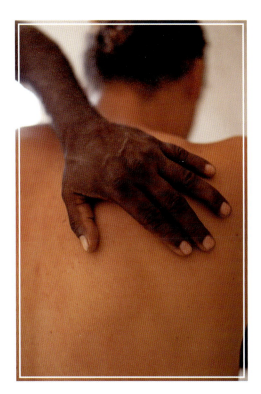

The healing touch. PHOTOGRAPH RHETT HAMMERTON

So I can get those stones which have been blocking the blood, blood that's turned to stone, and look at it and show the person and then give it to them. We show the person what we've removed and we give it to them so they can take it back to their place to show their mothers and fathers.

They have to flush it away afterwards to get rid of it. It's an important part of the process, of the Law, to get rid of it in that way, to finish it off. We say to people, 'Here, this is what we've removed. First put it in butter, and then put water on it, and in that way the stone is cooled down. And when it's cooled, that cools the person's head and in turn their body recovers. At times, ngangkari will remove those stones, show the person and then go and bury it, place it in wet earth and mud and in that way the person's head can cool down, they calm down and then they get better. After that, things are evened out and people recover.

Things which cause people harm, an illness like mental illness and other physical illnesses, can be removed in this way and shown to people and disposed of in various ways. Their heads cool down and their bodies become better, depending on the range of illnesses.

Andy Tjilari

*We can remove objects from the person*

When ngangkari are healing, we can remove harmful elements from the person who has had harm done to them. Our powers allow us to remove things that make people sick, and the way I work, my mapanpa takes the object from the person and later on it places it in my hand when it is visible and I can see it and then I can deal with it.

Ilawanti Ungkutjuru Ken

*Ngangkari can see inside people and see at night, see everything*

A person's spirit can be displaced by many things when they're frightened or startled or shocked. For example: a door slamming, a dog barking, sharp movements or people calling out – all these things can cause a spirit to be displaced, to move to where it shouldn't be. Ngangkari are the ones who have the capacity to help people re-centre the spirit and restore balance. When a person's spirit has been displaced it's only ngangkari who can put the spirit back in its right place.

Ngangkari have the capacity to see people's spirits and that allows them to restore the balance in those who have become sick. Not only can they see spirits but ngangkari can see inside people and see at night, see everything. What was given to me by my grandfather allows me to see inside, see what's causing various illnesses, to see the spirit, showing us what the cause of the problems are – to see straight and clear. In the same way that Western doctors use the x-ray, we have the power to see inside and it's come from Ngangkari Law. It's part of our Law. My grandfather placed this within me, that mapanpa – the special power – an object which has equipped me to see at night, to see inside and to understand the causes of people's illnesses.

Without ngangkari, without the power to heal being placed within people, you wouldn't be able to see the harmful spirit beings. You wouldn't be able to see them at night, you wouldn't be able to see them during the day – they'd be free to cause harm. Ngangkari have this capacity to see spirit beings and they have the capacity, which has been put within them, to heal people who have been harmed by them. Ngangkari have the knowledge and the skills to see these things. For example, if a harmful spirit being came into the camp at night and bit someone and caused them to become sick, a ngangkari could see this. They'd be able to see what had caused the illness and they'd be able to help the person recover. That was their role.

My grandfather gave me the tools and the capacity to see those harmful spirit beings and to help people in the same way he did. In his life he was an extremely knowledgeable man. He would look after his family and help his people. He would go out hunting and bring back kangaroo and give meat to the family. He'd heal people who had been harmed by the spirit beings, and when they recovered they in turn would go out hunting and give him meat. That was his life and that was his role as a ngangkari. That is the ngangkari role – to help to see these things and to help people who have been harmed by them.

Rupert Langkatjukur Peter

## This is ngangka_ri work

My work requires ma_ra a_la and ngalya a_la. This means that my hands are open and my forehead is open – and I can see things that are invisible to everyone else. If something comes towards me to do evil on me, I am ready and I can hit it. At night, I can hit it away with my powers. I see things that are invisible to others and I can banish them before they do harm. There are too many forms of these things to adequately describe. I use my hand to hit away or I get a stick and hit that bad thing that's coming towards me. I work hard all night, and then in the morning I come home for breakfast. This is ngangka_ri work.

Maringka Burton

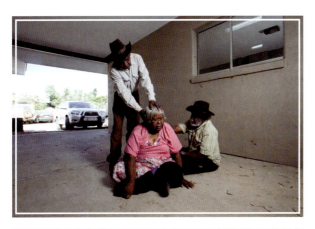

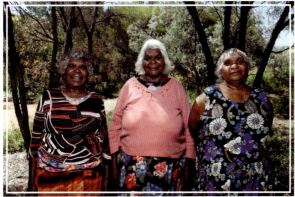

Top: Julie Anderson receives a healing treatment from Rupert Langkatjukur Peter and Toby Minyintiri Baker outside the NPY Women's Council office, Alice Springs, 2011.
PHOTOGRAPH RHETT HAMMERTON

Bottom: Three members of the NPY Women's Council Ngangka_ri Team: Ilawanti Ungkutjuru Ken, Naomi Kantjuriny and Maringka Burton, Alice Springs, 2011.
PHOTOGRAPH RHETT HAMMERTON

## Ngangka_ri work together

In essence all ngangka_ri have the same abilities and they are: to work with the spirit, to remove things, to stop blockages and a whole lot of other things to do with bush medicines and so on. But one ngangka_ri might decide a person needs another, so they will call in other help. They will call in another ngangka_ri. They will have a consultation about what needs to be done to the person or they will send that person to another ngangka_ri. Equally they might send the person to the hospital and to doctors saying, 'Look, you really need to go there'. They can work on a whole lot of different levels. Ngangka_ri should be able to work across the range of illnesses but with different levels of experience and specialities.

If we are unsuccessful in treating someone we will continue to give those treatments and we will go further and further. People won't say, 'Oh go away, you didn't do a good job!' They will say, 'Come again please, and help.' If I feel, or we feel, that it's beyond our ability, then we will advise that they see another ngangka_ri who can help them in that situation. We would call them in to work together.

If a junior ngangka_ri, someone who is just learning the work, is treating someone, they will have those same powers but they are just learning how to use them properly and they will call in some senior person to come and help them in a situation. If the person hasn't healed or they've become worse at the start, then we're asked to do more rather than less.

As a young boy living together with my father and my grandparents, I was unfamiliar with the work of a ngangka_r_i. I watched as they performed various treatments – they would give people massages and touch them and work with their spirits, replace their spirits or help people feel better in that way. So I watched. That was the first time I started to see those people at work. So I was watching and thinking about things. I wasn't a ngangka_r_i, I was observing their work, thinking they did really good work, especially with the kurunpa. I was thinking, 'I'd like to learn that.'

I have certain powers that are given to me in my hands. I am able to close off and heal those who have been treated by ngangka_r_i. I am a complementary ngangka_r_i in that way, working with other ngangka_r_i and following up on their work and using my hands in order to heal the open areas that are left after the ngangka_r_i work, and to complement their work.

The techniques I use in my area of ngangka_r_i work are using my breath and blowing and, as I have said, I heal and close off the wounds or marks left after my brother, Rupert, and other ngangka_r_i remove things from people. So that's the way we work together and they are my areas of speciality. Also part of my work is to get people's blood flowing properly within them, to level out or balance them in that way. So I work with ngangka_r_i who are removing things from people or putting things back in – I work to close off areas after that. I work to get things flowing well and get people feeling good again following treatment that they've had.

Toby Minyintiri Baker

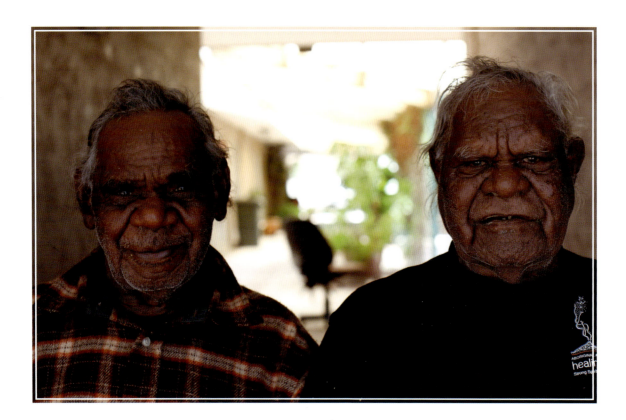

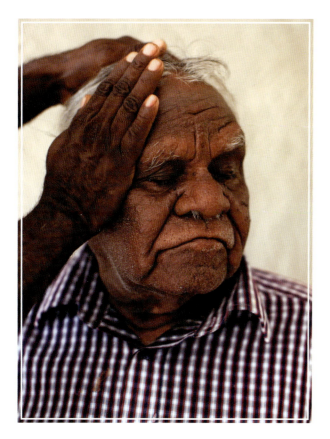

Above: Toby Minyintiri Baker receiving a ngangkari treatment from Rupert Langkatjukur Peter, Alice Springs, 2011. PHOTOGRAPH RHETT HAMMERTON

Opposite page: Rupert Langkatjukur Peter and Toby Minyintiri Baker at NPY Women's Council, Alice Springs, 2011. PHOTOGRAPH RHETT HAMMERTON

*It's been great to work alongside my friend, my brother Toby, together. It is important that we complement each other in the work ...* Rupert Langkatjukur Peter

## *We complement each other*

It's been great to work alongside my friend, my brother Toby, together. It is important that we complement each other in the work and we come across a whole range of issues we need to deal with.

Rupert Langkatjukur Peter

## *We work with the bodies but also with the mind*

We see people as a whole. Sometimes people will have physical illnesses but it will move up to the head. The treatments we can give could be related to clearing a person's head or removing the things that are causing harm there which have come from the illnesses in their body. We work with the bodies but also with the mind.

Often, if there is something that is making a person sick in their tummy, we can remove that, or blow and heal, or remove a blockage and then actually their head is also cleared after that. So we might be working on the body but the head also gets cleared that way as well. Similarly, working on the head might clear the body.

Toby Minyintiri Baker

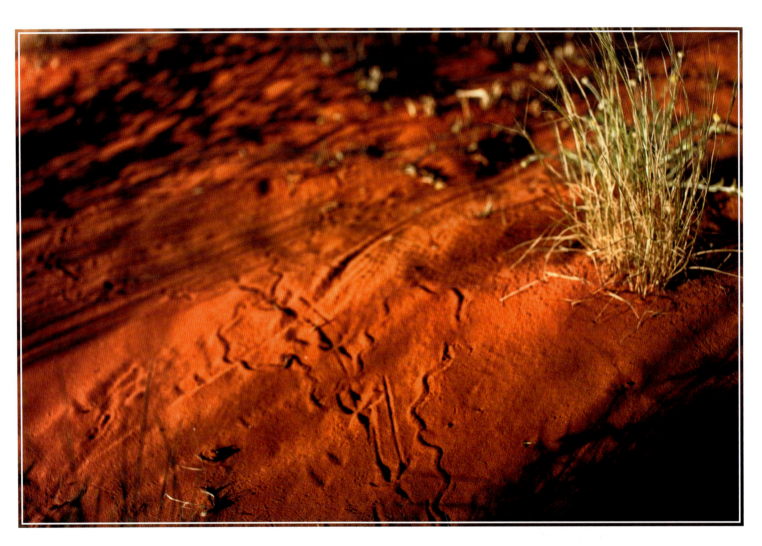

PHOTOGRAPH RHETT HAMMERTON

# Kurunpa – Spirits

## Only ngangka<u>r</u>i have the capacity to see spirits

As ngangka<u>r</u>i we can see spirits and if we are asked to give treatments we go and look. We can see the spirit. Only ngangka<u>r</u>i have the capacity to see spirits. You might know you have something wrong with you but the difference is that only ngangka<u>r</u>i can see where it is. You can't see where it is or how to get it and re-centre it. You might know you are not feeling good but ngangka<u>r</u>i have the capacity to see where and how that spirit is. So you won't be able to see your own spirit – it is invisible, in effect. They are not very big anyway, they are not as big as you are – they are actually quite small. Spirits are impossible to see if you are not a ngangka<u>r</u>i.

In essence the spirit is alive and it is you who gets sick and rundown without your spirit. But when a person is unwell the spirit is still alive, it's still well – it's just gone. If someone passes away, their spirit is still there, out there. It needs to be nurtured and looked after, but it is still alive even though the person has been placed in the earth, buried. So the spirit is not getting sick, it is the person.

Spirits are not particularly difficult to work with. If you can see them, then you can get them! They are not overly clever or trying to get away or escape you, they are just confidently themselves and they just need to be where they should be! This is where a spirit should be [Toby indicates below his sternum].

Sometimes you can see if someone's spirit has been displaced. It's still within them but it might go right up in the back or somewhere and that's when we would get it and put it back where it belongs. So things have taken the spirit's place there; for example, if the person has some other form of sickness. If there is something there that is causing a blockage, the ngangka<u>r</u>i will be able to put the spirit back, but again it will be pushed aside and will go to the wrong place so again you need to re-balance people, re-centre them in that way. So you have to deal with what's blocking it as well. Everyone has their own individual spirit. We've got ours, you've got yours, everyone has got their own. And it is only your own.

Toby Minyintiri Baker

## *Spirit is the most important thing*

Everyone has a spirit. Sometimes they can lose that spirit, become dispirited, and they can become really sick. You can see the signs of it in people vomiting and other forms of sickness or weakness. When people are sick their spirit gets displaced and they can become unbalanced because of that sickness too. We ngangkari have the ability to see that situation, to assess it, to see where their spirit's gone – often it will actually leave them or be out of place. We find that spirit and place it back within people in the right place so they are balanced again and centred. We do that with kids and also with older people too. Everyone has their spirit. It is the most important thing. Without your spirit it is really hard to get better.

Rupert Langkatjukur Peter

## *The spirit is in a relationship with the body. They are friends, they are together*

As ngangkari we really look at people's spiritual well-being – we look at how their spirit's going. If people are becoming dispirited or really exhausted, tired, unable to do things – we can recognise that in Anangu and work alongside doctors to help them.

Typically people will come to us – a mother or a father and ask, 'What do you think is wrong with my child?' A ngangkari will be able to see that that person has lost their spirit. They will be dispirited in some way and ngangkari have the capacity to see where that spirit is, where it has been displaced or gone from the person, get it and put it back within the person. It is a really important part of mental health work with people. You see, after their spirit has been returned to them and is in the right place, that they are feeling balanced, that they feel better again within their heads. They are happy and they feel good. Conversely, if we can't work on the spirit, you start to see sadness and depression and people feeling really lost.

In other situations if someone has lost their spirit and if you're giving them medicines or food, sometimes they'll just vomit the food up again or won't be able to take it down or aren't responding in that way. That's because they have lost their spirit. If we can work on that and give them back their spirit, then you'll see that food will stay down, they'll have their medicines and they will just feel a lot better about what's happening when they're ill.

If there are other things that are causing people harm we can remove them. But if we are talking about the spirit, ensuring that it's there helps people to be able to eat, to have their medicines, to hold down water, to just be a lot better. Often you'll see us at work centring people again, putting their spirit back where it belongs.

One of the reasons people lose their spirit is shock, and that can be on a whole number of levels. It can be as simple as being deeply asleep and people calling out. The spirit itself gets a fright when you are asleep and it leaves. The person wakes up and they've lost their spirit in that way. Spirits leave people because there are things that are scaring them, scaring the spirit. Also the spirit might leave someone or be displaced when they have other illnesses or are sick in some other way. And again their friends or others might come and get them and get the ngangkari and say, 'Look this person is really sick, could you have a look at them?' and we'll see that the spirit has been affected by the other illness.

The spirit is in a relationship with the body. They are friends, they are together. If the body is starting to get affected by something, the spirit feels that and feels really upset by that. Sometimes if the sickness or the disease is spreading through the body, in particular to where the spirit is, it will get displaced. It will actually go – it will leave. And that's when we need to come back and deal with the sickness as well, in order to create the room and the space for the spirit to be there properly again.

Toby Minyintiri Baker

## *Kurunpa need returning to the owner's body and this work keeps ngangkari busy*

Kurunpa travel around. Kurunpa call to people. A kurunpa calls out so people know where it is, to let them know it is close by, while they are sleeping. When people are deeply asleep, sometimes their spirit leaves their bodies, especially if they've had a scare. When this happens ngangkari hear the call of the spirit of the sleeping person, and they go to that person needing help. They help the person during the night using their specialised 'open head' technique. The ngangkari have special eyesight, like torches, and they can see in the dark. They see the kurunpa shining like a light and so they just go and capture it during the night. The kurunpa travel along at ground level, or they may ascend into a tree. Sometimes there are many kurunpa around, cut loose from their owners, lurking in the bush. All these kurunpa need returning to the owner's body and this work keeps ngangkari busy. They'll go and get them and restore them quickly. Everyone has a kurunpa. If the kurunpa departs the body, be it only briefly, it can bring on a bout of vomiting. As soon as it is returned, sickness departs. Ngangkari return it to the body, and when the kurunpa is correctly positioned, the person enjoys good health. Ngangkari know the exact spot and know what to do.

You know if your spirit has gone because there may have been a scare of some sort, which causes the kurunpa to jump out of the body, and the person to cry out. You can feel it. You'll not feel well, and you'll probably start vomiting and vomiting. We all know the dangers of vomiting. The call will go out for a ngangkari straight away: 'Here's someone in need! Quick, come and heal them!' Ngangkari will come over straight away and rectify the problem. If there is no vomiting, the kurunpa stays put. If the kurunpa has departed for whatever reason, vomiting will definitely follow.

Wakupi Clem Toby (Dalby)

*White doctors don't know about what the spirit does*

White doctors don't know about what the spirit does. I am able to pick up kurunpa. Oh yes, I catch those spirits too. White doctors don't know about what the spirit does. They don't know what it does.

People sicken through loss of spirit. They improve as soon as their spirit picks up. But loss of spirit weakens and weakens a person until they are dangerously frail.

Pantjiti Unkari McKenzie

## Mamu – harmful spirit beings

*We see mamu clearly with our ngangka̲ri eyes*

Some white people don't understand about mamu. A long time ago, a lot of huge mamu were around, before white people came. And today there are still mamu around. Like devils, they're in the sky, they travel around and they look down at us, yet they are invisible to most people. People don't see them but they're here. They're still here. We see them clearly with our ngangka̲ri eyes. They are visible to us ngangka̲ri. We can see them really clearly, whereas people without ngangka̲ri power can't see them. Those mamu, they're there all the time. They come and they take people's spirits away. Why do the mamu do that? Because they don't like people, that's why. They come and they want to destroy humans and they get angry and nasty for humans.

My family members and my father's brother, Nuyumpakunu, used to see mamu clearly. And when the mamu take something, or take off with a kurunpa, those old ngangka̲ri could break their 'string', meaning the stringy access tracks that mamu have. Ngangka̲ri can destroy its access track with their mapa̲npa and the mamu will fall down with the spirit that it's just stolen, and then the ngangka̲ri can retrieve the kurunpa and give it back. So with our mapa̲npa we can follow a mamu and be travelling along on its road and destroy its path ahead of it, causing it to fall and drop the spirit that it has stolen from someone. Mamu can come down from the sky on strings. Ngangka̲ri cut the strings and cut off their escape. Then we capture them and kill them with mapa̲npa.

Mamu have their own access ways, which are like their own roads, or tracks. They have their roads – mamuku iwara. That's why you have to destroy their roads so that you can decrease the numbers of mamu travelling around. Ngangka̲ri have fire too. The mamu access roads can be destroyed by a ngangka̲ri because we've got powers that we can use and fires to burn their way as well. We can throw a power that cuts off their road and burn it. It is better that we destroy the road, it's important. Healers can do that, ngangka̲ri can do that. They can destroy the roads. It's like a string, the mamu's road. It is similar to a man's headband, a pu̲tu̲ru, made of strings, which are easily cut.

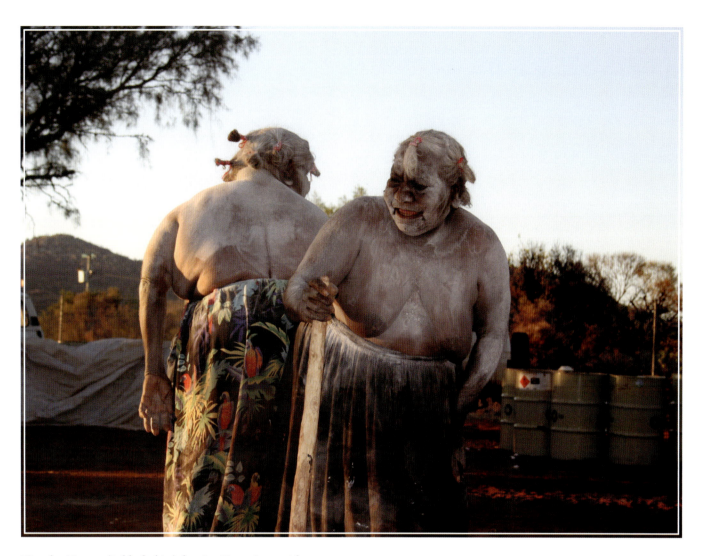

Tinpulya Mervyn (in black skirt) dancing Mamu Inma with her sister Wipana Jimmy, during the farewell for Amanda Dent and Brian Hallett at Nyapari, October 2011.
PHOTOGRAPH AMANDA DENT

In the Old Parliament House a long time ago there once lurked the spirit of a man who worked in the office there. He was nasty, and he didn't like Aboriginal people, in fact he didn't like whitefellas either. He was a nasty man. That person had a mamu spirit. Some people wanted to get rid of him, so they called ngangkari in to clear the area, which they did. They knew something was there.

In Adelaide, there are lots of mamu and ghosts. We have seen mamu in some houses. The spirits of the deceased hang around in the same house, in their own house. There are hundreds of spirits in Adelaide. Those people who bought a house, lived there and died and the others after them. We'd see all the spirits there. The spirits live around there because that's their home, and they stay there. Some people's houses are fine, but in other people's houses, where they are not Christians, they have a lot of mamu. There are a lot of mamu lurking close by. But people who are Christian don't have monsters lurking. A Christian household can repel mamu.

Toby Minyintiri Baker

## We have to rid our living areas of mamu

One of the most important tasks we have is to rid our living areas of mamu. We also have to deal with the dead and their departing spirits, make sure they do not go astray. We have to watch the winds. We realise that the hot western winds – the piriya – always bring new mamu in on the dust. They aggravate people's eyes and make them sick. Ngangkari are very busy during the hot, dusty, windy times. We use our hands to heal. Children cry in distress when they are not well. They are frightened of piriya winds because of the mamu, and we are always cautious of those winds because of that.

Andy Tjilari

## Mamu can take people's spirits away

Sometimes you can lose your spirit. There are harmful things out there which we call mamu which are causing harm. They are not your spirit, not kurunpa spirit. They are harmful beings which cannot be seen in the normal way, but ngangkari can see them.

For example, if there is a child, the mamu is seeing that child and it can take a child's spirit away. And that's another way you can lose your spirit. So this mamu has a path it travels to where it wishes to cause harm – it is thinking about doing that and it takes whatever it wants to take, the spirit of the child in this case. So the ngangkari that are called to deal with that situation actually recognise the way that the harmful force is coming into that person's life and, in effect, break the track of it. They physically cut the line so that the mamu, that harmful thing, can't get to that person. And then they deal with what needs to be done based on the problem that the mamu has caused. They will obviously get the spirit and put it back in the child if it was taken by that mamu. On one level it is spiritual, but on another it is physical. Then you will see the child heal and they will be able to feel good again.

Toby Minyintiri Baker

## What does it look like?

When we say we ngangkari can see the mamu – what does it look like, the mamu? Well, a mamu is a bit like a dog. It is a big size, like a big but skinny dog. A skinny dog-like mamu eats people and becomes fat. A mamu pussycat can also turn on people and become a big mamu and kill and eat people. The mamu cat and mamu dog can eat a person's spirit. However, a ngangkari is able to see a mamu over there eating the spirit of a person and that person's body can be still, not moving, because it's being eaten by a mamu.

Sam Wimitja Watson

## *Ngangkari have that role of getting people's kurunpa*

Right from the early days, mamu have entered camps and taken away the kurunpa of children. It causes the child to [Andy makes a puffing sound] like that. The kurunpa is crying out, the spirit cries out as it's being taken away, far away, during the night.

Ngangkari would traditionally block those mamu so they couldn't take people's spirits away during the night. Those mamu don't kill or hurt the person's spirit. They just put it down and leave it when the ngangkari block its escape route and then those ngangkari then hold on to the kurunpa, looking after it. They travel as spirit beings themselves to retrieve the spirit. The ngangkari then get that kurunpa and put it back in the child to straighten things up and bring them back to health again.

It can happen to anyone or everyone, older people, teenagers, men and women. For example, long ago when I was a child, I saw it happen to my grandfather. I saw my grandfather and heard him crying out – he nearly died! A ngangkari blocked the mamu from taking his kurunpa away, and he put his kurunpa back within my grandfather and he recovered. He was really well. This is a story from the really early days, the days before there were hospitals, aeroplanes or aerodromes. The ngangkari looked after people and cared for people and this was how things were understood. We hold onto that knowledge of how to look after the well-being of our people. It's knowledge that our fathers, our elder brothers and others held on to. This is the Law, knowledge and understanding that our grandfathers looked after. We hold onto that knowledge and Law, all of it.

When a child cried out as its kurunpa was being taken away, the ngangkari could see what was happening and obstruct the path of that mamu, get that spirit and place it back within the person, so that they'd get better again. When a child's spirit had been taken away the child became really sad, depressed, it would cry, be vomiting, lying there. If the child was given water they would vomit it up again because they didn't have their kurunpa.

If a kurunpa has been taken away by those mamu, the ngangkari from another place travel as a spirit being through the night and return that kurunpa to the base of a tree near the camp where the child is. Ngangkari travel as spirit beings and find and return the kurunpa and place it near the camp. Early the next morning the ngangkari in camp see that the kurunpa has been placed there at the base of that tree, and get it and place it back within the sick child.

Without its spirit a child becomes really sick, weakened, and becomes thin. The ngangkari places the spirit back within that child to help it recover and says, 'Let's really carefully and slowly give that child water, water and breast milk together.' Gradually that spirit settles back into its proper place within that child. There is a balance within that child again, they recover and are healthy. Ngangkari work like this.

Ngangkari have that role of getting people's kurunpa. It might be because they've lost their kurunpa or when someone has become really sick, incapacitated and is dying, the ngangkari have a role in getting that spirit and repositioning it in the person. Mamu haven't taken their spirit away in that situation – as the person has become more incapacitated and is dying, their spirit has left them and is nearby.

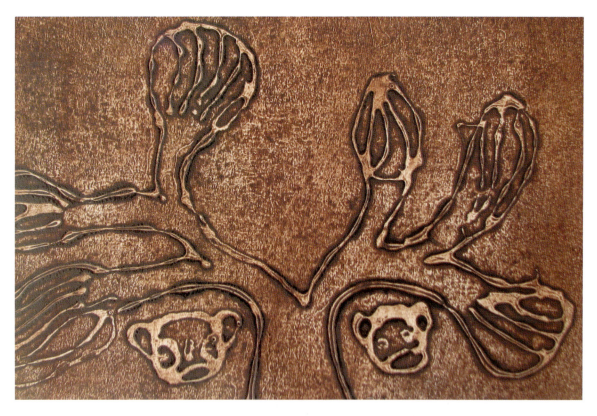

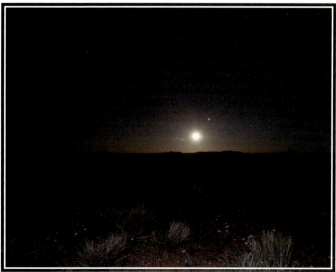

Top: Kanakiya Tjanyari, *Mamu*, 2007. Collograph on paper, 25 x 36 cm.
PHOTOGRAPH HELEN JOHNSON, © THE ARTIST, COURTESY IWANTJA ARTS AND CRAFTS

Bottom: Night sky at Wingellina, 2011.
PHOTOGRAPH RHETT HAMMERTON

When a person dies, at that time that the kurunpa leaves their body and goes to sit, we ngangkari have a role in capturing that spirit. The body is there and the kurunpa sits nearby, though the kurunpa itself is happy. As ngangkari we get that kurunpa and take it and place it within a close family member; for example, the brother or someone who can look after it. That close family member – brother, partner or grandson – has a good feeling about being the one to hold onto and look after the kurunpa of that deceased person. They hold it within themselves and they are happy and go about hunting, telling good stories and laughing and being with people, they feel good and proud to have it within them. They feel well and their thinking is good and the person who is holding onto the kurunpa of the person who has passed away nourishes that spirit. When they eat well, are satisfied and full, that kurunpa is also nourished with food, with water, with meat and feels good too.

Those mamu, those harmful spirit beings, can cause sickness and spoil things that have been really good and the ngangkari can remove them and things get better after that. Only ngangkari have the capacity to see these mamu, to get them and remove them. Sometimes those mamu can enter people's heads with the intention of spoiling the way that they think. The person can be thinking well, speaking well, be looking after themselves, and the mamu can enter their head and spoil their thinking with bad stories and thoughts. Their thinking has been hurt by a mamu. Ngangkari have a role in removing those things which cause a person's thinking to go bad. We ngangkari can work with these people to heal them and help them get better. After those harmful things have been removed, during the night the person's thinking improves, and in the morning they have much more clarity.

Andy Tjilari

## It scares a person's true spirit away

Mamu are harmful spirit beings that can take a person's spirit away, though a shock or being shaken by something can cause their spirit to go too. In these cases harmful spirits can enter a person's body. When those harmful beings go into a person's or child's body they can cause great sickness. When that mamu enters a person's body and goes to their belly it scares a person's true spirit away. It can go back behind and into the shoulder or to another place within the person's body where it sits, downcast, thinking and worrying about where it should be. And you can see the signs of this in a person's body – wasting away, they get thinner and, as that spirit becomes sadder and sadder, that person becomes more withdrawn and downcast.

When that kurunpa is back in its true place within the person, there's a great sense of relief and the spirit's happy again to be where it belongs. The person is happy, relaxed, taking in the fresh air again, whereas before they just smelt the really foul sweat of that mamu within them. That foul-smelling mamu causes the person's head to become really hot and they drip with sweat. When we feel their head we can feel how hot they are and we know that mamu is inside them. And when we re-centre their spirit and put it back where it belongs we can feel their head cool down. It's as if they're in a cool, fresh breeze again and their spirit is happy. When we ngangkari have re-centred a person's spirit, we feel their head cooling down and they're calm and we know that they've recovered their sense of self, that they're happy again.

Andy Tjilari

## Marali – Spirit Journey

### *Ngangkari have the ability to travel as spirit beings*

Ngangkari have the ability to travel as spirit beings. Only ngangkari have this knowledge of how to travel as spirit beings. I learnt how to do this. The knowledge of how to do this, for my spirit to be able to travel – not my body but my spirit – was passed down to me by all those old ngangkari in the old days. As a child, my spirit travelled, I was taught how to do it by that older generation of men. So my spirit travelled and travelled in those old days with those old men. As an older man I myself now can do many good things with this. We are doing many good things.

Andy Tjilari

### *We call it marali – our spirit body – and it travels*

The ngangkari travel and they also work together in groups. On another level ngangkari can heal someone by having their own spirit travel. The spirit of the ngangkari itself can travel independently or in a group, and they will go to heal or help someone and return to their bodies during the day. That's another way of travelling and helping people.

We call it marali – our spirit body – and it travels. Only ngangkari can do this and it's like being in a helicopter or an aeroplane. Vision is very clear and we go into the sky far, far away. We go to a sacred place, to a place where the ngangkari gather in order to make assessments and work out what's wrong. We consult each other.

We will fly to assess certain situations and see what needs to be done or treat someone by looking at them, but we will still have to go and do the treatment after this. We often go to that place where we consult and confer and see what needs to be done, but we still have to go and treat the patient in person afterwards.

Toby Minyintiri Baker

## My spirit was flying like a bird

Up in the night sky are many twinkling stars and the Tjukalpa – the Milky Way. Tjukalpa is like a ladder. It is made up of stars. Stars are kililpi. I went on marali with Mr Miller's grandfather. My old grandfather took me on marali. He took me on marali and taught me many things, gave me very valuable training. I was surprised at how much like a bird I felt. My spirit flew with my old grandfather. I was flying like a bird. My spirit was flying like a bird. That wonderful old man taught me so much on those journeys. Sometimes I would get nervous if I lost sight of the ground and the earth, and I would wonder how far or how high we would be going, but my old grandfather always gave me confidence to keep going. We would soar to and fro. My kurunpa would sometimes get scared but I held on. My grandfather always looked after me.

Tjukalpa is composed of thousands of kililpi, stars. Tjukalpa is made up of stars. Ngangkari go to that place. Everyone can see it but we go there. We are taken there by the hand by the senior ngangkari. It is exciting training but vitally important if we want to understand the way of the ngangkari. Mapanpa can look like little bits of bone. I had some bone mapanpa inserted into my forehead. Only after that could I go on marali. We give the appearance of lying down with our eyes shut, looking like we are asleep, but really we are flying in spirit up to the stars. We also collect kuuti. Kuuti are mapanpa.

Bernard Tjalkuriny

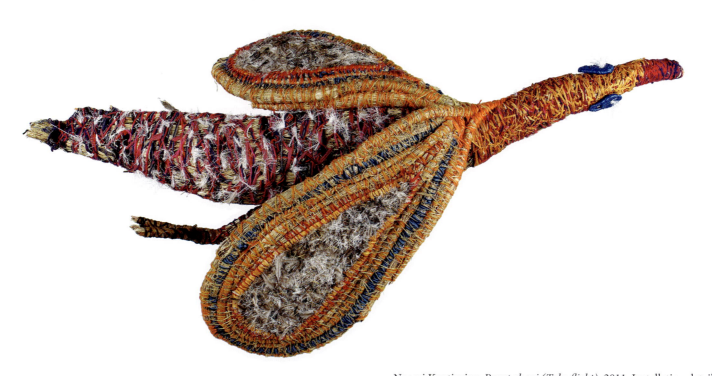

Naomi Kantjuriny, *Paarpakani (Take flight)*, 2011. Installation detail 'Deadly: in-between heaven and hell' exhibition Tandanya NACI and Adelaide Festival, 2012. Raffia, minnarri grass, poly-raffia, wool, emu feathers, wire, 30 x 65 x 150 cm. PHOTOGRAPH MICK BRADLEY, COURTESY THE ARTIST

## We travel to fantastic places

When we travel on marali journeys, it is really beautiful. We travel to fantastic places and sometimes after travelling a long way away, sometimes we come back too quickly – if, say, a dog barked, it may have disrupted our spiritual travel, which causes the kurunpa to suffer a minor shock. This may cause it to halt away from the body. That's how some people get sick, and how we healers can get sick ourselves. That's when my brother will come and heal me and say, 'Oh, your kurunpa is somewhere else!' So he works to reunite me with my own kurunpa. So that sort of thing can happen to us sometimes.

Many people travel on marali spirit journeys together. We travel up into the sky and journey to other places in the spiritual plane, and we meet other healers there. I used to travel with my brother a lot, and with other healers from other communities as well. Our spirits all meet and travel together high up, and for great distances. It can even be a bit scary, but when we are together we feel safe. I still travel on these spirit trips. We can travel and can see people going about their everyday life. You see, we travel to their homes. Sometimes it can be quite wonderful. You can't really tell whether it was a dream, or whether you really did go on that trip. It is a really good feeling. A lot of ngangkari people do that, and travel around together. It is a really beautiful thing to do. It is not my own skill or experience. It is an Anangu experience – a shared experience that binds us Anangu together.

Sometimes I'd say to my brother, 'You know, I just saw something?' and he'd say, 'Yes, I think you have seen it on your travels'. We can see things that others can't see. People who aren't healers can't see them, people who are not ngangkari.

Ilawanti Ungkutjuru Ken

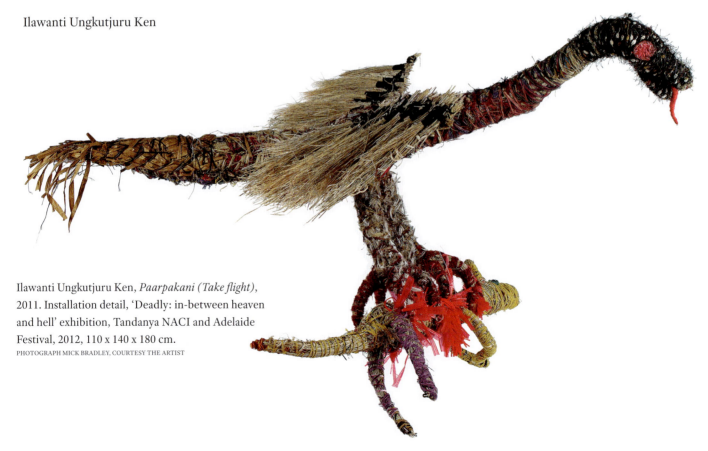

Ilawanti Ungkutjuru Ken, *Paarpakani (Take flight)*, 2011. Installation detail, 'Deadly: in-between heaven and hell' exhibition, Tandanya NACI and Adelaide Festival, 2012, 110 x 140 x 180 cm.
PHOTOGRAPH MICK BRADLEY, COURTESY THE ARTIST

*We perform a beautiful service to people while on our journeys*

We ngangkari always travel on spirit journeys. Our bodies are sleeping but our spirits travel on long journeys. We are invisible, as it is just our kurunpa that are travelling. We perform a beautiful service to people while on our journeys, because we find people who are unwell and in need of our help. We come back to our bodies in the morning and then we go around to see them and give the help that they require. What a beautiful thing to do! Sometimes I travel around by myself and other times I travel with other healers, including my sister Lynette, or other ngangkari.

Maringka Burton

*I can't help it ... my thoughts go out to them*

I go on marali journeys, absolutely! I go often. If someone near me is very ill, I can't help it – as soon as I fall asleep, my thoughts go out to them and I begin my marali journey. While on that journey I heal the sick person and I remove whatever thing is inside them, causing the sickness. Even dangerous illnesses I can heal. Even something rattling around in the body, like a loose bone, I can retrieve and remove as necessary. Sicknesses sometimes lodge in someone's bones, which is very dangerous, especially if it is close to the heart. In this case I work around their heart area. We always have good reason to worry if the heart is involved in some illness, in case it gets worse. This is when I go on marali, so I can deal with heart issues before they get worse. Women ngangkari go on marali, even child ngangkari go on marali, before they are even fully fledged. They all go on marali, mostly together. Their ngangkari grandfather will probably take them on marali, or their ngangkari father will be the one who will take a child ngangkari on a marali journey. They'll take young girls too. We all do this. I take my granddaughter and teach her about marali. I have taken my son. He did well, as I had taught him well.

Pantjiti Unkari McKenzie

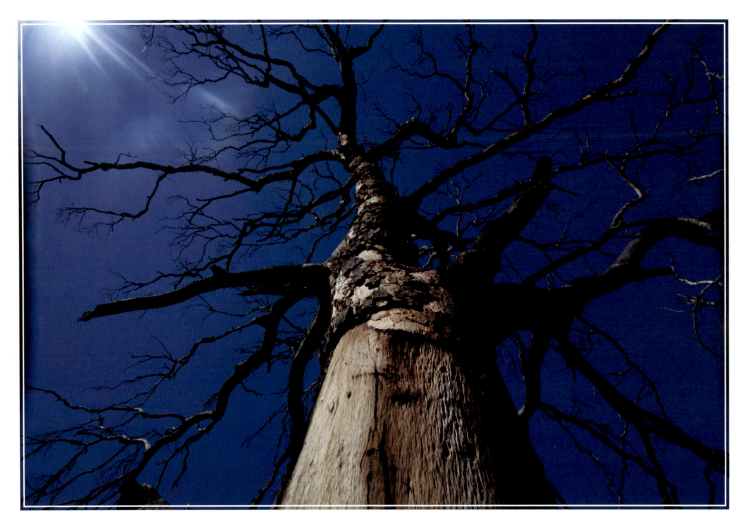

Kurkara (desert oak) near Warakurna. PHOTOGRAPH RHETT HAMMERTON

# Grief, Death, Dying

## *You are looking after it because it's family*

If someone passes away their spirit is out there, waiting, alone. The goal is to place it with the appropriate person so that it is nurtured and looked after. That could be, depending on the relationship of the person who passed away, an elder sister, mother or appropriate family member. They have to look after the spirit of that person. It is not something that displaces your own spirit when it is given to you, it sits in there with you. You are looking after it because it is family. For example, in the case where a partner has passed away you will see the person who is left behind, for example the wife, is just at home, really restless, not capable of sleeping, is really disturbed and really worried about things, unable to be comfortable. It is the spirit of the man who has passed away coming back and really trying to communicate with his wife. That's when the bereaved wife will come to us and say, 'Look, the spirit of my partner has come back. It's there. It's really unsettled and I am really bothered by it – could you do something?' That's when we will get that spirit and place it in the partner to be able to be looked after. So then the spirit is not bothering that person in effect, it is being looked after and it's happy again.

Toby Minyintiri Baker

## *It's important spirits are placed with the right person*

After accidents in which people have been killed the spirit will leave the body and go to a nearby tree, a place where it can shelter and find shade. It will be waiting there. Ngangka<u>r</u>i come at night to locate that spirit and bring it back. They might say, 'Can you see that? What is that up in the tree?' and then they can see it.

It might be that someone's partner has passed away. The spirit will be returned and placed within the spouse to be cared for and looked after. When that spirit is put inside the surviving partner then we say to them, 'For a period of time don't drink anything too hot, just have really warm tea and nothing that could hurt that spirit, because it has just come within you now.' This is because initially when the spirit is placed in a person it can be quite weak and if you have really hot drinks or things that could shock that spirit, it might 'finish it off.' So it's important to nurture it, let it settle in and become strong again. And so for a period of time it's important to have cool drinks and warm food, not really hot stews and things like that, until the spirit has settled and things have evened out. It allows the person's spirit to be balanced and that other spirit to be nurtured rather than to be shocked, to become stronger until things are even within that person again.

A spirit can become weakened and get really thin and this is when you can see hair growing on it – you can see that they're getting weak. The opposite happens when you look after it and place it to sit alongside in the spirit of the living person.

So in the case of a brother who is really sad, you place the spirit of his deceased elder brother within him, and he feels happy again and clear. He feels the same sort of way that he'd felt in the past when the two brothers played together as children and shared that one spirit of togetherness.

Those spirits of people who have passed away and of ancestors can't just be placed with any family member. It's important they are placed with the right person: those that they shared a bond with as children, those that are really close, part of their true spirit.

Rupert Langkatjukur Peter

## *The spirit is scared of what is happening*

If there is an accident, and there has been a death, a ngangkari will go and fetch that person's kurunpa from the area, but that happens a bit later at the burial site. The kurunpa goes into hiding. At the cemetery, the kurunpa stays around, hiding in nearby trees and bushes and there it remains for one or two months. After that time has elapsed, many people will go together to the cemetery and the kurunpa will be recaptured and placed inside the surviving spouse to keep inside his or her own kurunpa. This is an ancient practice of ours, coming from ancient times. In the past, people would gather together after two months had elapsed, in order to carry out this task. The ngangkari will be ready in advance and waiting and in position to carry out this special work, to locate and capture the kurunpa. He will have captured it already and will be there ready to place it into the surviving spouse when she arrives. He will be there, holding that kurunpa. The spouse will arrive and she will sit down and the kurunpa will quickly be placed inside her body. It happens quickly. We do this to hold onto the spirit and to keep it for all time.

When someone falls ill with a particular kind of sickness, or if something hidden becomes lodged inside them and makes them weak and ill and their health begins to fail, when a ngangkari on marali spots that, the next day they'll come as quickly as possible to see them. But sometimes it happens that they are too late. If they are too late, and the sickness is too deeply embedded and the ngangkari realises he is unable to see it, because it is too hidden, he'll never say the words, 'Oh dear, it looks like I'm too late. This person is going to die'. They'll never say that. They'll say, 'Your kurunpa is out of sight right now,' but they'll tell other people that the person is going to die very soon. The people, on hearing this, know it to be true, and that nothing can be done. This is how someone would die in years gone by, before hospitals came along.

Upon death, the kurunpa departs the body. It departs the body and moves to a location not far away. It won't return and the person is then dead, lying on the ground. The kurunpa has already departed and so the person dies after that. The person dies because the kurunpa has departed the body. All ngangkari treatments fail at this point. Too late. They'll be too late. This can happen at any time; in the middle of the night or the middle of the day, they'll just fall asleep and die.

The spirit is scared of what is happening and it will flee away and hide. Nobody can find it again apart from a skilled ngangkari, who will go and look for it shortly afterwards, usually at night. At night they'll find it and bring it back upon their shoulders. They'll bring it back home. They'll go on foot and find that spirit. They'll also dig the grave. That requires a lot of work, it is a big job, especially in the days before we had shovels. We only had wira to dig graves before, wooden dishes. They'd have to carry the body to the grave and place it in the hole. It used to be a lot of work. No shovels. Lay the body inside, place lots of tjanpi grasses and spinifex on top, and on top of that, a great pile of branches. They also put many strong branches inside the grave, to stop dingoes from digging it up. They block it up completely. On top of that the soil is put back and a large mound is made on top. This is an early-days cemetery. Our traditional graves were made like that. Our grandfathers are buried like this.

The kurunpa is nearby, hidden not far away. It is not far away but it is totally separated from the body now, and will never return to re-animate the body, that never happens. It is outside now. A ngangkari's job is to come and find that spirit later.

Wakupi Clem Toby (Dalby)

### It stays nearby in a tree

When someone dies their kurunpa leaves the body but it stays nearby in a tree, on the tree trunk. Nowadays we are churchgoers and the spirit departs with the body. But in the past, the kurunpa would stay around, attached to the trunk of a tree waiting to move into the surviving spouse. It is the job of the wati ngangkari – initiated male ngangkari – to put the kurunpa into the surviving spouse. He will take his miru, spear thrower, and pick up the kurunpa with his miru. This is men's business to do this, using his miru. He will take a woman's kurunpa and put it into the surviving man or take a man's kurunpa and place it into the surviving woman's body. She will receive her husband's kurunpa. It is usual for the spouse to receive his or her departed spouse's kurunpa.

Pantjiti Unkari McKenzie

### Many people suffer grief and we help them

Once a woman asked to see us who was having great difficulty sleeping after the loss of her partner. We spoke with her and her family, and we could see that the spirit of her partner and the loss of her partner was the cause of her grief and her worries.

Rupert was able to locate the spirit of that person, her partner. After death, the spirit will stay close to home, where the family is. After talking with the family it was agreed that Rupert should place the spirit back within the bereaved spouse so that she could look after the spirit of the partner in that way – she would feel good again, and did. They spoke with the sons and daughters about who would properly hold onto the spirit of that person. Rupert found where it was – it will always be close to home there – and placed it within the person and healed her grief in that way.

It wasn't just that one case – there are many people who have asked us to help them in situations of loss. There were sons and daughters too who asked us why they were feeling the way they were. We saw those people's spirits, found where they were and helped place them in the bereaved people as well. Many people suffer grief and we help them by looking after the spirits of those they love, or putting them back in those who can care for them.

The spirit is still part of the home after there's a death and often it will be close to that place, but it belongs there. But if it's not 'at home' in effect, if it's not being nurtured, then people are going to get sick. We heal them and get them better by finding it.

Toby Minyintiri Baker

## *Ngangkari try and help to bring about peace*

In the past, if someone in the family passed away, people were stricken by grief and they would be throwing stones and hitting themselves on their own pulyku, sinew. I did this to myself when I lost my own daughter. I shouldn't have, but I did. Too sad. It is too sad and we don't know what to do with ourselves, so we hurt ourselves. In the past we used to cut ourselves on the head in sheer grief. Our mothers used to do that. If you have lost a daughter you'll understand. Ngangkari try and help to bring about peace. They help to heal the wounds on the head. Sometimes people damage their own skulls, if they hit themselves too hard, and this is terribly serious. Ngangkari have to work hard then, fixing the crushed skulls. Women feel grief too keenly if they lose one of their own children, as I did. I can't talk about it any more. Too sad.

Pantjiti Unkari McKenzie

## *That was an important role of the ngangkari too, in helping that grieving*

In the old days, people would be really sad and depressed when they lost a family member through violence or if a mamu had harmed a family member. You could see them become weak and lying and sitting around, not moving, losing appetite. And it was only ngangkari that had the capacity to treat those people and heal them, to remove harmful spirits that had entered their body, banish them, to cleanse and to help them heal and recover.

If a man passed away, the whole camp, all the men, the women and the children that were living there, would move to another place and be crying tears and sadness. The men, the women and the kids would be crying through the day, crying through the night. It was a really sad time when someone passed away. The great sadness, the constant weeping when someone had lost a relative, lost a child or a niece, a young person. The whole camp would be really saddened and move.

In another situation when a man passed away who couldn't be healed there was great misery amongst the family in the camp. All the men, all the women and all the children would cry – they'd cry through the day, cry through the night, overcome with grief. They would leave that place where the person had passed away – for up to a year or more – over a summer. They would live in another place and still be grieving for that person.

After a period of time the in-laws would assess that it was right to return to the spot. And with ngangkari they would go back to where the person had died and they would look for the kurunpa of that person. The ngangkari would use a spear thrower to help them find it. It might be in a tree near where that person had been buried. They'd capture that kurunpa and they'd take it and put it in the partner of that person. And she would then look after and nourish the kurunpa of her partner who had passed away. And initially they'd have to eat cool foods and cold meats and cool water to help nourish that spirit and it would live healthily and well within the partner. And that was an important role of the ngangkari too, in helping that grieving.

If a young, unmarried person passed away who didn't have a spouse, immediate family members could hold onto and look after a spirit. So a younger brother's spirit might be placed inside the older brother to look after.

Ngangkari used spear throwers as part of their work. In returning to the burial place the two ngangkari would have a spear thrower and they would use it. The kurunpa of the person who passed away would come towards them and keep on coming and eventually sit in the hand of the ngangkari. It would be waiting to be put into the family member who had come back to that site. The ngangkari would call out to them – they'd be at a distance – and the family member who was to have and to hold the kurunpa of that man would be called over and he'd come and they'd place it within the person and say, 'Don't eat hot meats or have hot drinks for a few days. Only have cold water and cool foods so that the kurunpa can be well.' And that was the way that the spear thrower was used.

Rupert Langkatjukur Peter

## *We would hear the kurunpa calling out*

We have a very important task when someone passes away. There is a certain smell emanating from a dead body and the person has to be buried properly to deal with this. Their body has to be protected by a strong, good grave. We have to recapture their spirit, and then their spirit is bestowed upon a surviving close relative. As you can see, our culture is quite different. We have many interesting but important practices, such as capturing a kurunpa with the use of a spear thrower. We would hear that kurunpa calling out and my brother would hold his spear thrower, hoping to catch that spirit. When someone dies we leave everything of theirs behind. We do not touch it ever again. I work with mamu and I have had a lifetime of experience with mamu

Bernard Tjalkuriny

## *Our job is to capture that spirit*

Our job is to capture that kurunpa. We do it with our miru. Many ngangka<u>r</u>i will help to get that spirit. As many ngangka<u>r</u>i as there are around will all be involved in that family activity, capturing that kurunpa. Children see it as well. My brother and I would work together. We are there in the presence of our relatives, listening out for that calling of the kurunpa. We hold our spear throwers, hoping to catch that spirit, which we do eventually. A grave is the work of the relatives, but ngangka<u>r</u>i are always involved. Many people are involved in burials.

Andy Tjilari

## *Older people are cared for and looked after properly until it is their time to pass away*

As a person becomes older, and their kurunpa becomes tired, they lose the energy to be able to do things. He or she will be cared for in camp; given a good shelter: given meat and water, have firewood brought, and generally be cared for and looked after properly until it is their time to pass away. And at that time you see them as helpless as when they were young babies. As their time approaches and arrives they are quiet and calm, not angry and calling out, not thinking in a confused way, just clear and calm and they feel really free and happy – relaxed to be in that state, not critical nor blaming people – they feel free.

As a person gets older they become more and more dependent on their children and grandchildren to look after them. When those children were kids, that person looked after them, cared for them and helped them and gave them the things that they needed. In turn, as they get older, they are looked after and cared for, as they become more like a child.

Rupert Langkatjukur Peter

## *The family can all talk together and work through their feelings*

When someone has lost their partner they become really sad and depressed and think about all the circumstances that led to their loss. If, for example, the deceased was harmed by someone, and if their partner had said where their partner was and helped that person go to them (mistakenly thinking they were going to do something good but in fact they went and harmed that person) the surviving partner would be thinking about that a lot. And, over the weeks, they'd just become more and more worried and feeling bad about the whole circumstances. After a number of weeks, they might go and talk with the family and tell them how they're feeling about all those circumstances – all the things that they are blaming themselves for, as well as the sadness they feel at the loss.

After the surviving partner has talked to the family, ngangkari can be involved in finding the spirit of the deceased partner, getting it and placing the kurunpa within the grieving partner. This helps to clear the bereaved person's head after they've witnessed what's happened, after worrying about it then talking with the family about it.

Being able to talk about the whole situation, to bring it out into the open, to have that person's spirit back with them, allows them to feel better, to think properly. Having told their family about the whole situation, then those brothers, close family, talk with the brother-in-law and the broader family and explain the circumstances and what actually happened – for those who didn't really know what was happening – then they can all get a clear understanding of what actually happened.

The children of the person who has passed away really feel the loss of their father. They worry about it and think about it. And as they grow up, they feel deeply saddened by that loss. Family members – the broader family – explain what happened. The mother, the children and the broader family can all talk together and work through their feelings. So they have their understanding together and it's not the source of arguments, constant talking, constant worry – but they've come to an understanding.

Andy Tjilari

## *Older brothers, brothers-in-law and grandfathers have a really important role*

If your grandfather had come from a far-off place to marry a woman here, you would have relatives, a lot of relatives, that live over there. And you would have brothers-in-law associated with them, and brothers-in-law that had come from the woman as well. You would have family everywhere, over the whole place. This is the way that Anangu have family.

A man's brother-in-law – his wife's brothers or his sister's husband – is an extremely close relationship, a friendly relationship. They sit together and be together and are really happy like that. There's no fighting, they try and make things fair and level between themselves. That's why the brothers-in-law have an important role in supporting people when they're sad, because of that really close and caring relationship, which is characterised by giving to each other.

Older brothers, brothers-in-law and grandfathers have a really important role in supporting someone who has lost a relative and is grieving. They come to them, they sit with them and they gently talk with them to help them feel better.

Rupert Langkatjukur Peter

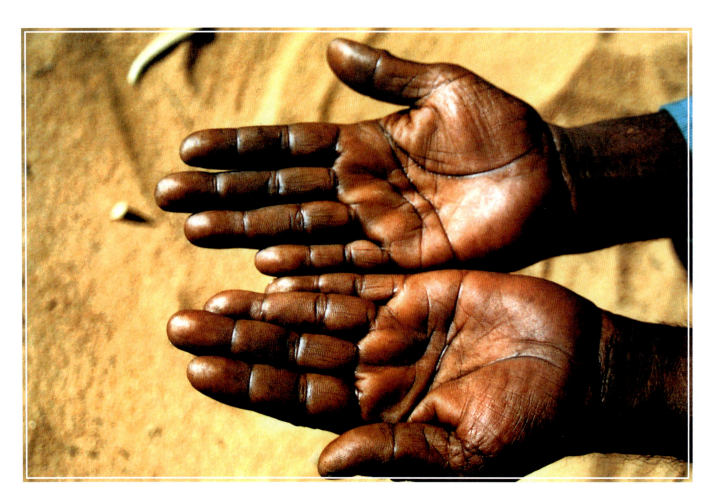

PHOTOGRAPH ANGELA LYNCH

# Substance Abuse

## *If you drink, then your spirit starts to leave you*

If you drink, then your spirit starts to leave you. That's what happens, the spirit starts to move away, and people are getting sick. In principle when someone is drinking a lot then they are going to get really sick. But their spirit is not being harmed – it is just being pushed aside, in effect, or displaced from where it should be, and changes how people should feel. But I don't drink – I never have – so I am not familiar with that. It is not the spirit that drinks!

Toby Minyintiri Baker

## *People's thinking was really clear*

In the old days there was only mingkulpa and people's thinking was really clear. The bush tobacco didn't cause people to waste away or become really thin. They were strong. Mingkulpa had properties like water, in that it could relieve thirst when people were without water. People would have mingkulpa when they had to travel great distances to where there was water. They would travel well and happily and not be thirsty and arrive safely in a place where there was water. You'd put the mingkulpa in your mouth and off you'd go! You could travel over two nights without water. So for trips when you had to camp out for two nights without water, mingkulpa was really important to help relieve your thirst. So people would carry it – it was like water, it helped them on those long journeys. Then when they arrived at a place where there was water to drink, then they could recuperate from the strenuous trip. Without water people can perish, get really sick, gradually get weaker and weaker, then collapse and be unable to go on, so mingkulpa was an important substance to have. On the other hand, if you see people smoking cigarettes and it comes out their noses and mouths, it actually weakens them, you know – it doesn't help them in the same way that mingkulpa does.

Rupert Langkatjukur Peter

## *You can't fix somebody when they are affected by marijuana*

Marijuana is like Maralinga – poison. Marijuana smoke is like that. You can't fix somebody when they are affected by marijuana! You can't grab smoke, you can't! And you can't grab water. You can't! That's what destroys the brain – the smoke. So when you go crazy from marijuana, that's it! You can never return to the normal, proper state, the healthy state. Marijuana and alcohol change a person's mind in a really different way that cannot be cured by a ngangkari healer.

People who smoke marijuana think about taking their own lives or just walking off somewhere and getting lost – that's their way of thinking. You can't cure that way of thinking – it cannot be cured by a healer. All the good ideas are blocked and they end up with bad thoughts. People who are alcoholics and marijuana addicts tend to think bad thoughts. And when people do that, they drink and smoke even more – and then they kill their spirit.

Toby Minyintiri Baker

## *People knowingly do this serious damage to themselves*

I remember once, doing a treatment, and I had to tell the person that I could not help them, because their string was too damaged and had all shrivelled up. Rupert and I tried but we couldn't help that person. We could not extract anything because it comes from smoke. People knowingly do this serious damage to themselves and destroy their pulyku, which ngangkari are powerless to heal, though we can give them some temporary relief, I suppose, in the neck and the head.

The effect of alcohol is very similar. It is not a mamu. It is not an illness. Alcohol is something else, that affects the body and makes people forget to eat, so they don't have proper meals, don't drink water and don't eat breakfast; they just start drinking alcohol as soon as they can. This causes irreparable damage that, again, ngangkari simply cannot mend. Alcoholism is not for ngangkari to fix. Young women who drink when they are pregnant give birth to babies that have Foetal Alcohol Syndrome (FAS). When their baby grows up with FAS, we cannot fix that. I am sorry, but we just cannot. We can't. We cannot fix that. We cannot help with that.

Wakupi Clem Toby (Dalby)

## *Marijuana, petrol, wine, and cigarettes are causing a lot of health problems for our people*

Many new things have come in from the outside, things like marijuana, petrol, wine and cigarettes – things that are causing a lot of health problems for our people. And with these things arriving we've seen a rise in incidents where people want to harm themselves, when their thinking becomes very confused and they're getting really sick. Mental health problems such as people wanting to hurt themselves are really new things for us.

Often we talk to people in vain about leading a balanced, healthy life and listening to the older people. If they don't listen and they go down that other path then it's really hard to help them. All the associated mental health problems are really terrible and it's very difficult to help people and look after them properly.

In the past when people got sick we were able to straighten them out, to help people live well, but with substance abuse people don't listen and it's really hard to help them find a balance in their lives.

As ngangkari we have the power to see when people are sad and sick and we can see some causes of those illnesses and sadness and can remove those things so people can be well again. There are many illnesses and mental health problems associated with substance abuse that have come into the Anangu world, and it's really difficult to work with these problems.

Rupert Langkatjukur Peter


## *They need to want that help*

In terms of substance abuse, if people drink a lot or smoke a lot of marijuana, they start to hear voices in their heads and hallucinate. They might think about going to hit someone or fight. I don't drink or smoke but I can see how this causes mental health issues for people. These substances are not something that was part of our culture, they were brought here by whitefellas and they have made a lot of Anangu very sick. People get sick from having too much of them. If they are not drinking or smoking, then they think really clearly.

Marijuana has caused a lot of problems, especially with our young people. It really disturbs the way that they think, upsets the way that they think. It's to do with the linkages, the blood flowing through their mind. There are blockages in the pulyku, the flow of the blood there. Those blockages can cause people to imagine all sorts of things and not to think straight, basically. They can't understand what's happening around them. We see that a lot and there are a lot of problems associated with it.

We can help if someone would like that help. But if they continue to smoke it's really hard to deal with. So they need to want that help and we have to work on it progressively over time, unblocking, unblocking, unblocking and getting the thinking straight again. But it is very hard and if they continue to smoke it's ineffective.

Toby Minyintiri Baker

## *We reinforce the A̱nangu way*

Once someone starts to smoke marijuana they really start to like it so much that it is all they think about. They don't think about going out hunting, they don't think about going out to the homelands to stay there, don't think about making camps in other places. They only think about marijuana and how to get it.

We ngangka̱ri now think that marijuana is the biggest problem in our area. A lot of mental health issues have now arisen with marijuana, alcohol and petrol coming into our Lands and into our world. And some A̱nangu have gone down that road which is familiar to many non-Indigenous people – substance abuse. And many non-Indigenous people are familiar with the harmful effects that we see today.

When people are obsessing about marijuana it's hard for them to understand what's being told to them about its harmful effects. It's really important that the old people continue to get people to give it up. It's important that parents and grandparents talk strongly and medical professionals reinforce that message and give a clear idea to those people so that maybe, over time, they start to hear it.

Marijuana smokers often resist those messages about its harmful effects and often get very angry and aggressive when they're being reprimanded. The smokers can get really resentful in those situations so it's important to talk positively with them and not to hurt their feelings, because often when they're chastised they'll want to harm themselves. That's because of the effects of marijuana and the way that it confuses their thinking.

We've witnessed situations where people have contemplated hurting themselves, or hanging themselves after being told off for using marijuana, when it's really the illness you have when you smoke marijuana. In the case that we witnessed, when the person responded in that way, we talked really calmly and carefully and gently with them and convinced them that suicide was the wrong thing to do and that they should live well. It wasn't just us who talked with that person but their whole family, their parents and grandparents and managed to help them feel good again.

The message we give is that smoking marijuana is not OK, that it does really cause illness, that it's the wrong way to go, your thinking becomes really confused. We talk about the importance of listening to the parents and grandparents and learning the proper Law – living well, learning Tjukurpa, learning Law, listening about the proper way to live and how to conduct your life with a clear head. Whereas, smoking marijuana causes a lot of mental health problems and can make you really sick.

Often people will respond positively to that and listen closely to their family and learn the Law. But other times people will resist and think exclusively about marijuana. When they are smoking a lot of marijuana is when we see people starting to think about hurting themselves or killing themselves.

A good way to talk to people is to talk about the importance of the A̱nangu way and of A̱nangu Law and A̱nangu culture, the importance of holding onto that and listening and learning about it – and smoking marijuana is not part of that way. It's really harmful and something that's come from the outside. It's a road that is familiar to a lot of non-Indigenous people. They see substance abuse in their world and now we are seeing it in ours. We talk to people in a gentle way and say, 'Look, we're not criticising you or making you feel bad! We are telling you because we want you to be able to think clearly and well again.'

Often people become a bit embarrassed by their actions and their behaviour and the things that they've done when they've smoked marijuana and so they begin to listen and learn from their families about good ways to do things. We reinforce the Anangu way, the beliefs and understandings and knowledge which have come from our grandparents and we hold onto today. That Law is the proper way to live and these things that have come from outside our world, the non-Indigenous world; they aren't right and are not good and they don't help you think straight and learn properly.

Andy Tjilari

## *We can work on the spiritual well-being of those people*

The health issues associated with heavy drinking and marijuana use are not something the ngangkari can really work with. We can work on the spiritual well-being of those people and our work is with the spirit: making people feel balanced, getting that flow going, removing things that are causing illness and helping people to think straight. But we can't work really well with people who are smoking marijuana or drinking – we can't get our hands on what we need in order to help them get better.

Wakupi Clem Toby (Dalby)

## *The blowing technique is very effective*

When people get mental problems from marijuana or something, I press the top of their head, pressing down on it and blowing on it. I press their head, blow on it and that calms them down. That makes them feel better instantly. The blowing technique is very effective.

Ilawanti Ungkutjuru Ken

### We can get through to people and try to give them the strength to reject those bad influences

A lot of marijuana that we see today in our communities comes from Mintabie, in South Australia, and that's the source of a lot of problems. We know the difficulties of trying to stop that flow. Marijuana comes from a long way away, right from the south, all the way through. Often it's carried on the highway, bypassing Coober Pedy. It's very difficult for the police – they try to stop that flow. We know that marijuana comes from a long way away. Originally people went to Mintabie and to dig for opal. Over time they brought in drugs and relationships developed between those people and Anangu. As those relationships developed, Anangu learnt about those new drugs and it spread from there.

For young people today there are a lot of negative influences. A lot of people get very bad advice, they are given the wrong information and people try to influence them in a negative way. Other people try to give them good advice and good ideas about how to live their lives. So it can be very confusing for young people and they think, 'Which way should I go, what should I do?' Many people are speaking to those young people and giving them good ideas and talking in a way that is designed to look after them. At the same time they are getting a lot of bad advice and negative influences and that's making it really difficult for other people to help.

If they are around bad influences then they often revert to bad behaviour and forget that what was told to them was designed to help them.

As a ngangkari I try to speak from the heart and from my spirit to help them understand things – to leave marijuana alone. When people are feeling good and their spirit's open, that's when they are really open to good ideas and listen and learn to leave marijuana. Substance abuse can have a very negative effect on people's spirit and close it off, depressing them. Our goal is to try and help their spirit be well again.

Over time there have been a lot of negative influences on Anangu and today we have a significant problem with marijuana. We can get through to people and try to give them the strength to reject those bad influences. When people go down the wrong path and take up smoking again we try to give people the strength to say, 'No, look, I don't want that – go away!' and continue to listen and to learn properly.

Andy Tjilari


### How people are affected with marijuana is totally different

We are often asked, why do people go mad? Well, it is quite simple really. People learn from other mad and crazy people! The head boils when a person gets silly in the head. If your head doesn't get hot and boil you're fine but if it does that's when you get silly, go crazy! But when people smoke marijuana that's a totally different story and a different kind of 'crazy' which is really hard to fix. That's a city and a town problem, but it's not a problem that can be fixed in town. But when people smoke marijuana they can see things that are not there. They see people who are naked and they say things that are quite silly. It's something that's unexplainable and you can't really fix it. How people are affected with marijuana is totally different, and with the alcohol as well, it's too hard to fix someone. We can't really heal a person completely when they are affected by alcohol and marijuana. But in the bush when people lived a lifestyle that ngangka<u>r</u>i could heal, people lived healthily, mentally and emotionally well. In the old days we treated illnesses that were healable.

Sam Wimitja Watson

## *They spend more and more time with those substances and less and less time with the older people*

You can see people's spirit change; they're not open, they're not listening and understanding, their character changes, they can't see things, can't do things, they don't go out. When the marijuana runs out they just sit.

The older men and women worry about younger people. The old men worry that the young men aren't learning – they worry for their mental health. They think about how they themselves were taught, what they learnt, and what a good way that was. Often older people will say this to young people and those young people will listen and respect that and come to be with them and learn.

At other times, because of the marijuana, people's spirit is so down that they just want to sit by themselves and they don't join in. Some people are asked to join in, to sit with and be with the older people and listen and learn – but they don't go. Maybe it's because they are not with them in spirit, their spirit can't join in. They feel really sad within themselves and they don't feel like joining in, talking with people, just sitting there.

A lot of young people's spirits have been affected because they've smoked marijuana. Their spirit is really sad, they are depressed and the spirit itself is hunched over. Previously they were happy people but over time as they've started to use marijuana or, equally so, alcohol or petrol, they become increasingly depressed. After that they spend more and more time with those substances and less and less time with the older people and a lot of that knowledge is lost to them.

A father, observing this process, might speak to his son and say, 'Why aren't you joining in with the others? It's good to go over there and sit with people, laugh and talk and share stories – it's a really healthy way to be. Why are you just sitting here sad? You should go over there and join in, you'll feel a lot better.' The son might say, 'Look, it's OK, I can see them over there, I can see what they're doing, but I might just stay here, I might sit here.'

It's because their understanding has been badly affected by marijuana and those other substances. They are not thinking straight, their heart and their head are not working together. If people have smoked marijuana for a long time or sniffed petrol for a long time or been drinkers over a long period of time –

then it really harms their thinking. It's like their brain shrinks, it gets smaller and they just don't think clearly. It's important that we ngangka<u>r</u>i help people get better, look after them in those circumstances and work with Western doctors and nurses and sisters to really care for those people.

Andy Tjilari

### *The first thing we need is for everybody to open their eyes and to face up to the fact that the problem exists*

We realise there are serious health problems caused by wine, petrol and marijuana. These drugs are now commonplace. We wish they didn't exist. They are causing very serious problems. We find dealing with these drugs very difficult. Sometimes we need additional help to deal with people who are affected. We can't ignore the problem. We hate seeing people succumb to these drugs. We need to know more about how they affect the body, because we are still learning about their effects. They are still new to us. We have got to find better ways to combat this problem. The first thing we need is for everybody to open their eyes and to face up to the fact that the problem exists. We need to look at the problem with our eyes and ears wide open, because I believe right now most of us have shut our eyes to the problem and refuse to acknowledge it. We try to forget about it, even, but we can't keep doing this for long, because it won't get us anywhere.

Arnie Frank

### *Alcohol, petrol and marijuana can have the effect of making people feel really paranoid and confused*

When marijuana smokers don't have marijuana, when it's run out, they can get really aggressive and angry and the smoker will get really bad headaches and feel really bad. That's because they haven't got the marijuana they crave – it's finished and they'll then criticise others and say, 'Why is it you're making me feel bad?' When they don't have marijuana they'll say a lot of things that aren't true. They'll speak in a wrong way that people aren't going to help them and they'll often just get really angry and say, 'Why aren't you helping me? Go on, get out of here! Go!' They are really missing and wanting marijuana and it makes them behave in that way.

If they are given a small amount, then they'll be OK for a short period of time and calm down but then it all starts up again – they get aggressive again and very angry with people and start blaming them. People who smoke together have arguments – especially if someone's run out of marijuana, or they don't have any. When other people come around, they'll say, 'Whenever you come around for marijuana I very generously and promptly give you marijuana! But when I need some you don't give me any! Just wait till you guys run out! I'm not going to give you any!' They talk like that. It changes week by week, they'll be up and down, up and down: sometimes thinking calmly and clearly and other times really confused and angry.

Alcohol, petrol and marijuana can have the effect of making people feel really paranoid and confused about how people feel towards them and how they feel towards other people. They are constantly having arguments about why they've done something or not helped someone or done something mean to them. Parents and grandparents – the family – will say to the marijuana smokers 'What that other person is saying is wrong! They're not thinking straight in their head, that's silly talk! This is the proper way to live your life. We'd like to teach you these good things – the Law, the proper way to look after people. If you go down that path and listen to those bad ideas, then things are really going to go downhill. But the way to get better and to live well is to listen closely. We want you to be able to get better, that sort of talk is rubbish and you are just going to go downhill with that.'

If that person is open to what they say, if their spirit is good and open, they'll start to listen. From the spirit the good ideas will go up to the head and they will be able to think clearly and live properly.

Marijuana is brought into the community by various people. For example, a man might arrive with marijuana and go back to his own place and all those other marijuana smokers will know that he has arrived with marijuana and they'll say, 'OK! Let's go and buy some!'

Once people have smoked marijuana a lot, they think about it and want more and more. It's really hard for someone who has been smoking to give it up. Their spirit and mind is saying, 'Go and get it! Go and get it! Why leave it?' And other people are saying, 'Let's go and get it! You should go and get some and we can share it'. There's that pressure.

People do give up though. For example, one man might say, 'No, I'm not going to smoke marijuana,' and set the example for others. Someone else will see the way that person is, that they no longer smoke, so they too might decide to stop smoking marijuana. They'll choose to spend time with that person and go off and do other things. But they'll also see that others are continuing to smoke. It's difficult for those individuals and they'll see more and more people going to buy marijuana, more and more young men smoking.

Over time we have seen a gradual increase in numbers of people smoking. It becomes more and more difficult for an individual to give up smoking marijuana when their peers smoke and put pressure on them to smoke. Gradually they spend less and less time with the old people.

In the past the younger men would be with the older people and they'd be learning about Tjukurpa and about Law, about stories, listening and sitting with them. You can see, now that more and more young people smoke, that they are leaving that behind. They are not spending the time listening to, and learning from, the older people. Fathers, uncles and others might come to a house and say, 'Oh, my son's not here. Where is my son?' but he'll be at home, thinking about marijuana and thinking about going to get marijuana when people arrive with it.

You can see people waiting at home, just waiting for their dealer so they can go and buy it again, and after that they'll feel more relaxed and happy, but otherwise just thinking about it and waiting and wanting it. You can see after they've got the marijuana, smoked it and again run out, they get depressed and sad again. They stay at home and become either very sad or resentful and angry with other people. They think that other people are not helping them – those arguments that we talked about before.

Andy Tjilari

## We work with our hands to remove the blockages

Traditionally we've used mingkulpa and that's been a good thing for people. But recently marijuana has come in from the side and really taken over. People have tried it and have developed a liking for it. They've become addicted and it's really affected people's thinking and caused a lot of mental health problems.

With the arrival of marijuana we are seeing a lot of different health problems. People might think at the start that it's good, but we've witnessed the harm that's been done. It adversely affects people's mental health. We as ngangkari can see where the blood flows through the veins and the arteries and we can see where marijuana has caused it to be blocked and the blood not to flow. Marijuana stops the blood getting up into the brain. We can, if not too much damage has been done, remove these blockages when we see them and help people's thinking become clear again. If we can intervene early enough we can remove those blockages and talk to people and say, 'Look, you have to leave that marijuana, don't keep on using it. If you use it again it will cause long term damage.' We're strong in talking to people about that. If people don't heed that advice it can cause serious damage and it's really hard to fix it.

So we ngangkari can see and feel those blockages, they are often around the throat where the blood flows up through into the head there. Instead of going up into the head and around it just gets blocked there and goes back down again. Ngangkari have a role of removing those blockages so blood flow can continue to work properly and go right round. We work with our hands to remove the blockages, to open up the flow of blood again through the veins and the arteries, to allow it to flow through to the head and for people's thinking and brains to be clear and well. Petrol has the same effect as marijuana at times and also cigarette smoking can cause blockages. You can add wine to that too – alcohol does a lot of harm to the brain in the same way.

Rupert Langkatjukur Peter

## It's very difficult work

We ngangka<u>r</u>i work with petrol sniffers and try to help them get better. But sometimes we can't. It's very difficult work. Often they don't want help and will verbally abuse us. Other times when petrol sniffers get really sick, they become out of control and very difficult to work with. You can feel in touching their heads that the elements which are causing harm are like smoke. It's difficult to see what's causing the harm or to get our hands on it. Their heads become really hot and there are blockages in the way the blood flows to the brain.

We work with the petrol sniffers, giving them treatments where we are primarily trying to get their blood flowing well again and removing blockages to their brains. So we can help them in this way, to get the blood flowing, but in terms of removing the harmful things that are causing their illnesses and causing the mental health problems, it's very difficult, because it's like smoke – we can't see it or feel it or get our hands on it.

So we can help them to some extent but often after that, people go back to sniffing petrol and cause further harm. Others will be able to leave it and start to get better but it's very difficult. It might be that, over time, those that go back to sniffing will listen to their grandmothers and grandfathers or their parents who are encouraging them to leave petrol sniffing, but they've really got their own thoughts and often resist that advice.

Andy Tjilari


## It's a process of working together

Doctors play a really important role in caring for people who have been harmed by substance abuse, supporting and looking after them. They use various tools and equipment to assess the damage caused both in people's brains and to their bodies by smoking marijuana. They can work to help people to recover too.

As ngangka<u>r</u>i we too can see the changes that take place. It's very difficult, but we can help to get people's blood flowing well again. You can see changes take place where people's veins will join together and blood will no longer be able to flow freely to the brain and that's causing a lot of the harm and damage to people's intellect. We try and clear those out and get the flow going again. Both of us, Andy Tjilari and I, work side by side but it's very difficult work and often things can't be done to help people. We've been able to work with a whole series of people to help get their blood to flow freely to their brains again, to help them think properly again, and they've managed to leave marijuana and become men and to learn again.

So the blood isn't getting properly to the brain again, and things have joined together or become really twisted and broken. Our goal is to separate them and straighten out those paths so that people's brains can work clearly again. We can be successful in this, at times, but at other times it's very difficult to get our hands on those things. When that natural flow is stopped, blocked or broken, people have difficulty learning, listening and thinking properly so that's why we focus on that.

You can see at times people's blood turns to stone, to black stones, in effect, and we can remove those and help the flow go again. This is what we do and doctors in turn do their work to help look after people. It's a process of working together.

All ngangkari help to look after their people, help them recover from these things, and doctors work together to help look after people too. And through the work of the doctors and the sisters and ngangkari a whole series of people have been able to stop smoking, to stop sniffing petrol, to stop drinking. Some will leave it and get back on with their lives.

Sadly, though, there's a group of people who have not been able to recover or quit. They've resisted the efforts and are just thinking inside themselves about those things. Their spirits have become hardened and they've not been able to give up those substances. If people can't give up marijuana and continue to smoke, you see them go less and less frequently to be with the older people. They spend less and less time laughing and talking and learning about life in the company of others. They become more and more isolated and their spirits become more and more hardened. If we can't get through to people, then we can't help them. They're always thinking about marijuana. That is the way that they think.

Rupert Langkatjukur Peter


## *If you have ngangkari powers and you drink alcohol you can't do healing*

Ngangkari wirulymankupai – means we can 'smooth' a person to heal them. Wiruly means to smooth, but it also means to heal. We touch a person on the head, just touching the head also will heal, when ngangkari do that. Karalymankupai is like wirulymankupai – is to become smooth, healing, or become good or healed well. We couldn't do that if we drank alcohol. If you have ngangkari powers and you drink alcohol you can't do healing. You lose that power.

Marijuana is also really bad. It's really hard to heal a person for life if they smoke marijuana. You can only ease their pain. They have a bad head and you can ease the situation in the head for a bit. People who smoke cigarettes, they look unwell and it shows in their face. If a person is sick then you can put their spirit back in their body, that's it. Most people are happy but some people are sad or worrying. When they've got a lot of things worrying them or if they're drinking, they've got a lot of problems. There are a lot of young fellas smoking marijuana and it's really hard to get rid of that. The one and only time when I tried alcohol, my mouth went funny and I fell and my son threw a rock at me and I never tried it again.

Sam Wimitja Watson

## *Ngangkari cannot be drinkers*

Ngangkari cannot be drinkers. If they are drinking just a little bit, then they are probably OK. Ngangkari may well drink a little bit just to be sociable, but they won't be big drinkers. They can't drink. They really can't. Other people might drink, and some people like it too much, but not proper ngangkari. If a ngangkari does drink, he renders himself impotent. His hands close off and he is impotent. His hands shut off. After a while they'll open back up again. If you are a big drinker, you can't be a ngangkari. Their power is shut down. If they've had too much to drink they are probably talking in a drunken way and maybe they believe their hands are open, when really they are not, and they are just doing it for the money. They just want the money. The hands close up and the mapanpa goes back inside. The hands close up behind the re-entering mapanpa. It doesn't re-open. No way would a ngangkari smoke marijuana either. It just wouldn't happen. He'll just lose it if he does. He'll lose his power totally.

Wakupi Clem Toby (Dalby)

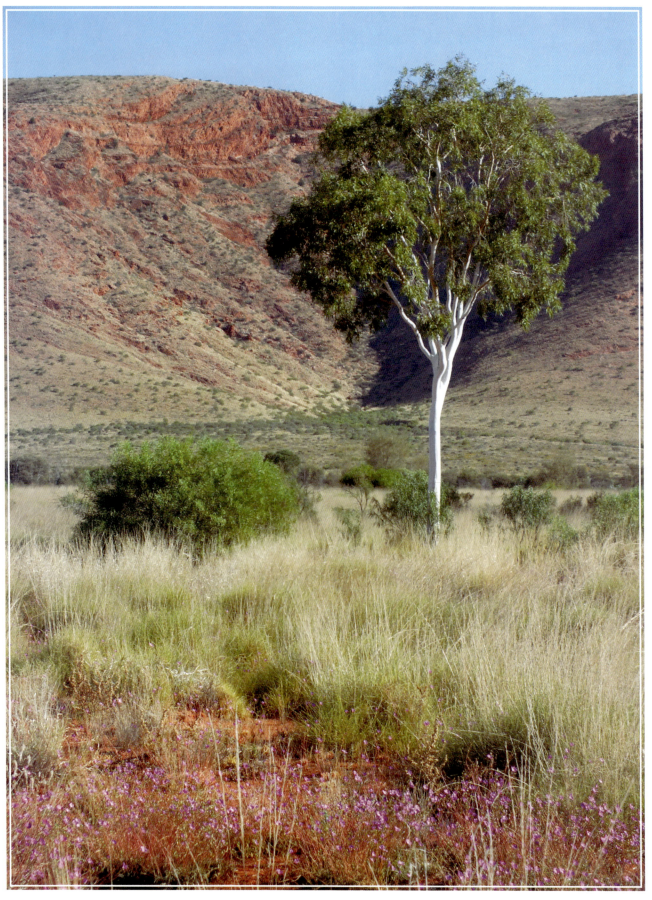

PHOTOGRAPH MAGGIE KAVANAGH

# Mental Health

### *The relationship of the head to the body*

We see a link between mental health, how people are thinking, and a link to the stomach, where there are 'strings.' There are links there. If people have mental health problems you can see them getting sick there. And conversely, if you are sick here too, it can really affect the way you are thinking. So we look at that and assess how people are going. I am talking about the relationship of the head to the body and how the blood flows through the body. We can see where there are blockages.

Toby Minyintiri Baker

### *There are many people who are affected by sadness and need the help of ngangkari*

At times you can see a person who appears to be constantly tired and not able to do very much – they can't set up their camp or make a windbreak, find shelter or prepare food. They just seem to be constantly feeling tired, not really moving or having much energy. It's because their spirit is really sick and it's affecting their ability in all things to move to work and they just don't have the energy to be able to do things. They just lie there.

Ngangkari have an important role helping these people recover and get well again. No amount of drinking medicine is going to help you get better in this situation. The role of the ngangkari is to remove and throw out the things that are causing the illness within someone – something that's harming their spirit. The ngangkari's role is to remove those sicknesses, release them, get them out of the system and that person will be happy again and be able to do well.

The family have a really important role to play here in looking after the person while they are sick. Being with family is a really important part of being happy. When someone's spirit is down and they are feeling sick, losing their energy, the rest of the family group come together and help that person by giving them food and meat and caring for them. In turn when that person has recovered and another family member might become sick, they'll look after them too.

When someone's sick they can be far from family too and when they're recovering or well again they return to their family and often say something like, 'Gee, I was nearly lost to you all there, now I'm getting better!' and they're happy to all be together again and to care for each other again.

When someone has lost their mother or their father, is feeling lonely and sad because of the passing of relatives, ngangkari have an important role in caring for those people and bringing in other family members to help look after them. When a person has lost their parents and is feeling very lonely it's really important that the rest of the family support that person. For a man it might be their elder brother, their brothers-in-law or their grandfathers who rally around them and get close. The father's sisters' sons also play an important role; they talk with them, bring them water and meat, share, laugh and help them get well again. In that way they work on helping someone to be happy and to be amongst other people. It's a really important role for those people.

There are many people who are affected by sadness and need the help of ngangkari in the Lands. I see them sad and depressed and feeling very lethargic and we have an important role in caring for those people and helping them get up and about again. In some cases people can be feeling really sad, feeling empty within themselves, feeling hopeless. And other Anangu will see this and come to me and tell me that person needs help.

As ngangkari we go to those people and touch them and feel them and feel how weakened their spirit has become, how it has lost that ability to get up and go and do things. That person will be thinking a lot within themselves, be worried about themselves being sick, and that sickness starts to spread through their body until it touches the heart. When it touches the heart people can pass away. Ngangkari play an important role in removing those things that are causing the sadness and the sickness, helping people become strong again so they can go out and fend for themselves and cook and do things for themselves again.

When a person is sick or has an illness, sometimes that can really affect their spirit, where they just feel really sad about everything. Ngangkari can play a role not only healing that person when they are sick but working with their spirit as well. Sometimes if someone is really sad, depending on the condition that they are in, many ngangkari can come together to help that person as well, not just one person.

There are various ways that a person can become sick or sad. People can be affected by a range of things. At times when there are really big winds and there is a lot of dust around, there are many harmful things that can enter people's bodies in the forms of sticks, stones and objects which are causing harm and making people sad. We ngangkari can recognise those things and help that person by removing them and help them get well again.

In one case we saw a person in Adelaide who was really hurting himself: smashing his feet into rocks, banging his forehead against hard things to the point that he was bleeding and really injured. He was really isolated and depressed and uncertain where his family was. He thought maybe his mother and father had passed away and that he too should pass away. He just didn't know what was going on and was very isolated.

So the doctors spoke with us two ngangkari and asked if we could go and see him. When we arrived we could see that he was really apprehensive when he saw us. The doctor explained that we were two healers – two ngangkari that had come to see if they could help. We said to him, 'Sit here.' We sat next to him and we held him and we explained that we were two ngangkari that had come to see if we could help him and we asked if he would like to be treated by us. He said, 'Yes,' and we gave him a range of treatments that evening. We worked with him and now he is healed and well again. But at the time his hands were bloodied and beaten and his forehead equally so. He was deeply depressed, but now he lives happily.

We went back and saw him again the next morning and we saw that he was already feeling better. He came and hugged us and said, 'Thank you for seeing me and giving me that help.' He understood that his parents were coming to visit him, they were close. And when he was better he was able to roll his swag and go and be with his parents again.

The heart of his problem was that his spirit had become too depressed, he was really sad inside. We could see that his spirit was really down and when we questioned him and asked why he was beating his forehead against the wall and smashing his fists into it, he said he just didn't know what was happening with his family. He was really alone and didn't know where his mother and father were. He explained that he was continually worrying about his family, about where his parents were and what was happening with them. This was what made him so desperate – to the point where he started to think that he'd kill himself. We could see that his spirit had been hurt and we worked with him to help him find balance again, help him find his sense of self.

We noted that his spirit was up in his back and had been really pushed aside. We re-centred it so he had that balance again, so he was the way he was when he was born. That's what we talk about in giving people a sense of balance again and levelling things out – it's re-centring their kurunpa and putting it back where it belongs so that people can be well. That's a really important role for ngangkari.

Rupert Langkatjukur Peter

## *People who are in gaols or mental health institutions are always thinking about their family*

One case that we worked with, we went to help a person who was very unwell, who was in gaol. We arrived on the first afternoon and we observed the person. He was moving around a lot, obviously very unsettled and upset. Previously he had been hitting himself in the head, just hitting, hitting, hitting, until blood was coming from his head. He was really hurting himself, really upset. We could see where the wounds hadn't healed and see that he was really sick. We worked with this person for two days and by the third day we felt that he was improving. I would like to tell you a bit about that.

Initially we observed him that afternoon and the next day went back and began our work with him. He was really scared at the start. He was unsure about what we were doing as ngangkari there. When he first saw us we could see he was shaking and upset but we sat down with him and explained that we wanted to talk with him. We said, 'Look, we'd like to be able to talk with you. If you say that's OK, after that we can give you some treatments to try to help you.' The police and the doctors explained the same: that we were there to help him if he would like us to and, if he agreed, then we could go ahead. He thought about that and then the following day we returned to give those treatments.

The process involved sitting with him, holding him and listening to what his concerns were, and a variety of treatments to remove objects that were causing him harm, causing his illnesses. We removed those and showed the doctors and the police what we had done as well. So we asked – 'Is it OK if we can see you?' and he said it was OK, so we saw him a series of times and we helped him a great deal.

Initially we sat with him. We held him in our arms, held him like a child, like his family held him when he was a child and we did this to calm him and make him happy so that we could talk together. That next day he told us how sad he was, how deeply despairing he was. He was suffering from a sense of hopelessness. His whole spirit was really sad. To see us, he said, made him really happy, he was really relieved to have someone to be able to talk to. He felt really crushed by the experience of being in gaol.

After those initial conversations we returned again in the afternoon to continue the treatments that we've mentioned and again we held him and talked. He said again how relieved he was that we'd come and he talked about his desire to see his family, to be able to talk with his family and to be with his family. He was getting weaker, despairing at his situation of not seeing his family. You see that with people in gaol. They lose their strength, their spirits weaken, and they are basically worrying about family. They are thinking within themselves, their thoughts in their heads just going round and round all day, all night: 'Where are my family? What are they doing? Why aren't they visiting me? Have they forgotten me? Maybe they don't care, maybe they've just left me here.' That's what they think and it really makes people despair and that's what's making them weak.

When family come to visit, inmates become really happy. It clears the head, allows them to get a perspective on things. Not seeing family – things become confused, their thinking becomes distorted, and it really affects people. They are not thinking clearly. Initially, they might think, 'Hmm. Why isn't my sister or my mother coming to visit? Why aren't they here? What's happening?' The gaoled person doesn't know what's happening so they think 'Maybe my family doesn't care. I'll be in here forever and not see them.' They get sadder, become sick and they get weaker.

People who are in gaols or mental health institutions are always thinking about their family. When they are discharged or released they go back to their families and to the places where they used to live, to be with their families, and everyone's really happy to see them. There's joy that they've returned. They go out hunting, eat meals together, after dinner sit around talking and laughing, wake up early together and go about things together. It's a really happy time.

On the other hand, sometimes people can lose connection with their families. They'll go back to where they used to live and they'll ask, 'Oh, where has my family gone? Where have they moved to?' Because they live in different communities doing different work in different places and people would be able to say, 'Look, they went there,' and that person can join up with the family and be with them again. But some people arrive back in the places where they used to live and they don't know where the family has gone and people can't say where they've gone. They might be spread out in a whole range of places. It is really difficult for those people who have lost that connection there. They're very despairing and very sad.

People who are separated from their family are always thinking about their family. Thinking about when they'll be able to see them again, where they'll be, what they can do together. And equally the family is thinking about them, when they'll return, how they're going and what they're doing. So when people are released from gaols or discharged from mental health institutions they want to go back to their families. Sometimes, however, they might arrive home to find that their family has gone away for work, just for a week or two to another community. If the family has left word about where they have gone or how long they're going to be away, that's fine – people can understand what's going on and wait for them. But other times there's confusion. People don't know how long they're going to be away for or where they've actually gone. So all of those things are part of people's worries when they're separated from family.

Andy Tjilari

## *People all over the world get really sad and depressed*

I do what I can to help people with mental health problems. I counsel people if they have got problems. I help where I can. People all over the world and in the cities get really sad and depressed, they can't talk, and they feel bad. I saw someone like that in Alice Springs hospital. I put my hand on him but he shouted at me to go away. Depression is not madness, it is sadness. It comes from the pulyku. When the pulyku are not working properly it causes problems all through the body.

Pantjiti Unkari McKenzie

## *Depressed people start to lose a sense of perspective about what's going on*

When people are really sad it's important to talk with them really gently. It's a process of listening and talking together over time, being together day after day. Slowly people's thinking becomes more balanced, they start to feel happier and after that their thinking becomes clearer. They're not just feeling worried the whole time.

The brothers-in-law of that person, their uncles, their grandparents, sit with that person and look after them really well. It's they who can see when someone's really worried by something. They are sitting by themselves and thinking and they can see that that's going to lead to problems if they don't go and help that person. That's why they look after the person. They can see they're really worried and problems will inevitably develop.

They go and sit with the person and begin that gentle process of talking and listening. The person will understand that they are cared for, they'll think, 'My brothers-in-law, my family, my grandfathers are caring for me well.' And because they feel cared for and they're being listened to, they think they should behave well, therefore preventing a lot of the problems that can come when people aren't being looked after and their worries continue. Those brothers-in-law, the grandparents and the uncles all sit with the person and do it in a really considerate way. Gradually people start to talk about funny stories and they laugh together – they speak in a way which makes the person relax. That sitting together, laughing together and being cared for in that way helps people forget what they were worried about. It allows them to have a much more balanced view of things rather than lose perspective and do things that might not be good for them and for others.

After that initial phase of sitting together the person feels more comfortable about leaving the place which has caused them to become sad, or where they are sad, and go and visit some of those relatives, the brothers-in-law and grandparents and stay at their places and leave the sad place behind for a while. So they go and do that and that helps in the healing process.

On their return, because they're feeling much better about the situation, much more balanced in their thinking, they don't fight, there's no spearing or swearing. All the things that were building up in that person when they were first seen to be really worried have gone – they're much clearer in their thinking.

If someone is really worried about something and they're sitting by themselves, their thoughts going round and round, they can become really confused in their thinking. They see people passing, going this way and that, beside them, but not being with them. Sitting there thinking about things by themselves and seeing all these things going on around them, depressed people can get really confused in their thinking, really mistaken. He might see two people laughing in the distance and think, 'Oh, they are laughing at me, talking about me.' A lot of problems come up that way, people just get the wrong idea and get really sick thinking like this. They start to resent people and get annoyed by things. For example, if two people are passing by and the person sees them laughing they'll think, 'Oh, they're talking about me and they're laughing about me.'

But if those people were to go over and sit with them and explain, 'No, we're just talking between ourselves,' then that person feels that they know what's going on and they don't get the wrong idea, they don't get angry because of that. They can start to lose a sense of perspective about what's going on but when they are cared for and looked after in the way that we described, then they don't feel like being aggressive towards those people, they understand what's going on around them a lot more, and they recover. People recover their sense of perspective and feel happy again. None of the fights and the violence that could come from misunderstanding and worrying too much occur.

Rupert Langkatjukur Peter

## *Treating and healing people who are fearful and have anxiety*

Some A̱nangu suffer from depression and anxiety too. You can see, for example, a person who will eat very little and will drink very little. They're sad inside, their spirit is sad. They won't drink much water or eat much meat, they are not well. Over time their spirit becomes weaker and weaker and makes them much more vulnerable to other sicknesses too.

People can become anxious, for example, if they have witnessed an accident. After seeing an accident they might be really afraid of travel and certain situations. They won't go to different places they'll stay at home a lot. It's because of what they've seen that they've got a certain knowledge, or think, 'Maybe the same thing could happen to me' – an accident in that way – they're fearful. Seeing those bad things happen, seeing people being hurt, their thinking is affected. They start to think bad things and worry about things and their thinking is harmed.

We ngangka̱ri can help give treatments to those who are depressed. When we see that people are depressed we understand that their kurunpa has been saddened. Their spirit is affected. Sometimes we might have to find their spirit, it might be lost, and so we follow it and see it at the trunk of a tree, see that it is really weakened, hungry. Sometimes we see hair sprouting from the spirits and they're thin and emaciated, they haven't been fed and nourished, with water or food. We get that kurunpa and take it back and place it in the person. Ngangka̱ri, when giving treatments, have the power to see where those spirits are and are able to put them back into people.

When people are anxious it can be because they have witnessed something happen to their family members. And that's what's teaching them that fear or anxiety. They can think that the same thing might happen to them, that they might be harmed or die, and in turn that can lead to people harming themselves. We give treatments to help people's spirit.

The person might explain to us, 'Oh, I don't know what's going on', 'I don't understand things' or 'I'm not feeling myself' – they'll talk like this. We ngangka̱ri listen to that person and hear all the different things they're thinking and hear their uncertainties. In giving them a treatment we can say, 'Ah yes, here is the cause of their problems', or 'This spirit has entered them.' It's this *other* different spirit which has entered them which is causing them to think in these different ways and to be anxious and worried about things, thinking about harming themselves. So it's our responsibility to get that spirit out of them and throw it away and then, in turn, go and find that person's true spirit, bring it back and position it within them in the right place.

Their true spirit has been displaced by that other spirit, pushed aside or forced to go, so we put back the spirit that people were born with, the spirit which gives them their true character. And that's what we put back within them. And when that true spirit is put back, they get a clear sense of themselves again. They feel much more balanced and their thinking becomes clear again. That different spirit – the one that's not theirs, the one that's causing the harm, and, forced their spirit to go – is removed and sent away.

We can see people's spirits go when they have witnessed accidents and other traumatic events. In the old days, before cars, still people's spirits left them when they were worried by things or had seen things. So in the past, for example, anxiety might be caused when someone had witnessed certain events – say, a group of men left the camp and speared and killed a person. And this person had followed that group and witnessed it at a distance, then seen them by various means revive that person and send them back into the camp where they'd then die in innocent circumstances. And the person had seen this and had come back to camp but didn't say anything or tell anybody what he'd seen because he was scared about the repercussions of talking about it. So inside their own heads they're getting more and more worried about things and feeling guilty that they haven't told anyone at the same time. And they've witnessed the killing of someone and they're very sorry for that and they're also thinking that they should've talked about it and let people know what they'd seen. In the process of thinking about this and thinking about it and thinking about it more and more, those thoughts going around in their head, that's when their thinking goes bad. They have really disturbing thoughts at night, can't sleep well and wake up with nightmares, reliving what they've seen. They suffer from great anxiety and also live with the fear that they too will be harmed by those people.

It's this constant anxiety which really weakens a person's spirit. It makes their thinking go bad and, over time, they develop serious mental health issues. Ngangkari could give treatments to these people. They would touch their heads and see inside and see that their brain had been harmed by what they'd seen. It was akin to a small ball that had shrunk and become narrow. They could also see the various blockages which had caused it to close off, a lot of heat coming from certain places. We can see the things that are causing people's thinking to become bad and see the blockages which can be caused in different ways that can lead to people wanting to 'finish themselves off' . The anxiety can lead people to think about suicide.

So we will talk to people, and family members will talk with the person who is feeling really anxious, if they've witnessed, say, the death of a family member in a car accident. Over time they'll talk, until the person is thinking a bit more clearly. So it is a gradual process of talking with the person until they're comfortable again about going to the scene of the accident. And, there, ngangkari have the role of assessing the situation and they'll see where the spirit of the person is who has passed away, get that spirit and put it back inside a close family member – a person who is part of that true family. They might put the spirit back into the brother of the person who passed away so that it can be looked after. And after that the surviving brother's thinking becomes clearer again and he recovers. The spirit is placed with the family member so that they can keep it. In that way the spirit continues to be nourished and fed. So the brother's spirit can be looked after and nourished by a brother – in turn, family look after each other's spirits.

When people have anxiety and are mistaken in their thinking it spreads down to their spirit and a whole range of illnesses can come from that. Those illnesses can in turn cause further anxiety. Ngangkari have an important role in treating and healing people who are fearful and have anxiety.

Andy Tjilari

### *When someone is talking about harming themselves, the first time that it's said it's really important to listen and to sit with that person*

Sometimes, when people are sad, they think about harming themselves. They might be upset and they are thinking along these lines. They'll say to someone, 'Oh, OK! You're always saying bad things about me, always upset, irritated and annoyed with me! Right! Now I'm going to do something and later on you're going to cry!' Often these thought processes are the result of smoking marijuana and things that have come from outside Anangu culture. Smoking marijuana can really distort your thinking. Their thinking becomes really confused and they often think that people are angry with them and are out to get them in some way – not caring for them and irritated with them. Consequently they might think they'll do something so people will really think about them and be really saddened by what they do.

We see a range of people who have been affected by substance abuse: smoking too much marijuana, drinking, and other things which are causing them to become ill.

When someone is talking about harming themselves, the first time that it's said it's really important to listen and to sit with that person and treat it seriously. It's important not to give them a hard time, but care for them, slowly talk with them, not say bad things about them, and try to help them think straight again about things. When they think people are saying bad things about them, or that people are irritated and annoyed with them because of their behaviour, they are under quite a bit of pressure. But if they are given a chance to just sit quietly and be cared for, over a period of time they can start to feel good again and their thinking straightens out.

But, on the other hand, the pressure builds up on that person if one person, then another, and another, keeps on saying bad things about them, or says that they're crazy, or is irritated and annoyed with them. If that pressure builds up and a whole lot of people continue to say those things, that's when the person starts to think, 'Alright! If all of you are thinking that way, then I might finish myself off.'

It is important to tell people about the proper way to do things – to encourage them to listen and to learn about Law and to be with family. It's important to tell them that if they go down that broken road of smoking lots of marijuana they're going to get sick and it's a dead end there, it's a very unhealthy road to go down.

If you can see that someone wishes to hurt themselves you are in a position to be able to stop them, to talk with them and help them get through that time. But it's really hard to look after those people who do things in a way that you can't see – at night or in places where they are not being observed.

When we see people are in trouble and are suicidal we know that it's hard to look after them all the time. It's really important they get that help. As ngangkari we say that it's important that they can get to a hospital, be treated and helped. When we're aware of problems like people wanting to harm themselves, then we can work with them and help get their blood flowing properly, help them think more clearly. We also think it's really important that they get professional help in the hospitals and are put there to be looked after at times when they can't be looked after or monitored in the communities. So ngangkari can help those people and in the hospitals they can get good help too.

Rupert Langkatjukur Peter

## Mental health problems are recent phenomena

If people have mental health problems the first thing that happens is their ears cease functioning properly, but you have to understand that mental health problems are a very recent phenomena for us. We never suffered like this in the past, you know. We were all mentally healthy and strong once. What has happened to people today is that they are failing to understand what is going on around them and then they lose the ability to understand things properly. This leads to lack of understanding and getting ideas all mixed up. Much of the problem comes from marijuana and ngangkari are unable to assist with problems of this sort. All we can do is to recommend that the person go and see a doctor and get some tablets.

Wakupi Clem Toby (Dalby)

## I counsel the parents

I don't know why some people develop serious mental health issues and not others. I guess some parents have children who have certain physical disabilities, or mental disabilities – everyone is different. They work hard caring for their families and children. I ask the mothers or the carers, 'How is that person getting along?' and they say to me, 'Good thank you, he (or she) is fine.' But we always keep an eye out for those patients who are disabled and we talk to the families and keep in contact and make sure that everything's OK. I counsel the parents and do what I can and recommend they stick with their doctors and their medication plans.

Maringka Burton

## Kata kura tjuta – people with mental health problems

If the government gives funding it can help to develop and support ngangkari work and assist them to get around further and give treatments to more children. We will also be able to get around more and see young petrol sniffers and ex-petrol sniffers, and marijuana smokers, to try and help unblock their nervous system. My son and I work on the pulyku, tendons and nervous system. Pulyku get blocked and cause mental health problems, and this is caused by smoking and sniffing. People can't talk about it and suffer misery and upset for that person. They become isolated and just sit down by themselves, not talking to people.

Most ngangkari can't help people who are damaged from exotic outside products like petrol and marijuana but we can at least help them with their nervous systems and tendons. So we help to soothe and ease the pulyku by strong massage and help by loosening it and encouraging an improved flow. I am always going into the Mental Health Unit at Alice Springs hospital, doing exactly that, working with people with mental health problems. They are always really happy after I go in there. People are in there for all sorts of things. I'm never frightened of going in there. As soon as I enter I see things with my ngangka_ri vision.

Our people may have some mental health problems. My auntie had problems with her mental health once. She would cook rabbits but give them to us completely underdone. Blood would come flowing out! She had mental health problems at the time. My uncle gave her a good ngangka_ri treatment and she got better. But previously she would give the meat to us, quite red and fresh, instead of properly cooked through. She just didn't understand, she was not in a good space. She wasn't old at all, she was still quite young. She became mentally unstable. It manifested in this raw meat thing. She would say, 'Eat the meat!' and then she'd run off, shouting.

My mother was her sister-in-law, and the two of them would sit together while we children played elsewhere. My mother would sit and look after her sister-in-law. She was my father's sister. She became cranky and we were scared of her and would run away from her! She was mentally ill. We would run away from her when she shouted. Later, I would help her and I'd tell her, 'Come here and sit down!' Something had happened to her a long time ago. My father worked on her to keep her going.

It is possible that there is blood leaking into the brain when someone is mentally ill. When people get old, ngangka_ri can help with dementia. Ngangka_ri can help a bit but when people get really old their tendons get worn out, but their spirits are good. When women and men get old their bodies and minds get worn out.

Pantjiti Unkari McKenzie

## Using those substances leads to self harm

In so many different communities today you see a lot of problems associated with using marijuana, drinking alcohol and petrol sniffing. People will be thinking about going and getting marijuana, they'll be asking, trying to get it the whole time, and not thinking about other people or how they relate to other people there. It's a different way of thinking. Using those substances leads to self harm and people thinking about suicide. This different way of thinking is something recent that's come about. It's just come up through the use and abuse of those substances.

Rupert Langkatjukur Peter

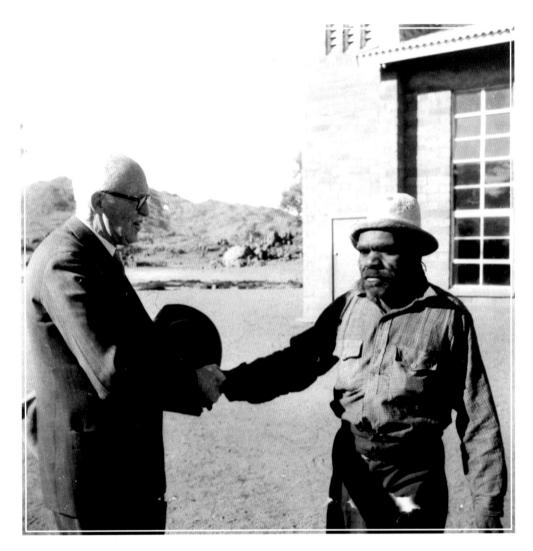

Dr Charles Duguid shaking hands with Jacky Tjupuru Baker, possibly during the official opening and dedication of the new Ernabella hospital, Pukatja (Ernabella), 1958.
PHOTOGRAPH JOHN FLETCHER, JOHN FLETCHER COLLECTION, ARA IRITITJA AI-0012956

*Duguid worked in his own way using needles and what have you. Meanwhile we were working in our way battling mamu and removing negative spirits, protecting our children from danger.* Andy Tjilari

# Working Together

### *Doctor, ngangkari. Ngangkari, doctor. Same thing*

Back in the days before white people moved to this land, ngangkari worked purely amongst their own people. Ngangkari have only recently been working with white doctors. White doctors have only recently begun to trust ngangkari. They used to think we were strangling people! So ngangkari never used to work openly. They always hid their treatments from white people. Since the days of Nganampa Health Council and the Mental Health Unit, though, ngangkari have performed their treatments in the presence and sight of white people and doctors.

Previously ngangkari didn't want to be seen giving treatments because they thought that white people would think they were killing their patients by lirintananyi – strangulation! Throttling them! That's what they thought back in those early days, 'Hey! Hey! Wait!' we would say. 'A white person is approaching! Wait! Wait!' So the treatment would stop until the white person had passed by, and then the treatment would be resumed. That's what we would do. But today it is recognised that a ngangkari is a doctor too. Doctor, ngangkari. Ngangkari, doctor. Same thing.

Pantjiti McKenzie

### *He did his doctoring and so did we*

Doctor Duguid arrived on our Lands and we saw him when we were still children. He was very keen on Anangu retaining their old traditional cultures and working in grandfather's way. So he encouraged us to work in the same style as grandfather, but he didn't know about ngangkari or understand what we did. He did his doctoring and so did we, but separately. Our older ngangkari never stopped working after he arrived. Just because he was there we had no reason to stop working. We worked as we always had done back in our own homes and camps.

Bernard Tjalkuriny

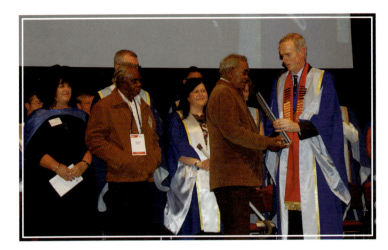

Professor Ken Kirkby, (now former) President of the Royal Australian and New Zealand College of Psychiatrists (RANZCP), presenting the 2009 Mark Sheldon Prize to Andy Tjilari and Rupert Peter (left) in recognition of the NPY Women's Council's Ngangkari Project's 'noteworthy contribution to Indigenous mental health'. Also present are Sharon Brownie, (now former) CEO of the RANZCP, and (centre) Dr Maria Tomasic (now former) Honorary Secretary of the RANZCP. The ceremony was held in Adelaide, South Australia, 2009. PHOTOGRAPH ANGELA LYNCH

*One time when we were at the hospital for a meeting with the doctors we told them we're doctors too. And now look at us! We are all level.* Rupert Langkatjukur Peter

## *Duguid had an open door policy*

I used to live at Ernabella Mission. Doctor Duguid and his contemporaries were there, but he was still a young man back then. My grandfather would watch Doctor Duguid working, using his style, but he was still very close to Anangu, he was like their own kin. He was very knowledgeable. Our traditional ngangkari doctors all went into his hospital to look around and they liked it very much. He had an open door policy and ngangkari were welcome to come in and work alongside him. Often he would wait until the ngangkari did their work before he looked at patients. He would give the patients tablets and medicines afterwards. The ngangkari were happy for him to work there, and they were welcome do their own work openly as well. It was open and the different doctors worked together.

Wakupi Clem Toby (Dalby)

## *Ngangkari work is varied and vitally important*

Duguid worked in his own way using needles and what have you. Meanwhile we were working in our own way battling mamu and removing negative spirits, protecting our children from danger. Our ngangkari work is very varied and vitally important.

Andy Tjilari

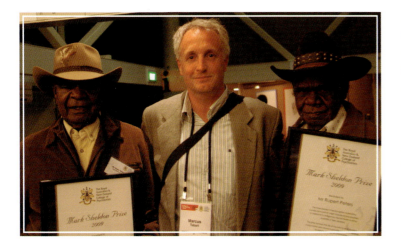

Andy Tjilari, Dr Marcus Tabart (Senior Consultant Psychiatrist, Central Australian Mental Health Service) and Rupert Langkatjukur Peter at the ceremony where the Royal Australian and New Zealand College of Psychiatrists awarded the Mark Sheldon Prize to the ngangkari, Adelaide, South Australia, 2009. PHOTOGRAPH ANGELA LYNCH

*We have formed a really good bond with doctors in hospitals and we work together as one. It's a really strong relationship where we work as one. That working together involves different techniques with the same purpose in mind.*
Andy Tjilari

### *Our fathers continued to be the leading, practising ngangkari*

Doctor Duguid didn't simply take over the delivery of health services. Our old fathers never stopped being in charge of our health. Doctor Duguid didn't come until much later. He was only a recent visitor, while our fathers continued to be the leading, practising ngangkari.

Pantjiti McKenzie

### *This level of cooperation makes us very happy*

One time, when we were at the hospital for a meeting with the doctors, we told them we were doctors too. And now look at us! We are all level. We had a meeting there on the other side. We went into an area and were questioned. We are level with them now. Nurses go to university and learn through books. We said, 'Can you see all those black people? This hospital is full of black people. It is our job to look after those people. They are our family members. You are mostly all white people and you are doing a good job looking after our people but there are times when our people want one of their own to treat them, and that's the truth of it. So sometimes you need to stand aside while we step in and perform what is, sometimes, dangerous work. It is fine for you to observe us working but please don't interfere. After we have given our treatments our family members are happy and relieved, and then we are only too glad for you to resume your own style of patient care. This level of cooperation makes us very happy and satisfied as opposed to us wandering around outside feeling miserable.' So we go there now and explain what we do. We are not here to kill anyone! Of course not!

Rupert Langkatjukur Peter

## *We are now working alongside doctors and sisters*

There is mamu in his kurunpa! With our mapanpa we remove that mamu in the form of a stone or a stick or a bone, because ngangkari can see inside a person, whereas a doctor will take their pulse and give medicines, while a ngangkari will look into their kurunpa and recognise that they may have no spirit, poor things.

Andy Tjilari

## *Working together involves different techniques with the same purpose in mind*

Often we work alongside Western practitioners and share the responsibilities for looking after people. For us, our ability to see the spirit and to recognise what has happened comes from within our minds, within our heads – we can see things that they can't see.

Our work as ngangkari takes us not only to communities within our world but also to cities where we see people as well. In our work in the cities, in the hospitals, we have formed a really good bond with doctors and we work together as one. It's a really strong relationship where we work as one. That working together involves different techniques with the same purpose in mind. Whereas doctors might use operations and provide medicines and things like that, we look at the effect of that illness on the spirit. We see when someone's lost their spirit. We can find the lost spirit and place it where it should be. And that is part of healing and looking after people properly, ngangkari way.

Recently I moved to a city where my daughter, Inawinytji, is on dialysis and I've been able to continue to work as a ngangkari there. The doctors have often called on me to come and help them in many situations. When I was a child both my grandfather and my father taught me how to be a ngangkari and I have continued from that time to heal and look after people. They gave me the ability to do that. My grandfather gave me the power to recognise the spirit, to see it, to hold it and to place it back in people.

When we went to Canberra we talked really strongly about the importance of working together and respecting each other's abilities. It is important to know that we ngangkari do our work, to recognise the work we do, and know that it's important to call us so we can work together. We really encourage those working in the hospitals and the Western medical systems to call on us and to utilise us.

Our work is not hidden. It's important that I work in a transparent way – people can see what I do. It is important work, we are proud of our work, we are not embarrassed about what we do and we are confident in working alongside Western practitioners. We think it is really important that we work together openly in that spirit.

Andy Tjilari

## I still am confident in the hospital situation

My father and all the other ngangkari of his generation never worked with whitefella doctors. We are the first generation of ngangkari to work like we do, openly in clinics with white people. We are the first ones to be working alongside doctors. The work my father did, and all the other ngangkari who lived in his time was never recognised. It is only us modern ones who are working like we do now, appearing in books and on videos and DVDs, talking about the healing.

We go into the hospitals and do healing, too. I remember going into the hospital to see Kunbry's granddaughter and I healed her. One day I came into Alice Springs for an NPY Women's Council executive meeting, and Kunbry told me, 'My granddaughter is really sick. Can you go in there and see her?' That poor little child was there a long time with a bad burn, and she would cry all the time. So I went to the hospital and I marched straight in. I was confident in myself and I still am confident in the hospital situation. They let Kunbry and I in and we went straight in. I walked in empty-handed. The doctors know me and they know I get people out of hospital quicker. Nobody tried to stop us from doing our work. When I entered the ward, I saw that child lying there with a hot fever, and miserable, and I saw her kurunpa quite separate from her, cowering in the corner of the room. I captured her kurunpa and straight away I replaced it where it should be, and she instantly improved! When I saw her, she was still a little girl, but she's all grown up now. At meetings I follow up on her and ask Kunbry, 'How's your granddaughter getting along now?' and she tells me she's really good! 'She's fantastic, she's great! She's a big girl now!'

I'd really like to get an ID tag, you know, that identifies who I am and acknowledges my skills and my work. I have worked in Adelaide hospital as well as Alice Springs hospital. So, yes, our work there is important work and it's good work and it would be good to have a photo ID tag for us, just so that the sisters and nurses and the medical staff can see us, and see our ID, and know that we are traditional healers.

And that's what we do, you know, we get the person's kurunpa and we reposition it back into the body. We work together, our ngangkari team, we all work together, Andy, Rupert and Martin. When there's NPY Women's Council Women's Law and Culture gathering, Kanakiya is another ngangkari, she and I work together. Kanakiya has gone back to Adelaide now, but when we are together we are a really strong team. What a great woman she is! She's marvellous!

Maringka Burton

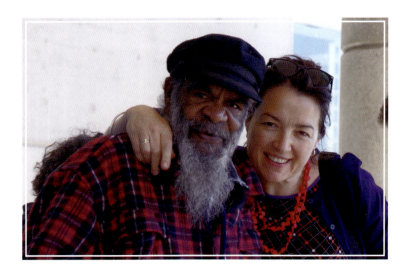

Andy Tjilari and Angela Lynch in Sydney, New South Wales, 2011 (with the rest of the team), to collect the World Council for Psychotherapy Sigmund Freud award for 'contributions to psychotherapy,' bestowed by the city of Vienna.
PHOTOGRAPH AIDAN HOOKEY

### *The two treatments complement each other*

Modern Western doctors prescribe medication and tablets in the clinic, while our work takes place in the open air. Many of our healing treatments happen outside, and theirs happen indoors. That's OK. That works fine. We find that the two treatments complement each other. Doctors have recently started consulting with me and other ngangkari. This is a recent change. Before that they had no idea about our work, yet before then there were no other doctors but us. Nowadays, however, the doctors are getting to appreciate the way ngangkari work and understand us a lot more.

Wakupi Clem Toby (Dalby)

### *Hopefully we'll work out good ways to support each other, the doctors doing their work, we doing our work*

So, you have learnt about some of our understandings, our observations about how and why people get sick. Western doctors often have difficulty understanding these things and the way we work. And so we hope the way we're talking now helps those people understand something of our work, see how we do things. We hope the doctors will be able to understand something of Anangu Law, of traditional healing, the things that we can do, and see the ways that we can work productively side by side, in harmony with each other. Hopefully we'll work out good ways to support each other, the doctors doing their work, we doing our work.

We understand that Western medicine has a whole range of good ways of helping people get better – really intelligent ways of being able to help people by conducting operations, seeing what's causing the harm inside and removing things. And we as ngangkari, too, have the knowledge to be able to remove things that are causing harm.

When doctors perform operations and see what's causing the problem they remove things and close people off again and you see a scar from where the operation took place. When we remove things that are causing harm from people, there is no scar and no wound that you can see. When the object that's causing harm is removed it's only on the inside that you see that wound. It doesn't cause a wound as it comes through the skin and we take it out.

Andy Tjilari

## *Sharing knowledge*

And so we tell you these things so you can understand something of our Law and our knowledge and of the work that we can do. We work as ngangkari in this way. This is our body of knowledge – it's the important things that we do to help people feel well within themselves and stay well. There are many ngangkari that do the same sort of work that we do. We are just two working here but there are many ngangkari who help work with Anangu. Ngangkari have that role of finding a spiritual balance and well-being.

Rupert Langkatjukur Peter

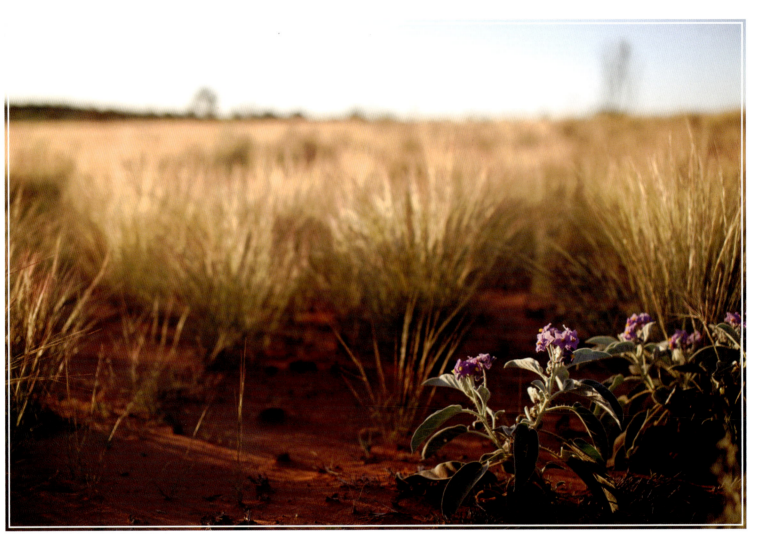

PHOTOGRAPH RHETT HAMMERTON

# Recognition and Equality

*We ngangkari are asking for proper recognition of our special skills*

We are talking about the way ngangkari think and work in order for others to understand. Ngangkari are talking especially for the people who work in health in other ways. Ngangkari work differently from doctors who prescribe medicines. People are eager to learn more about us ngangkari. We are cooperating with other people's desires to learn about ngangkari. However, we wonder what they might do with these stories. They are our stories. They are just for listening to. Remember that they belong to Anangu and they are full of our Tjukurpa. Tjukurpa nganampa Ananguku. Tjukurpa ngangkariku. This means, 'Our Law – Aboriginal people's Law. Ngangkari Law.'

We know a lot of people are looking forward to hearing what we ngangkari have to say, and we are obliging by telling them what they want to know. But we ngangkari want recognition and understanding in return for talking clearly and revealing our names and our work. We'll be telling the truth, of course, and our names will be attached to our stories. So you'll know who we are and we'll be more out in the open. If this brings about a greater demand for our services, then we want an improvement in the way our services are used. We need to make a living. Many of us go hungry a lot of the time, and so if we have got a skill that is in demand, and is respected as it should be, then we would like to start making enough income to improve our living conditions and to stop having to go around hungry all the time.

Who else can talk about ngangkari but us? We are the only ones. There are very few of us left these days. Yet we are still working, which is good, because it is important and valued work in our community. It should be. Who else can refer to ancestral ngangkari power in the sky for help?

We ngangkari love our work and all we are asking for is a better deal. There are quite a few people who are having such a difficult time in life that they are starting to say that they won't be able to continue working as ngangkari any more despite the special gift that they have. We are hoping that by telling people about our work that we will become able to be qualified to receive a proper amount of payment for our work, an amount that will give us enough to live on, like so many other people who are specialists. People like to see us work. It is a special thing. I know white people are fascinated and interested. We know this because we are being asked to talk into this cassette recorder.

When I do my healing work I really appreciate it if someone buys me a kangaroo tail or some meat, or gives me enough money to get a tank of petrol. Don't forget what I said though, ngangkari work is mostly a labour of love because everyone is our kin. But we've got to live on something. No point in going around hungry. It's a terrible thing if we are starving hungry and we have to refuse to help someone. Nobody can work on an empty stomach, can they?

This book will have stories from all of us. We are ngangkari and we are putting our stories down for the record. Once you have gone over all the stories you will have something to think about. I hope you enjoy all the stories you read, which we ngangkari have given, in order to help not only the ngangkari, but also the sick people who rely on ngangkari for spiritual healing. We are hoping that other good things come from this book too. It is a teaching book. We have already done a lot of teaching, but we are prepared to do more, as much as it takes to get ourselves properly listened to, instead of sidelined as we are sometimes. We sometimes find ourselves bypassed and forgotten, which is a shame for the sick people who could benefit from seeing us. We find ourselves being treated suspiciously, as if we were charlatans. Treated suspiciously as if we were charlatans! As if we were absolute charlatans!

It is for all these reasons that we ngangkari are asking for proper recognition of our special skills. Better pay and a better working life isn't really asking for much, considering the job we do. We are all asking. I am telling you this now, because you asked me to talk. I am advocating on behalf of all the other ngangkari because it is a topic of conversation among us. Ngangkari do a lot of talking, especially now that we are making a book. So when the book is finished, with a bit of luck all, the workers in our communities will have heard our stories and will be a bit more aware of the problems we face and the issues we want to raise.

Arnie Frank

## *People cannot survive on medication and needles alone*

If there were no ngangkari, Anangu would all die. All Anangu would die if we had no ngangkari. Nobody would be left, without ngangkari. This is why we need ngangkari programs to be supported. People cannot survive on medication and needles alone.

The government needs to support ngangkari because ngangkari work with their bodies. Their bodies are their tools. They do not use needles and tablets. They heal people with their hands, in people's own homes. Ngangkari is an ancient skill handed down to us by our ancestors.

Anangu have got much worse health statistics than non-Anangu. We are all renal patients. Ngangkari cannot change renal failure. They cannot use the healing touch on renal failure or extract the disease. They are unable to help renal patients. The only ones that can help are the renal dialysis nurses and the doctors with their drugs and machines.

Our old men and women were the ultimate survivors, living without illness, living on wild food and wild meat and no butter.

Pantjiti Unkari McKenzie

## *Ngangkari want to be recognised as specialist doctors*

I don't worry about money as much as some people. It is more important to me to keep up my skills as a ngangkari and a traditional healer and to keep practising them. I worry more about helping sick people and using my ngangkari powers. We are specialist doctors and ngangkari want to be recognised as specialist doctors. Because of that we would like to get the pay of a specialist doctor. We already get other kinds of specialists who come in from distant places from all over Australia, but don't forget that there are us specialists who live here.

The specialists come in and are able to diagnose particular illnesses and recommend particular treatments. We ngangkari do exactly the same. We are specialists and have had a long training, too. Not everybody has the training and ability to be a ngangkari. We have a certain power in our hands. We have the ability to capture sicknesses and heal people. The way a non-Anangu specialist works is to diagnose an illness, say, inside the body, and then recommend an operation. They'll perform the operation by cutting open the body and removing a part of the body. The skin will be cut and blood will be spilt. Healthy spilt blood is wasted blood. Ngangkari do not cut open the skin nor spill blood. They touch, massage and knead the skin and the body. They can extract sickness and bring about rapid healing and relief. This is all done in a pain-free way, which only a specialist doctor can perform. We are specialist doctors – there is no doubt about it.

Everybody has their own specialities. The men certainly have strong power and special abilities. They are generally at the top, they are number one, the men. They have a special power. We see white men doctors who are specialists who earn a lot of money. Well, our wati ngangkari are just the same, but we, too, should receive equal pay. They do equal work. Government people, please listen to us, as this is such an important issue.

We would like the Government to try to understand us more and give us better recognition. We would also like to receive better pay. I'd like to see the Women's Council get better funding to help all us ngangkari. We could do with more money. They could employ more women ngangkari and men ngangkari.

I would like to keep talking up about this because it is the lack of recognition that is the hard part. As I said, I specialise in treating women and children. I work as a ngangkari. I don't get paid for ngangkari work, as apparently there is no money to pay ngangkari. This is big Tjukurpa, ngangkari Tjukurpa. We are specialist doctors, just like other specialist doctors. That just about sums up what I want to say.

Josephine Mick

## *Why should I do all this work and not get paid?*

I used to work as a ngangkari but I didn't receive any pay and that's why I didn't work for a while. I didn't do any healing work because there was no money and I didn't have any ngangkari payment. That's why I refused to work. If I know that I'm getting a cheque I'll work really hard through the clinic doing healing work with the clinic. Now I'm still not working as much because I'm not being paid a wage. So I say, 'Why should I do all this work and not get paid for the work?' Maybe Nganampa Health Council should pay my wages so that I can do my work full-time. I get paid by the clinic. It's big, important work, that ngangkari work. I join up in the clinic and do healing work. And in the clinic you'll see all the stones, all the objects, sticks and stuff, with the names of the people on the bottle. The objects that I've removed from the sick people, they're there in bottles there, labelled with people's names.

Sam Wimitja Watson

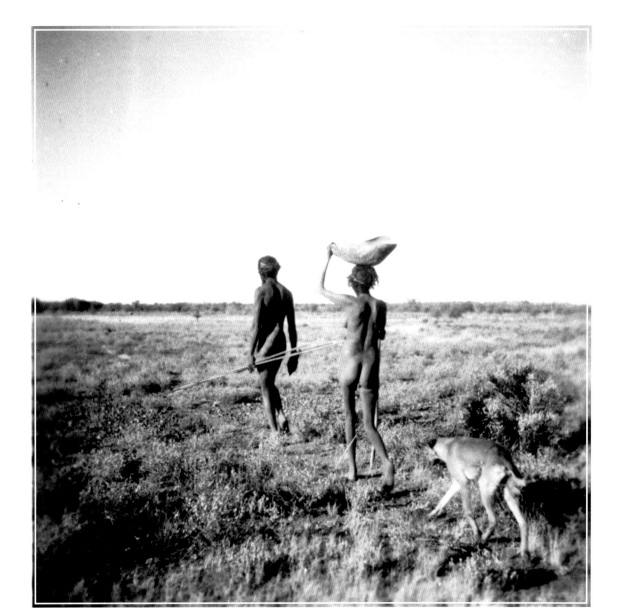

Tommy Urutjakunu and Anawari Inkgatji (Andy Tjilari's parents) carrying water in a piti – wooden bowl, Atila (Mt Connor), Northern Territory, 1940.
PHOTOGRAPH CHARLES MOUNTFORD, MOUNTFORD SHEARD COLLECTION, COURTESY OF THE STATE LIBRARY OF SOUTH AUSTRALIA, PRG 1218/34/1302B

*I reflect on how well my mother and father looked after me. In those days my father would go hunting and bring back kangaroo. My mother and sisters would go and dig up rabbits and bring back that meat. They really looked after me well and gave me a strength that I have today.* Andy Tjilari

# Children and Youth

*Today you see a lot of children weakened and not having strength and not being cared for*

When I was a child my mother and father gave me a great education in life and that has helped me today. I reflect on how well my mother and father looked after me. In those days my father would go hunting and bring back kangaroo. My mother and sisters would go and dig up rabbits and bring back that meat. They really looked after me well and gave me a strength that I have today.

I think about how hard it is for children when their parents have left them or aren't looking after them – it weakens their spirit – and how difficult it is for them. Today you see a lot of children weakened and not having strength and not being cared for.

If the child has been left and the mother and father aren't looking after them, it often falls to the grandparents to care for those children. As people get older, it's really difficult for them to take on that full responsibility – they are getting tired themselves. You can really see the children's spirit getting weaker and weaker in those situations, when they are not being looked after by their parents. When I say they are getting weak, I am talking about their spirit getting weak. You can see a shift from where it should be – their sense of self and balance – it goes somewhere else. As ngangkari that is one of our key roles with children: to look after their spirit and help put it back where it should be, to give them the strength to cope.

When someone is sick their spirit can leave their body and you can see it somewhere; for example, in a tree or somewhere nearby. It has left the person – they are dispirited – and as ngangkari we recognise where that is and we put it back where it belongs. That's a really important part of people getting better.

In the case of children, when their parents have left them and are not caring for them properly – neither their mother nor their father – and they are with their grandmother and she is getting tired, she is not in a position to be able to look after them. We give them treatments and we help them and we strengthen them. But again and again they'll continue to get sick. At night they will cry and their spirit will leave them because they're really sad – it's an ongoing thing. When they are crying that's when their spirit goes and they start to get sicker and sicker.

Many things affect people's spirit. If that child is left by themselves and they are with other children, they can get into fights and disputes. They get a bit upset if they are hit – their spirit will be displaced from fear or other things. The spirit should be here [Andy touches centre of his abdomen] and it might be up here, for example, but they don't feel centred. They have lost their sense of self and as ngangka<u>r</u>i we can see where it's gone to. We just put it back where it belongs and that's a way of helping them heal.

It's been a really satisfying process working with healers and other doctors to try to care for these children who have been left, who aren't being cared for – say, if their parents are drinking, or not thinking about them or not being close by. We observe that these children get really sad – they cry and cry and cry. We observe the effect on their spirit, we think about their situation and talk a lot with doctors about how best to help them. Doctors have a good understanding about what we can do and we work together to try and help those children.

It's not only the spirit side of things for these children. Often their parents will leave them and their grandmother will be the sole person looking after them. They might not have a blanket, they might just be sleeping on the ground. They are open to getting sick in so many different ways and not being cared for properly.

The problem is, if all the responsibility falls on the grandmother or grandparents to look after those children, they are getting older and older and it's really difficult. What can they do? It's a really bad situation at times. They get older, eventually they pass away, and then the children are really lost. Then there's no one to look after those children so they're in a very difficult situation. We observe that a lot. The grandparents are placed under extraordinary pressure and they're getting older and older and it's increasingly difficult to look after those children.

So when that's all happening, that's when you see children being taken from their families and put in foster care. Then the kids are not living with their own families any more. That's happening all the time. That's the cycle you see going on now. If that happens and there's no one in the extended family who can look after those children, that's when they need to be looked after and are taken and cared for properly. But it's only when there is no one else who can look after them within the family. You see that happening quite a lot.

Andy Tjilari


### *Today it's really difficult for a lot of children ... It's not as clear as it was when I was growing up*

Today we work as ngangka<u>r</u>i over a really extensive area of Central Australia. We do it together because we care. We want to look after people. That's what we were taught. So in our work we see a lot of children and you can see their spirit getting weaker. As ngangka<u>r</u>i we can see their spirit, see where it is, know where it should be and put it back where it belongs so they can regain a sense of self. That's the primary way we care for and look after those children.

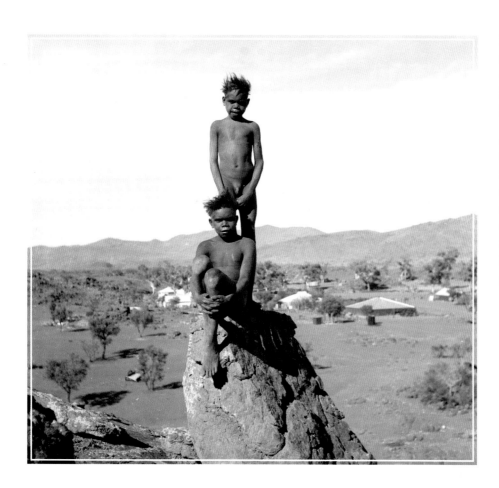

Rupert Langkatjukur Peter (standing) and Mungkuri (sitting) on a rock, with Pukatja community buildings in background, Pukatja (Ernabella), 1950.
PHOTOGRAPH RICHARD SEEGER, COURTESY MUSEUM VICTORIA (XP617)

*I grew up in a time when things were really clear. Ngangka__ri__ had the sole responsibility for healing and caring and we lived in the bush without clothes and that was our way. Today it's really difficult for a lot of children – they find themselves in a really difficult situation. It's not as clear as it was when I was growing up.* Rupert Langkatjukur Peter

We can see them really sad if their parents are neglecting them or are not with them. We can see at night, see them crying and getting really upset. We see that happening and our work is to treat their spirit to help them feel better.

For us, we are continuing a really long tradition of healing within our world, the Pitjantjatjara world. The skills, the way that I do my work, I was taught by my father and grandfather. I grew up in a family that was really strong and clear about the proper way to do things. And that is the way that I work today as a ngangka__ri__.

I grew up in a time when things were really clear. Ngangka__ri__ had the sole responsibility for healing and caring and we lived in the bush without clothes and that was our way. Today it's really difficult for a lot of children – they find themselves in a really difficult situation. It's not as clear as it was when I was growing up.

In these times there are clinics within the communities and we work really closely with the clinic staff. We respect what they are trying to do and they respect what we are trying to do. We know there are a lot of problems and we work really closely together.

Rupert Langkatjukur Peter

*Children and Youth*

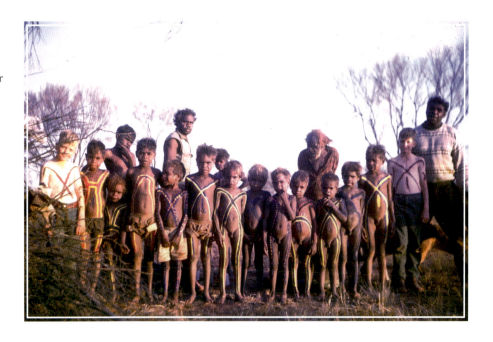

Boys decorated for Inma Matukupiri Nyiinyii with Rupert Langkatjukur Peter (adult in back row, left) and Rupert's brother (on his father's side) Windlass (far right), Kaltjiti (Fregon), South Australia, 1970. PHOTOGRAPH BOB CAPP, ARA IRITITJA AI-0010479

## *In our area our children are all doing really well*

I only work with children who are sick – physically sick with sore feet, ears and eyes and so on – but we don't work with those children who are witnessing, on a day-to-day basis, family fighting, and who live with alcoholic parents and are seeing fighting and violent behaviour. We can't prevent lifelong trauma and mental health problems from that. We only work with children and adults who are ill, with sickness or sores or aches and pains in their body, hands, ears, eyes and feet.

Sometimes I work with the puuni blowing technique. I do that on the foot, blowing on the foot. That's for when a child gets poked in the foot by something sharp. That's what we call the puuni blowing technique. Blowing seals up the wound cleanly. It is great to see it work so well and to see the children later on running around happily. I go and check them out later and it is very satisfying to see them well again. We grandmothers care for our grandchildren sometimes and we find our children are happy where we live. Maybe in other places, children are not so well cared for but in our area our children are all doing really well. It is great to see the children in the school yard playing so happily, and I know I helped to get them there. We have a very strong community spirit where I live.

Maringka Burton

## *No mother or father*

Nowadays there are a lot of children in the communities with no mother or father. If there is no mother, the aunts and the grandmother will care for the children. They will look after them if they are not well and take them to see a ngankgari and after seeing a ngangkari, they will take them to see a doctor.

Pantjiti Unkari McKenzie


## *All the family have a responsibility*

When a baby is born it lives with its mother and father, it sits there listening, mother and father talking, it sees the other family members around, and as the baby grows up it starts to walk, it will start to get around.

As the young child goes around, its mother will be keeping an eye on it, and might call out, 'Hey! Come over here my child!' And the kid, being young, will come straight away, responding to the mum. It's really only listening to its mother. If the child hears its mother or father calling out, it comes immediately because that's who it's listening to – its family. The child is only being influenced by the family. The mothers and fathers and family will see their child grow up. As they grow up they start to spend more time with a range of different people and have other influences on their lives.

As teenagers, they start to become more and more independent, they hold onto the understanding that their parents gave them. They also start to learn a lot more things and you see a whole series of people growing up really well, living well, and having that one story that was given to them by their parents.

So some kids grow up and as teenagers they have a really good understanding of life. Their parents have looked after them, they've given them a good story, they hold onto that story and you can see in their brain their blood is working well. It's flowing really well and they are thinking really well about things.

On the other hand, this is the time when a lot of teenagers are really vulnerable to other influences. If someone who has been thinking really well takes up marijuana smoking or petrol sniffing, this is a time when that good understanding can be finished. Their blood gets blocked, it doesn't flow well, and it's like having a lid put on their brain. It's like they don't listen any more, their mind is closed off, there are blockages blocking the blood from flowing through – stones, pieces of wood or things that close their minds off. They become really confused in their thinking. When their family is talking to them they don't understand what's being said to them. They get confused, they get the wrong idea, and they don't understand what's really happening.

Others are OK. They grow up to become men with a really good understanding of life, clear in their thinking. They begin at this stage to help others: sons and grandsons and other young people. They begin to help them develop their understanding of life. And so the person's world view continues to grow and their understanding of life develops. We grew up in this way. Our parents gave us a really good understanding of things. Then we learnt from others. That's why we are alive and well today. Previously, this was the way we grew up and continued to learn as we got older. You see us now – we hold onto a good understanding of things.

So the way we grew up previously was along a really straight line, as I've outlined to you – through from being a baby, to becoming a teenager, to becoming a man and the influences on your life and thinking as you grew up. With petrol sniffing and marijuana smoking, that line is no longer there. It's finished. Instead of having the one clear straight line, it separated out into all these different ways and all these different paths. And all these other harmful things have come in on the side and started to cause that one line to be split up and divided.

We've been talking about how open-minded children are. They are open to influences and those influences initially are of their parents and immediate family – people they see and listen to. They are really responsive to that. As they grow older, especially in those teenage years, you start to see they're being influenced by other things and that's when they are most vulnerable to things like marijuana, and to petrol. You see a number of people, their mind's been really harmed by those things. As teenagers they might start smoking or sniffing petrol and they might think, 'Oh, this is pretty good!' But they are damaging themselves, harming their mind in doing that. In drinking and sniffing and smoking, that's when they start to lose that clear understanding of life. Their blood starts to become all mixed up rather than flowing through in one clear, good line. In the process their thinking starts to become confused and they harm their minds. Their thinking changes – that's when we say it's 'blocked' and not flowing through properly.

Previously, when petrol and marijuana weren't part of the world, a good understanding of things came from your mother and father, from your older brothers – this guidance through life. But now marijuana and petrol have caused a lot of problems. They are spoiling a lot of things and causing a lot of harm to people everywhere. And there's no longer that clear and straightway of growing up, and of thinking well. It's not straight any more.

We've got to work out how to block those things to stop them coming in and we've got to keep on caring for those who've been harmed by marijuana and by petrol. Stop them and then care and keep on caring, for those people, continue to look after them, continue to give them good understanding, talk with them well and after that they will be able to become more balanced and things will level out within them. All the family have a responsibility with this.

Rupert Langkatjukur Peter

## *The kids I've healed are really good*

Last year we did a big healing with all the children at Iwantja. When children are unwell mentally we work with them, we do the wirunymankupai.

There are kids who have parents who don't care for them and what happens to them emotionally and mentally. A lot of the kids from Docker River get sent to me and I heal them.

I heal people if they've got sore tummies or sore heads. And the kids I've healed are really good, they're really well now.

Sam Wimitja Watson


## *They start to lose contact with those positive influences*

Obviously there's an important role for grandparents and parents, uncles and aunties and the whole family in caring for people when they're saddened and depressed, especially young people. There's an important role for mothers and fathers, grandparents and older brothers and sisters to look after children, to help them be happy, to support them. When they are cared for in that way they are happy. You see a child play during the day, at night as well, they're happy.

A lot of young children you see play all the time, they're really happy. It's as they get slightly older and become teenagers that they come into contact with marijuana and other things and it's from that time they're at great risk of their happiness finishing. As teenagers, when they come into contact with marijuana, that's the time we often see them becoming really depressed and sad, a time when they start to lose contact with those positive influences of their older brothers and sisters and family. They become more isolated and more and more sad as they smoke. They start to think more about marijuana. You can see great harm done to their spirit and also to their heads and to their thinking during this process. There are a whole lot of really harmful changes that take place, both within their spirit and within their minds.

Rupert Langkatjukur Peter

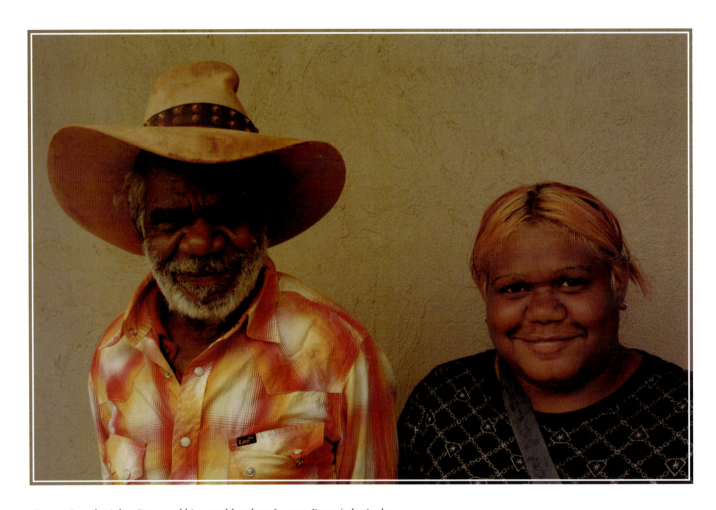

Rupert Langkatjukur Peter and his granddaughter Loretta Peter (who is also Tinpulya Mervyn's granddaughter), Alice Springs, Northern Territory, 2011.
PHOTOGRAPH ANGELA LYNCH

*In my case, now that I am a senior man, there are four grandsons and three granddaughters who I have given powers to and begun their training. They are doing really good things.* Rupert Langkatjukur Peter

*There are many new young ngangkari coming up. I am passing my ngangkari knowledge on to two of my granddaughters, Loretta and Rosemary, who have been given their healing tools by Langkatjukur.* Tinpulya Mervyn

# Future Ngangka*r*i

*The skills of the ngangka*r*i are handed down through the generations*

I was young, a young fella, unfamiliar with the work of a ngangka*r*i when my grandfather approached me and asked me if I was interested in learning about being a ngangka*r*i.

He was getting older and reaching the end of his working life. He was looking at being able to pass those skills and knowledge on. He asked if I would like to be involved in that and after that he began my training and giving me the capacity to do things. Part of that process involved times at night when he placed certain things – tools and abilities and skills – within me, things that were his, which belonged to ngangka*r*i and which were important to enable me to look after people. So these tools and abilities and skills were placed within me, but I still had to learn how to use them.

My grandfather began to teach me how to use them properly and to ask me questions and test how I was going. For example, he would ask if I could see and recognise a spirit or something that was causing people harm. He said, 'Can you see what's there?' And I said, 'Yes I can see that.' I began to be able to see things and recognise things. I had said yes I could see it, but he was keen to test me further, so he said, 'Look, can you really see it? Go over there and get it, if that's the case!' And he watched me as I did, I got it. In that way he started to develop my ability. It was a harmful thing that he wanted me to take hold of and remove and I got the right one and gave it to him and he said, 'Good, this is the start now, now we'll really get on with things.'

In those early days I was growing up still, I was still young and I followed in my father's, grandfather's footsteps as a ngangka*r*i. I am talking about in the days before hospitals. We were looking after our people in the bush and that was the role of the ngangka*r*i. And obviously in those days we weren't getting paid for our work, it was something we did – not for money; it was part of looking after our people. I grew up continuing to work as a ngangka*r*i.

Just getting back to what I was talking about with my grandfathers with what he was saying and the way that he tested me there, the next phase of that was working with the spirit and he said to me, 'Can you see that spirit over there?' and in this case the spirit of a person, not a harmful thing. And my grandfather said, 'Go over there and get it because this is the sort of thing you are going to have to do.' I did – I went over and I got it and held onto it. And so I was able to hold that spirit that had been there – it was up on a tree. My grandfather said, 'OK, now it's time to place it back in that person, that young fella nearby. I did that and the person felt really good again, their spirit was back within them, they felt invigorated again.

This is working with the spiritual well-being of our people, looking after our people. The knowledge of how to do that and the skills of the ngangka*r*i are handed down through the generations. We have held onto that knowledge. It's just natural, it's the way it was. My grandfather, for example, as he was getting older and coming towards the end of his working life, would look at passing on those skills. The older ngangka*r*i would start to bring us up in that way so that we could continue to hold onto it and look after it too. That's the way that Ngangka*r*i Law is held onto.

In my case, now that I am a senior man, there are four grandsons and three granddaughters who I have given powers to and begun their training. They are doing really good things. For example, just this morning I rang in and one said they had just treated someone who would be able to go home now.

You've got to remember that this is the tradition, this is knowledge and Law. It's something that has been held onto which came from the days before there were hospitals and other forms of doctors. We were responsible for looking after all the people. We have held onto that knowledge and it was something that was part of living in the bush. That's where it has come from. Today we work in the clinics and work together but it came out of that tradition, out of the bush, and there was no one else.

Rupert Langkatjukur Peter

## *We still do that work and people still are learning to be ngangka*r*i*

Ngangka*r*i work has come out of a really long tradition. It comes from a time when we lived in the bush and there were no hospitals or other things. Obviously everyone is seeing and understanding the work ngangka*r*i do and relying on us to look after the people. Today we've got hospitals also. But we still do that work and people still are learning to be ngangka*r*i. Obviously there's a great demand on our services.

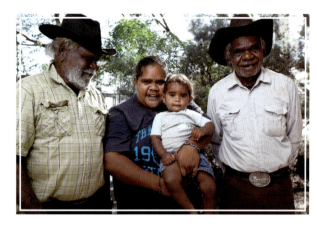

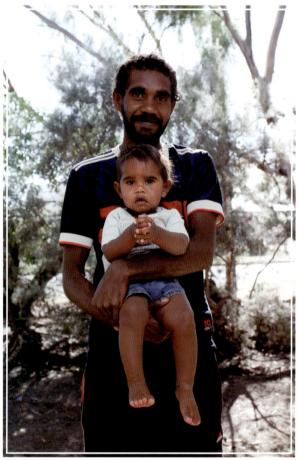

Top: Toby Minyintiri Baker, Marresha Luckey, Jimarcus Mumu Luckey and Rupert Langkatjukur Peter, Alice Springs, 2011. PHOTOGRAPH RHETT HAMMERTON

Bottom: Simon Mumu and his son Jimarcus Mumu Luckey, Alice Springs 2011. PHOTOGRAPH RHETT HAMMERTON

People still want to learn it and people are always asking for treatments. People are always looking for us, looking for ngangka<u>r</u>i if someone is sick – a kungka – a young girl, or a young man. They might say, 'let's go down to the ngangka<u>r</u>i now, we'd better go and see a ngangka<u>r</u>i'. They will come and sit down and explain how they are feeling and we give treatments in that way. People are always looking for us, that's really what's happening today. The network is very broad and there are a range of different people asking for our services. There are many ngangka<u>r</u>i and many people wanting their services.

Toby Minyintiri Baker

## *At the right time*

At the right time, when we are really senior, that is the time to give our particular skills over.

Wakupi Clem Toby (Dalby)

## *Ngangka<u>r</u>i have to assess whether a person is in a position to use the powers properly*

I'm teaching four of my grandchildren at the moment. There are four grandchildren and I began the process some time ago where they began learning. They are actually giving treatments now – they are helping children and still learning now. It has happened before, earlier.

You can't just talk to people about it, you can't just tell them to go and heal someone. It's about the mapa<u>n</u>pa, the powers, about being given the ability to see, to assess the situation and have the powers to heal people. Mapa<u>n</u>pa are placed within our hands, within our forehead and they open up so we can actually see – see where the spirit is. We use those powers. Without mapa<u>n</u>pa, without being given those particular powers, they can't just talk to people and they can't just do it. They need those mapa<u>n</u>pa and they need to learn how to use them properly.

Before passing on mapa<u>n</u>pa, ngangka<u>r</u>i have to assess whether a person is in a position to use the powers properly. When you receive the powers it's like being hit – you get knocked over to have them. It is a very powerful experience.

It is really something that is within our culture. Our children and grandchildren will see when we are getting older and in need of support and if they have a real interest in becoming a ngangka<u>r</u>i they will actually ask. They say, 'Look, I'd really like to learn how to do that', in the same way medical students might learn how to inject people and do that properly. They'll be watching someone and learning from that. They'll ask if they can try and then they'll have a go.

So grandchildren approach us if they have an interest. We talk about it and, over time, start to teach them if we think they are going to be good ngangka<u>r</u>i. One of the first things is to take them on that spiritual journey – that's the beginning of the learning.

Rupert Langkatjukur Peter

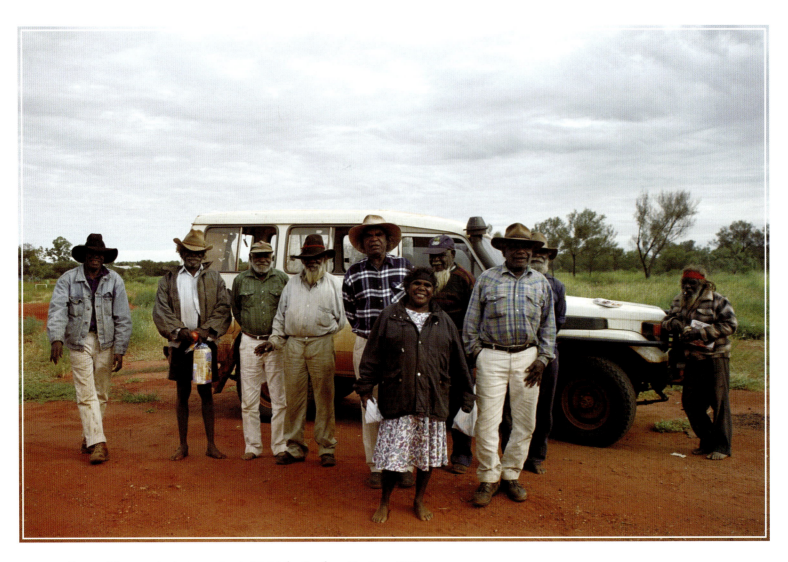

Some of the ngangkari at a meeting in Mutitjulu, Northern Territory, 2000. From left: Arnie Frank, Jacky Giles, Barney Wangin, Tiger Palpatja, Andy Tjilari, Josephine Mick, Jimmy Baker, Bernard Tjalkuriny, Harry Tjutjuna and Nakul Dawson. PHOTOGRAPH ANGELA LYNCH

# *About Ngaanyatjarra Pitjantjatjara Yankunytjatjara Women's Council Aboriginal Corporation*

Ngaanyatjarra Pitjantjatjara Yankunytjatjara (NPY) Women's Council was formed in 1980 and was separately incorporated in 1994. The idea for a women's organisation arose from the South Australian Pitjantjatjara Land Rights struggle in the late 1970s. During consultations over land rights the women felt that their needs were not being addressed so they established their own organisation.

NPY Women's Council's region covers 350,000 square kilometres of the remote cross border region of Western Australia, South Australia and the Northern Territory. Anangu and Yarnangu – Aboriginal people – living in the Ngaanyatjarra, Pitjantjatjara and Yankunytjatjara Lands (Western Desert language region) share strong cultural and family affiliations. What began as an advocacy organisation is now also a major provider of human services in the region.

NPY Women's Council represents women in the region, which has an overall population of around 6,000. The members' determination to improve the quality of life for families in the region drives the organisation. Its existence gives members an avenue for participation in the decision-making processes that affect them and their families. It is a permanent forum where they are able to raise issues and make their opinions and decisions known. It also provides opportunities for Anangu and Yarnangu to learn, share knowledge and keep informed about relevant issues.

NPY Women's Council's success is largely due to its capacity to provide a decision-making process steered by the members. One of the major advantages of its existence is the development over time of members' ability to consider and analyse policy issues, deal with government agencies and advocate on their own behalf.

## *History of the Ngangkari Project*

The Ngangkari Project began in 1998 when NPY Women's Council was approached to develop training and education about mental health. In response, NPY Women's Council's Executive Committee felt that whilst they were interested in learning about mainstream concepts and strategies for emotional and social well-being, they strongly believed that it was more important to support and promote traditional Anangu and Yarnangu healing practices and cultural values. As a result we employed two well-respected ngangkari, Rupert Langkatjukur Peter and Andy Tjilari, and a project worker, Angela Lynch, to establish and co-ordinate what is now the Ngangkari Project. The main aims of the project have always been to provide healing treatments to Anangu and Yarnangu and promote the value and importance of ngangkari to non-Indigenous health professionals who work in this region.

For a decade ngangkari Rupert Langkatjukur Peter and Andy Tjilari worked closely together in remote communities, hospitals, nursing homes, gaols, hostels and health services in the region until 2008 when Andy Tjilari retired, at which time Toby Minyintiri Baker was employed. In 2011 the team expanded to include women ngangkari when NPY Women's Council received funding from the Aboriginal and Torres Strait Islander Healing Foundation. Maringka Burton, Pantjiti McKenzie, Naomi Kantjuriny, Ilawanti Ken, Tinpulya Mervyn and Josephine Mick are all ngangkari employed part-time by NPY Women's Council and are based in their home communities throughout the region. The women's team has a particular focus on the well-being of children and women, and also a strong interest in producing and promoting bush medicines.

The ngangkari believe that collaboration and mutual respect between western health professionals and ngangkari lead to the best outcomes for Anangu and Yarnangu. They say western and Anangu practitioners have different but equally valuable skills and knowledge and both are needed to address the significant problems Ngaanyatjarra Pitjantjatjara and Yankunytjatjara face. The ngangkari of NPY Women's Council's Ngangkari Project have worked hard for over a decade to have the importance and value of their work recognised by mainstream health systems, and have successfully established strong relationships with local health and mental health services. Rupert Langkatjukur Peter illustrated this concept with a gesture of bringing two hands together, fingers outstretched, gradually interlocking the two sets of fingers, thus representing the two ways or systems coming together.

In 2009 the effectiveness of the work of the NPY Women's Council ngangkari in Indigenous mental health was acknowledged with a prestigious award from the Royal Australian and New Zealand College of Psychiatrists, and also with the Dr Margaret Tobin Award for Excellence in Mental Health Service Delivery. In 2011 the ngangkari were conjoint recipients of the World Council for Psychotherapy Sigmund Freud Award for Contributions to Psychotherapy, bestowed by the city of Vienna. These accolades have been a wonderful acknowledgement of the tireless efforts of NPY Women's Council's Ngangkari Project workers, who serve, arguably, those with the greatest health needs in this country.

The deserved respect and esteem for the ngangkari and the raised profile of NPY Women's Council's unique Ngangkari Project have led to even greater demands on the ngangkari. Regular requests from seriously ill people interstate and overseas wanting healing treatments unfortunately have to be rejected by the ngangkari, whose first and foremost priority must always be to serve the health needs of their own people. The increased national and international awareness of who and what ngangkari are has also regrettably resulted in the cultural theft of the title and concept by others. Disappointingly, people not of this region or language group have taken this Western Desert language word to describe traditional healer and used it in relation to their own methods of practice. Misuse and theft of Anangu culture in this way causes profound distress to the ngangkari and NPY Women's Council members, because it is interpreted by Anangu as an attempt to imbue others' practises with the hard-won credibility and respect achieved by the ngangkari of the NPY Lands.

## The Ngangka_ri Book

In April 2000 a large group of ngangka_ri from all over the NPY Lands came together to attend the first ngangka_ri meeting at Ulu_ru. From this meeting, which was proposed by ngangka_ri and facilitated by NPY Women's Council, it transpired that the ngangka_ri wanted to educate non-Aboriginal health practitioners, as well as the wider community, about ngangka_ri ways, with the aim of encouraging greater collaboration and understanding within the mainstream health system. These discussions culminated in the idea of a book being produced. Ngangka_ri from all over the NPY Lands recorded stories in their first language (Pitjantjatjara, Yankunytjatjara or Ngaanyatjarra) which were then transcribed and translated into English. This resulted in the book *Ngangka_ri Work — A_nangu Way*, self-published by NPY Women's Council in 2003 and reprinted in 2004. By 2008 all copies of this publication had been sold and the ngangka_ri decided it was time to update the original book with the stories you find here and publish a new edition of the book. The ngangka_ri trust you enjoy and respect the knowledge contained in this book, this knowledge is generously shared with you in the hope that it will lead to greater respect for their culture and practices, and better outcomes for their people.

NPY Women's Council, our members and indeed the wider community were dealt a devastating blow in early 2012 when our colleague, friend and number one ngangka_ri Rupert Langkatjukur Peter died in a car accident. Rupert was a founding member of our ngangka_ri team and his vision shaped the direction of the project. His incredible contribution to A_nangu health through healing and education, whilst maintaining cultural integrity, is honoured and continued to this day by our organisation. All of the ngangka_ri employed by NPY Women's Council continue to be greatly in demand to provide treatments for A_nangu and Yarnangu throughout the NPY Lands, as well as share their knowledge nationally and internationally.

Rupert Langkatjukur Peter made an enormous contribution to the production of this book and to *Ngangka_ri Work – A_nangu Way*. He saw these books as a way of increasing understanding of ngangka_ri to improve health outcomes for A_nangu, whilst maintaining A_nangu authority on which issues were talked about, how and by whom. This book reflects his vision. He passed away just as the book was being completed. It is testament to his life's work and acknowledgement of his central role in the book project that his family and the NPY Women's Council Directors decided to honour him by retaining his images and his words in this book. As the Directors so eloquently put it: 'This book is filled with his spirit and his dreams.' It is to him we dedicate this book.

Yanyi Bandicha, Chairperson of NPY Women's Council

# Spelling and Pronunciation

The consonant sounds of Pitjantjatjara/Yankunytjatjara are set out below in the spelling system in use in the Aboriginal schools of South Australia. Note that some sounds are spelt by a combination of two letters and that the spelling system makes use of a 'diacritic', or special mark – namely the underlining found beneath some letters. There are three vowels, which may be short – *a, i, u*, or less frequently long – *aa, ii, uu*.

| | | | | | |
|---|---|---|---|---|---|
| stops | *p* | *tj* | *t* | *ṯ* | *k* |
| nasals | *m* | *ny* | *n* | *ṉ* | *ng* |
| l-sounds | | *ly* | *l* | *ḻ* | |
| other | *w* | *y* | *r* | *ṟ* | |

At the beginning of a word, *p*, *t* and *k* are pronounced almost as in English, except that they are unaspirated, meaning that they lack the puff of air released as the corresponding sounds are pronounced at the beginning of an English word. In the middle of a word, *p*, *t* and *k* generally sound like English *b*, *t* and *g*: in fact, the difference between *p* and *b*, *t* and *d*, and so on (what linguists call the 'voicing' distinction) is not relevant to distinguishing meaning in Pitjantjatjara/Yankunytjatjara.

There are two kinds of sound pronounced in a way quite different to English. The laminodentals or 'teeth' sounds *tj*, *ny* and *ly* have the tongue thrust forward in the mouth, touching both sets of teeth. You can find the correct position by putting the tip of the tongue at the base of the lower teeth and pushing the tongue forward. *Tj* sounds something like the underlined part of the word T<u>u</u>esday, *ny* something like o<u>ni</u>on, and *ly* something like mi<u>lli</u>on. The retroflex sounds *ṯ*, *ṉ*, *ḻ* are made with the tongue curled back slightly in the mouth to give an r-like colouring, something like the way most Americans pronounce wa<u>rd</u>er, co<u>r</u>ner, and su<u>r</u>ely.

*Ng* represents a single sound, as in the English word si<u>ng</u>ing. In Pitjantjatjara/Yankunytjatjara, this sound often occurs at the beginning of a word. The *r* is tapped or rolled, as in some European languages and Scottish English. The remaining sounds *w*, *y* and *ṟ* are pronounced as in English <u>w</u>et, <u>y</u>ellow and <u>r</u>oad. Stress is always on the first syllable of a Pitjantjatjara/Yankunytjatjara word.

REPRINTED FROM CLIFF GODDARD (ED.), PITJANTJATJARA/YANKUNYTJATJARA POCKET DICTIONARY, © INSTITUTE FOR ABORIGINAL DEVELOPMENT 1997.

# Glossary

alani = opening

alatji = in this manner

alpiri = morning news, early morning community speeches

alu = liver

anangu = person, human

Anangu = Western Desert language speaking Aboriginal people

anangu maru = dark skinned people, Aboriginal people

anangitja = of the body, of Aboriginal people

anumara = edible grub

arnguli = wild bush plum *Santalum lanceolatum*

ara = tradition, style, way, method, story

auru = camel

butter = healing fats, bush medicine ointments, butter

bush medicine = typically irmangka-irmangka

hub cap wira = a dish fashioned from the metal hub cap of a car

ilani = to pull out, to draw out, to remove

ili = wild bush figs *Ficus platypoda*

Ili Tjukurpa = Wild Bush Fig Dreaming

ilytji = abundant food-bearing bushlands

inma = song, ceremonial song

intjanungku ungkupai = given as a gift without need for reciprocity

ipilypa = healthy, in good health

irati = venom, invisible poisonous power, epidemic, venom, nuclear radiation

irmangka-irmangka = a powerful medicinal bush, *Eremophila alternifolia*

iwara = way, route, track, trail, road

iyani = send, send off, banish

kalaya = emu

kalaya kanpi – emu fat, fat

kalpari – medicinal rat-tail grass *Dysphania kalpari*

kaltu-kaltu – edible native millet *Panicum decompositum*

kami = grandmother, granddaughter

kampurarpa = bush tomato *Solanum* spp

kanti = sharp stone blade, stone chisel

kanyala = euro, hills kangaroo *Macropus robustus*

kapi = water, liquid

kapi piti = waterhole

kapi piti wala = a natural spring-fed waterhole

kaputu = small round ball, knotted hard ball

karalymankupai, karalymananyi = to make smooth, smoothing

Karpirinypa = powerful Emu mamu spirit

kata kura / kata kura tjuta = people with mental health problems

kata kuraringanyi = developing mental health problems

kililpi = star

kipara = bush turkey, bustard *Ardeotis australis*

kirkinpa = bird of prey, brown falcon, *Falco berigora*

kuka – meat, meat animal

kukaputju = a skilled, accomplished hunter

kulata – man's hunting spear

kumpilpa = hidden, out of sight

kuna = faeces, droppings

kunakanti = edible seed grass *Brachiaria miliiformis*

kungka = girl, woman, female

kungkawara = tall girl, teenager

kuniya = woma python *Aspitites ramsayi*

kuntili = father's sister, aunt

kulypurpa = edible wild gooseberry *Solanum ellipticum*

kupi-kupi = whirlwind

kura = bad, not good

kura mulapa = very bad, evil

kurulpa = grave mound, grave materials such as logs and sticks, grave

kurunpa = spirit, will, self

kurunpa nyinakatipai = spirit come to rest

kurunpa ultu = spiritless or empty of spirit, deeply depressed

kurunpa wiyaringanyi = spirit fading away, fainting with shock

kuru pati = blind, eyes shut

kuta = older brother

kutatji = executioner, 'feather-foot'

kuurtjananyi, kuurtjankupai = ngangkari suction technique, draw out by suction

kuuti = vital energy, life force, tektite

lipulankupai = from the English 'to make things level', harmonise, equalise, balance

lirintananyi = throttling or choking

mai = food, non-meat food

maku = witchetty grubs

makura = golden bandicoot *Isodon auratus* (now locally extinct)

mala = rufous hare-wallaby *Lagorchestes hirsutus* (now locally extinct)

malpa, malpa wiru – friend, best friend

malparara = with a companion, with a colleague

malukurukuru = Sturt's desert pea *Swainsona formosa*

malypanypa – tendon, ligament, sinew, 'string'

mama = father, father's brother

mama nyuyurpa = stepfather

mamu = harmful spirit being, dangerous spirit force or energy

Mamu Karpirinypa = emu-shaped dangerous spirit creature

mamuku iwara = pathway of mamu, track or road

manguri = cushioning headring for carrying items on head

mapanpa = ngangkari sacred tools

mapantjara = holder of mapanpa, ngangkari (Pitjantjatjara)

maparntjarra = holder of maparnpa, ngangkari (Ngaanyatjarra)

mara ala = open hands, healing hands

marali = spirit journey undertaken by Ngangkari

marali katipai = ngangkari taking apprentices on spirit journeys

Maralinga = location of British atomic bomb tests, now used generically to describe all the atomic bomb tests from that area

maru = dark, black, or dark skinned people

miilmiilpa = secret and sacred

milpatjunanyi = storytelling wire which is used as a rhythmic tapping and drawing device to tell stories in the sand

mimpu = deep wooden bowl for carrying water

mingkulpa = wild bush tobacco *Nicotania* spp

miru = spear thrower

mulapa – true, real

muturka = prized fat around the innards of kangaroo, euro and other animals

ninti pulka = knowledgeable, experienced

ngaalypa = breath, breathing, sign of life

Ngaatjatjarra = a dialect of the Western Desert language, spoken around Blackstone Ranges

ngalya ala = having the powers of spiritual perception, open mind, open forehead

nganamara = mallee fowl *Leipoa acellata*

nganamara ngampu = mallee fowl egg

ngangkari = healer, traditional healer, Anangu doctor

ngangkariku iwara – the ngangkari way of life, sacred route taken by ngangkari

ngangkari pulka = important ngangkari, ngangkari of great stature

Ngangkariku Tjukurpa = Ngangkari Dreaming Law

Ngangkari tjutaku Tjukurpa = Ngangkari people's Law

ngangkarinanyi = giving a healing treatment

ngaya = feral cat

ngayulu ngalturingkupai = I feel sympathetic, I feel sympathy

ngalturingkupai = sympathetic, sympathy

ngintaka = perentie lizard *Varanus giganteus*

ngulytju = friendly, known, familiar

nguratjunu = made camp

nuunpunganyi = throbbing, twitching in muscle, indicating something happening to a relative

nyiinka = pre-initiated boy

nyuma = seed cake

nyumpu tjutaku = people with disabilities

pakuringanyi = becoming tired, weak, exhausted

pampa = older lady, elderly lady

pampuni = touching, healing

pampuntja = one who is touched or healed by ngangkari

papa = dog, dingo *Canis lupus dingo*

pii = skin, outer skin of a caterpillar nest (yuunpa)

pika = pain, sickness, argument

pila = spinifex plain

pinpanyi, pinpantja, pinpapai = flashing, sparkling, lightning

piriya = hot, dusty springtime winds from the north and west

piti = source, hole, wellspring, creation place

Pitjantjatjara = a dialect of the Western Desert language

pulka = big, large, important

pulyi = umbilical cord, belly-button

pulyku = tendon, sinew, ligament, 'string'

punti = the bush, *Cassia* or *Senna* bushes

puntu, puntutja = body, of the body

punu = tree, wood, splinters, objects which cause sickness, thing

puti = the bush, bushes

putjitja = from the bush

puturu = headband made of string or yarn

puulpai = blowing upon

puuni = to blow on, ngangkari healing blowing technique, ngangkari closing technique

puunkuninypa = tektites, similar to kuuti

puyu = smoke, fallout from nuclear bomb

rama = serious mental health problems, insanity

rama-rama = mental health problems, dementia

rirra, rirrangka ngaranyi = rocky gravelly ridge, on a rocky, gravelly ridge (Ngaanyatjarra)

tali = sand dune, sandhill

tarka = bone

tarka mapanpa = ngangkari bone tools

tawal-tawalpa = edible wild gooseberry *Solanum ellipticum*

tektite = small, dark, natural glass rocks formed by meteorite impact, used by ngangkari

tili = flame, firelight, torchlight

tiwilpa, tiwilarinyi = stiff, cramped, cramping up

tjala = honey ant *Camponotus inflatus*

tjanpi = spinifex grasses *Triodia* spp, grasses

tjamu = grandfather, grandson

tjilira = bundle of spears or sticks

tjilpi = grey hair, old man

tjina, tjinangku = foot, by foot

tjitji = child

tjitji ngangkari = child ngangkari

tjitji tjiranka = child, youth or pre-adolescent

tjiwa rungkani = grinding on a grindstone

tjukalpa, Tjukalpa = ladder, the Milky Way

tjukurpa, Tjukurpa = story, history, Aboriginal Law, 'Dreaming'

Tjukurpa nganampa = our Aboriginal Law

Tjukurpa wirunya = a good story

tjulani = to make soft, to make flexible

tjulpu = bird

tjuta = many, plural

uliringanyi = fainting, close to death, slipping into unconsciousness

ultu = empty, hollow

urkuni = to draw out, to pull out

wakalpuka = dead finish bush *Acacia tetragonophylla*

wakati = inland pigweed *Portulaca* aff. *oleracea*

walatjunanyi = release, set free

walawuru = eagle

walkalpa = emu poison bush *Duboisia hopwoodii*, highly poisonous

walkatjunanyi = making marks, writing

walupara = white woman

walypala = white people, white men

walytja = kin, relation, own

wama = sweet nectar, honey, alcohol, sweet wine

wana = woman's digging stick

wanampi = rainbow serpent

wanka = spider, itchy grub

wangkanyi = talking

wangunu = naked woollybutt grass *Eragrostis eriopoda*

warmala = vendetta, revenge party, traditional army

Warmala Inma = song and dance associated with dodging spears from revenge party

waru = fire, very hot

Waru Tjukurpa = Fire Dreaming Law

wati = initiated man

Watiku = men's business

wati ngangkari = initiated male ngangkari

wati putjitja = a man of the bush

wati tjilpi ngangkari = senior elder male ngangkari

Wati Tjukurtjara = Men of the Ancients, Men of the Creation Times

wayanu = quandong *Santalum acuminatum*

whitefella = white person, non-Aboriginal person

wilki-wilki = neck muscles just below the ear

wiltja = shade, shade shelter

Wiltjantjatjara = Pitjantjatjara dialect from east of Pipalyatjara

wilu = curlew

wipiya = emu feathers

Wipukarpilypa = a being that has its tail tied together

wira = all-purpose wooden dish primarily used for digging or winnowing

wiriny-wirinypa = edible bush tomato *Solanum cleistogamum*

wirunya = beautiful, lovely

wirunymankupai = ngangkari healing treatment, laying on of hands

wirunymankula waninyi = to declare someone well and to banish illness

wirulymankupai, wirulymananyi = ngangkari healing treatment, laying on of hands, massaging, physiotherapy

wiyaringanyi = finishing, ending, dying

Yankunytjatjara = dialect of the Western Desert language

yarnangu = person, human (Ngaanyatjarra)

youngfella = young man, young person

yuunpa = processionary caterpillar nest

# Acknowledgements

The project was initiated, shaped, advised and directed throughout by:

NPY Women's Council Ngangkari Team: Rupert Langkatjukur Peter, Toby Minyintiri Baker, Andy Tjilari, Naomi Kantjuriny, Ilawanti Ungkutjuru Ken, Maringka Burton, Tinpulya Kangitja Mervyn, Josephine Watjari Mick, Pantjiti Unkari McKenzie and Angela Lynch.

NPY Women's Council Directors 2011–13: Yanyi Bandicha (Chairperson), Margaret Smith, Kunbry Peipai, Tjawina Roberts, Carlene Thompson, Nyurpaya Kaika, Janet Inyika, Nyunmiti Burton, Roslyn Yiparti, Julie Porter, Janet Jennings and Ingrid Simms.

NPY Women's Council Directors 2009–11: Margaret Smith (Chairperson), Yanyi Bandicha, Janet Inyika, Ingrid Treacle, Pantjiti McKenzie, Julie Anderson, Elsie Wanatjura, Rene Kulitja, Olive Lawson, Valerie Foster, Martha Ward, Anawari Mitchell.

This book project grew upon foundations laid by a previous book: *Ngangkari Work – Anangu Way,* Ngaanyatjarra Pitjantjatjara Yankunytjatjara Women's Council Aboriginal Corporation, 2003. The authors acknowledge the work of the following people on that project: Julia Burke, Andy Tjilari, Rupert Peter, Elsie Wanatjura, Angela Lynch, Linda Rive, Jo Boniface, RedDirt Graphics and the Office for Aboriginal and Torres Strait Islander Health.

Thanks also to:

The families of those ngangkari who have passed away for allowing the continued use of images, artworks and words of those people in this publication. These families have acknowledged that this book is a testament to the skill of ngangkari and their important place in history.

NPY Women's Council Co-ordinator Andrea Mason and Deputy Co-ordinator Liza Balmer

Marita Baker and Clive Peter, Julia Burke, Mick Bradley, Dr Alex Brown

Suzanne Bryce, Alex Craig, Belle Davidson, Andrew Duguid, Angus Duguid, Elizabeth Marrkilyi Ellis, Paul Exline, Rhett Hammerton, David and Margaret Hewitt, Sally Hodson, Patrick Hookey, Shivaun Inglis, Maggie Kavanagh, Pantjiti Lewis , Dr Helen Milroy, Steven Oxenbury, Kunbry Peipai, Loretta Peter, Linda Rive, Margaret Smith, Steve Strike, Dr Marcus Tabart, Bernard Tjalkuriny, Clem Toby, Daisy Ward, Margaret Whiskin, John Wischusen

Galleries & Arts Centres:

Art Gallery of NSW: Michelle Andringa and Nicole Kluk; Ernabella Arts: Julian Green & Ruth McMillan; Gallery Gabrielle Pizzi; Iwantja Arts and Crafts: Helen Johnson; Marshall Arts: Karen Zadra; Ninuku Arts: Claire Eltringham, Vanessa Patterson; Tandanya National Aboriginal Cultural Institute: Fulvia Mantelli

Tjala Arts: Skye O'Meara, Joanna Byrne; Tjanpi Desert Weavers: Marg Bowman, Michelle Young, Rebekah Osbourne Ken; Tjungu Palya: Amanda Dent, Brian Hallett, Joanna Byrne

Legal: Ashurst Australia: Anita Cade, Lisa Ritson and Maya Port

Magabala Books: Margaret Whiskin, Tracey Gibbs, Jacqueline Wright

Our Funders:

Aboriginal and Torres Strait Islander Healing Foundation

NPYWC gratefully acknowledges the long standing support of the Ngangkari Project by Country Health South Australia and the Government of South Australia

Archives:

Ara Irititja: John Dallwitz, Linda Rive, Julia Burke and Dora Dallwitz; Museum Victoria: Dr Heather Gaunt; State Library of South Australia: Suzy Russell http://www.ministers.sa.gov.au/; South Australian Museum: Lea Gardam; Strehlow Research Centre: Michael Cawthorn.

# NPY Women's Council Region Map

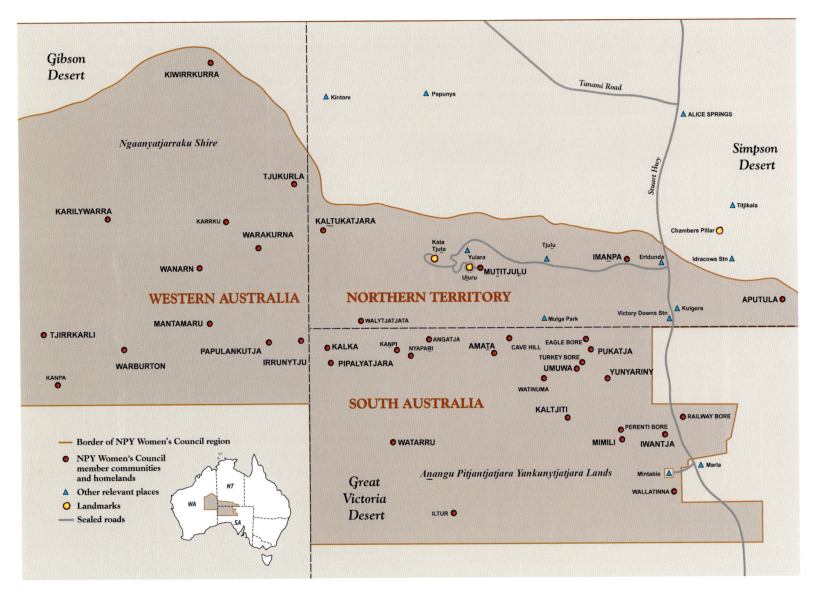

Ngaanyatjarra Pitjantjatjara Yankunytjatjara Women's Council Aboriginal Corporation

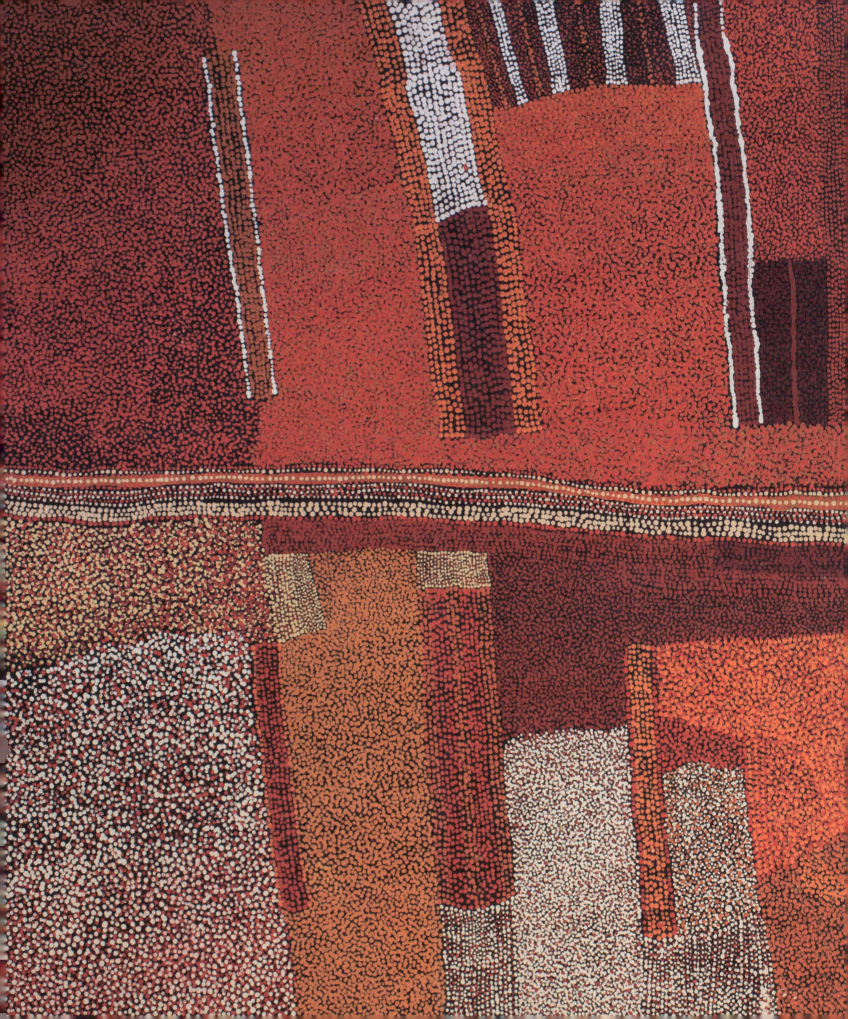